Speech-Language Pathology Assistants

A Resource Manual

Speech-Language Pathology Assistants

A Resource Manual

Jennifer A. Ostergren, PhD, CCC-SLP

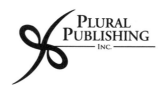

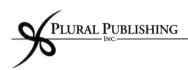

5521 Ruffin Road
San Diego, CA 92123

e-mail: info@pluralpublishing.com
Website: http://www.pluralpublishing.com

Copyright © by Plural Publishing, Inc. 2014

Typeset in 10.5/13 Palatino by Flanagan's Publishing Services, Inc.
Printed in the United States of America by McNaughton & Gunn, Inc.
19 18 17 16   3 4 5 6

All rights, including that of translation, reserved. No part of this publication may be reproduced, stored in a retrieval system, or transmitted in any form or by any means, electronic, mechanical, recording, or otherwise, including photocopying, recording, taping, Web distribution, or information storage and retrieval systems without the prior written consent of the publisher.

For permission to use material from this text, contact us by
Telephone: (866) 758-7251
Fax: (888) 758-7255
e-mail: permissions@pluralpublishing.com

Every attempt has been made to contact the copyright holders for material originally printed in another source. If any have been inadvertently overlooked, the publishers will gladly make the necessary arrangements at the first opportunity.

Cover artwork courtesy of Gwen A. Ostergren.

Library of Congress Cataloging-in-Publication Data

Ostergren, Jennifer A., author.
  Speech-language pathology assistants : a resource manual / Jennifer A. Ostergren.
      p. ; cm.
  Includes bibliographical references and index.
  ISBN-13: 978-1-59756-500-4 (alk. paper)
  ISBN-10: 1-59756-500-8 (alk. paper)
  I. Title.
  [DNLM: 1. Allied Health Personnel. 2. Speech-Language Pathology—methods.
3. Language Disorders. 4. Professional Competence. 5. Professional Practice.
6. Professional Role. WL 21]
  RC424.7
  616.85'5—dc23
                                                            2013039987

Contents

List of Appendices		*vi*
Preface		*ix*
Acknowledgments		*xi*
Contributors		*xii*

Part I. Defining Roles: Speech-Language Pathology Assistants (SLPAs) — **1**

Chapter 1.	Defining Roles: SLPAs	3
Chapter 2.	Defining Roles: Supervision and Mentoring	73
Chapter 3.	Ethical Conduct	89
Chapter 4.	Professional Conduct	127
Chapter 5.	Cultural and Linguistic Diversity *Carolyn Conway Madding*	155
Chapter 6.	Health and Safety *Pei-Fang Hung*	171

Part II. Skills Development — **191**

Chapter 7.	Deciphering Lesson Plans and Goals	193
Chapter 8.	Data Collection	247
Chapter 9.	Note Writing	271
Chapter 10.	Implementing Treatment	287
Chapter 11.	Group Therapy *Jennifer A. Ostergren and Sarah Guzzino*	317
Chapter 12.	Incorporating Play and Literacy in Treatment *Sara M. Aguilar*	339
Chapter 13.	Speech Sound Remediation *Lei Sun*	355
Chapter 14.	Augmentative and Alternative Communication *Margaret Vento-Wilson*	381
Chapter 15.	Autism Spectrum Disorder (ASD) *Jodi Robledo*	413

Index	*429*

List of Appendices

Part I. Defining Roles: Speech-Language Pathology Assistant (SLPAs)

Chapter 1. Defining Roles: SLPAs

Appendix 1–A.	ASHA Speech-Language Pathology Assistant Scope of Practice	16
Appendix 1–B.	Audiology and Speech-Language Pathology Associations Outside of the United States	30
Appendix 1–C.	Relevant ASHA Documents	35
Appendix 1–D.	A Day in the Life of an SLPA: Interviews/Advice From SLPAs	36
Appendix 1–E.	A Glimpse Into the World of Speech-Language Pathology Assistants (SLPAs) in the Health Care Setting	54
Appendix 1–F.	Sample Job Description—Medical Setting	57
Appendix 1–G.	Sample Job Description—Educational Setting	59
Appendix 1–H.	Example of Competency-Based Assessment	61
Appendix 1–I.	Technical Proficiency Checklist	66
Appendix 1–J.	Direct Observation Skills Brief Checklist—Medical Setting	69
Appendix 1–K.	Direct Observation Skills Brief Checklist—Educational Setting	70
Appendix 1–L.	Skills Proficiency Checklist	71

Chapter 2. Defining Roles: Supervision and Mentoring

Appendix 2–A.	Supervisor Log of Direct and Indirect Observations	85
Appendix 2–B.	SLPA Weekly Activity Log	86
Appendix 2–C.	SLPA Weekly Activity Record	87

Chapter 3. Ethical Conduct

Appendix 3–A.	ASHA Code of Ethics	104
Appendix 3–B.	Ethical Principles, Rules, and Guidance Pertinent to the Supervision of Support Personnel	109
Appendix 3–C.	Sample SLPA Ethical Decision-Making Worksheet	112
Appendix 3–D.	ASHA Confidentiality Statement	117
Appendix 3–E.	SLPA Ethical Dilemma Scenarios	125

Chapter 4. Professional Conduct

Appendix 4–A.	Common Medical Abbreviations	141
Appendix 4–B.	Common International Phonetic Alphabet (IPA) Symbols	143
Appendix 4–C.	Commonly Misused Words and Phrases	145
Appendix 4–D.	Commonly Misspelled Words in English	150
Appendix 4–E.	Self-Evaluation of Intervention Sessions—Educational Setting	151
Appendix 4–F.	Self-Evaluation of Intervention Sessions—Medical Setting	153

Chapter 5. Cultural and Linguistic Diversity

Appendix 5–A. Chapter Review Self-Test 169
Appendix 5–B. Cultural Consciousness Activities 170

Chapter 6. Health and Safety

Appendix 6–A. CDC Cleaning and Infection Guidelines (Schools) 189

Part II. Skills Development

Chapter 7. Deciphering Lesson Plans and Goals

Appendix 7–A. Educational Setting—Sample Reports 204
Appendix 7–B. Private Practice—Sample Reports 219
Appendix 7–C. Medical Setting—Sample Reports 226
Appendix 7–D. Sample Goals and Objectives 241

Chapter 8. Data Collection

Appendix 8–A. Mean Length of Utterance (MLU) and Age Equivalent 268
Appendix 8–B. Common Morphological Features and Age of Mastery 269

Chapter 9. Note Writing

Appendix 9–A. Data Sheet Incorporating SOAP Format 283
Appendix 9–B. Sample SOAP Notes 284

Chapter 11. Group Therapy

Appendix 11–A. Social Skills Group Activities 334
Appendix 11–B. Group Data Collection Sheet 337

Chapter 12. Incorporating Play and Literacy in Treatment

Appendix 12–A. Summary of Play Stages 351

Chapter 13. Speech Sound Remediation

Appendix 13–A. Sample SSD Homework Sheet 378
Appendix 13–B. Sample SSD Treatment Data Collection Form 379

Chapter 14. Augmentative and Alternative Communication

Appendix 14–A. Example of Communication Book 400
Appendix 14–B. Eye-Gaze Board: SpeakBook 401
Appendix 14–C. Example of Alphabet Boards 402
Appendix 14–D. Example of Choice Board 403
Appendix 14–E. Example of Clock Communicator 404
Appendix 14–F. Example of Switch Communicator 405
Appendix 14–G. Speech-Generating Device: GoTalk Express 32 406
Appendix 14–H. Text-to-Speech Device: LightwriterSL40 407
Appendix 14–I. Visual Scene Display: Speaking Dynamically Pro 408
Appendix 14–J. iPad Tablet with the Proloquo Application 409

| Appendix 14–K. | Eye Tracking Device (Mouse Control): Enable Eyes Control Bar | 410 |
| Appendix 14–L. | Eye Tracking Device (Keypad Access): Enable Eyes Control Bar | 411 |

Preface

Speech-language pathology assistants (SLPAs) are "support personnel who, following academic and/or on-the-job training, perform tasks prescribed, directed, and supervised by ASHA-certified speech-language pathologists [SLPs]" (American Speech-Language-Hearing Association [ASHA], n.d., para. 2). The use of SLPAs and support personnel is not new. As early as the 1970s, support personnel in the field of speech-language pathology were being used and regulated by different states in the United States (ASHA, n.d.). ASHA has had guidelines for the use of support personnel since 1969. According to ASHA, attention to the use of SLPAs has increased as professionals in the field look for ways to contain costs and expand clinical services (ASHA, n.d.). ASHA maintains and periodically updates formal policy and guidelines on the training, use, and supervision of SLPAs. Recognizing national inconsistency in SLPA use and training, ASHA also created an optional associates program in 2011 (Robinson, 2010). This program extends ASHA affiliation to qualified support personnel who agree to follow all ASHA policies and guidelines pertaining to the use and supervision of support personnel (*McNeilly, 2010*).

CONTENT

This book is written specifically for SLPAs, addressing their unique needs. It is intended to be a practical resource on a wide range of topics that SLPAs may find of value. It does not cover in depth the areas of normal processes of communication or communicative disorders. Rather, it is intended as a "what now" or real-world perspective in offering suggestions in the area of technical and clinical procedures for an SLPA, including professional issues and ethics of an SLPA's duties, and instruction in workplace behaviors of SLPAs, such as implementing treatment and collecting and summarizing data. Specialized topics applicable to SLPAs, such as augmentative and alternative communication, cultural and linguistic diversity, play and literacy in therapy, speech sound remediation, and autism spectrum disorder, are also included and are meant to extend an SLPA's foundational knowledge in these areas to real-world applications. This book is written for individuals with a variety of SLPA experience and training. It is my hope that SLPAs with all levels of experience and background will find tools and resources of value to them in this book. If you are an SLPA who has been in the field for many years, this book may offer you a fresh perspective on your role as an SLPA and ideas in continuing to refine your skills as an SLPA. If you are an SLPA just starting your career, this book will offer you important information to take with you on your journey. If you are an SLPA in training, this book will provide you with information relevant for your training, particularly to your clinical practicum and future employment as an SLPA.

ORGANIZATION

The first six chapters of this book cover broad topics in the area of SLPA practice, including an overview of the roles and responsibilities of SLPAs and their supervisors. The initial chapters of this book also cover topics such as professional conduct, ethics, cultural and linguistic diversity, and topics important to the health and safety of SLPAs and the individuals they serve. Within these sections, ASHA documents are a cornerstone when referencing policies, procedures, rules, and regulations applicable to SLPA practice. At present, there is considerable variability between states in regulations applicable to SLPAs. As such, ASHA as the sole national professional organization in the United States serves as an important and primary resource on the topic. That is not to say that SLPAs should ignore state regulations. Rather, as will be discussed, SLPAs must be cognizant of both ASHA and individual state regulations. As such, references and suggestions for accessing state-specific information are provided. Furthermore, given the dynamic nature of policies and procedures, readers should view the information in this book as an overview of regulations and policies in place at the time of publication. The reader is referred to ASHA's website, at http://www.asha.org, for the most recent information in this area.

The final nine chapters of the book are organized as "skill development" chapters. These chapters cover a specific set of skills needed by SLPAs in working *clinically* with individuals with communication disorders. Throughout each skill development chapter, helpful tips and applicable references and resources are provided, with the major emphasis on providing information that will be of value in actual clinical work as an SLPA. It should be noted that these chapters are meant for a reader who has knowledge about normal process in communication and communication disorders, as would be covered in coursework to become an SLPA.

CD MATERIALS

A CD is provided with this book. This CD contains important forms that readers can use in their clinical work as an SLPA. These forms can be freely modified and copied. Explanations about the content contained on the CD are embedded within the written material. The following symbol denotes where the content of the CD is referenced.

REFERENCES

American Speech-Language-Hearing Association (ASHA). (n.d.). *Frequently asked questions: Speech-language pathology assistants (SLPAs)*. Retrieved from http://www.asha.org/certification/faq_slpasst.htm

McNeilly, L. (2010, November 23). ASHA will roll out associates program in 2011. *ASHA Leader*. Retrieved from http://www.asha.org/Publications/leader/2010/101123/ASHA-Will-Roll-Out-Associates-Program-in-2011.htm

Robinson, T. L., Jr. (2010). Associates in ASHA: A new initiative. *ASHA Leader*. Retrieved from http://www.asha.org/Publications/leader/2010/100803/From-President-100803.htm

Acknowledgments

Foremost, I would like to acknowledge and thank my loving husband and my wonderful daughter for their patience and unwavering support. Without your words of encouragement and gifts of time to focus on my writing, this book would not have been possible. A special thank you as well to my daughter, Gwen, whose beautiful artwork graces the cover of this book. I would also like to thank my colleagues who contributed chapters to this book. Their names and accomplishments follow. Your expertise has added greatly to the depth of information available to SLPAs on very important topics. I would also like to thank all the students who completed their clinical practicum within my SLPA course at California State University, Long Beach (CSULB). You have positively shaped the content of this book through your experiences as SLPAs and SLPAs in training. A special thank you, as well, to Ben, for his wonderful illustrations, which add additional insight and detail to each chapter of this book. I would also like to acknowledge Plural Publishing and my publishing team for their commitment to excellence and constant support from start to finish.

Contributors*

Sara M. Aguilar, MA, CCC-SLP
Chapter 12
Sara M. Aguilar is a school-based speech-language pathologist in Southern California who currently provides services to children with severe disabilities. Her professional areas of interest include augmentative and alternative communication, early literacy intervention, and supervision and training of support personnel. She has published and presented research on the training, supervision, and use of speech-language pathology assistants in California. Sara was a recipient of the Contemporary Issues in Communication Sciences and Disorders Editor's Award at the 2012 American Speech-Language Hearing Association Conference.

Carolyn Conway Madding, PhD, CCC-SLP
Chapter 5
Carolyn Conway Madding, professor and chair of the Department of Communicative Disorders at California State University, Long Beach, is a Fellow of the American Speech-Language-Hearing Association (ASHA) and an ASHA Minority Champion. She received the Diversity Award from the California Speech-Language-Hearing Association and has published and presented nationally and internationally on bilingualism and linguistic/cultural diversity within the profession of speech-language pathology.

Sarah Guzzino, BA
Chapter 11
Sarah Guzzino is a graduate student studying communicative disorders at Califor-

nia State University, Long Beach. She is a licensed speech-language pathology assistant in the state of California, currently working at an elementary school, treating speech and language disorders within group settings. She is also an advocate for individuals with traumatic brain injury and has profound interest in neurogenic communication disorders.

Pei-Fang Hung, PhD, CCC-SLP
Chapter 6
Pei-Fang Hung is an assistant professor in the Department of Communicative Disorders at the California State University, Long Beach. She received both her MS and PhD in communication disorders and sciences from the University of Oregon. She has more than 10 years' experience working with patients with aphasia, dysphagia, motor speech disorders, and cognitive impairments after a traumatic brain injury. Her areas of expertise are acquired cognitive-communicative disorders, cognitive rehabilitation, and language deterioration related to normal aging and dementia.

Jodi Robledo, PhD
Chapter 15
Jodi Robledo is an assistant professor in special education at California State University, San Marcos and the program director for the Applied Behavior Analysis Certificate of Advanced Study. She also teaches courses in the Communicative Sciences and Disorders Department. Prior to this appointment, she was K–12 autism specialist and education

---

*Contributors are listed in alphabetical order.

specialist in an urban multicultural school district. Dr. Robledo currently teaches courses with a focus on autism spectrum disorder (ASD), supporting individuals with moderate/severe disabilities, and inclusive education. She has joint refereed journal publications, several book chapters, and numerous national conference presentations. She also cofounded the USD Autism Institute with Dr. Anne Donnellan and has ongoing presentations there as well. Her research interests focus on ASD, supportive relationships, sensory and movement differences, building self-advocacy skills in youth with ASD, and inclusive education.

Lei Sun, PhD, CCC-SLP
Chapter 13
Lei Sun is an assistant professor in the Department of Communicative Disorders at the California State University, Long Beach. She worked with Dr. Marilyn Nippold and received her doctoral degree from the University of Oregon, focusing on lexical and morphosyntactic development in typically developing school-age children. Her expertise is in the area of morphosyntactic, semantic, metalinguistic development in typically developing children and children with language learning disabilities.

Margaret Vento-Wilson, MA, CCC-SLP
Chapter 14
Margaret Vento-Wilson is a speech-language pathologist currently working at an autism spectrum disorder–specific program at an elementary school in Southern California. Her areas of interest include narrative language and augmentative and alternative communication (AAC), as well as their correlative effect for children with significant language impairments. Her published research and presentations involve motor speech disorders and the use of AAC with patients in the acute care setting. She entered the field of speech-language pathology because of her core belief in the power of language to allow individuals to share their worlds and shape their futures.

ILLUSTRATIONS

Ben Philpott
Chapter illustrations were provided by Ben Philpott. Ben Philpott lives in Long Beach, California, and recently earned his BA in communicative disorders from California State University, Long Beach (CSULB). He currently works as a speech-language pathology assistant intern at CSULB's Child Language Clinic.

PART I

Defining Roles: Speech–Language Pathology Assistants (SLPAs)

CHAPTER 1

Defining Roles: SLPAs

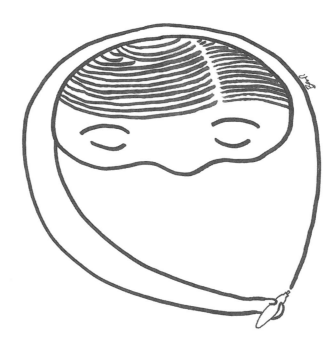

*Confidence, like art, never comes from having all the answers;
it comes from being open to all the questions.*

Earl Gray Stevens

The American Speech-Language-Hearing Association (ASHA) defines speech-language pathology assistants (SLPAs) as "support personnel who perform tasks as prescribed, directed, and supervised by an ASHA-certified speech-language pathologist (SLP)" (ASHA, 2013, Executive Summary, para. 1). SLPAs are not independent practitioners but rather work specifically under the direction and guidance of a qualified speech-language pathologist (SLP) to increase the availability, frequency, and efficiency of services provided by the SLP. SLPAs provide services in a wide variety of settings. These settings include but are not limited to the following (ASHA, 2013, Executive Summary, para. 1)[1]:

- Public, private, and charter elementary and secondary schools

- Early intervention settings, preschools, and day care settings
- Hospitals (in- and outpatient)
- Residential health care settings (e.g., long-term care and skilled nursing facilities)
- Nonresidential health care settings (e.g., home health agencies, adult day care settings, clinics)
- Private practice settings
- University/college clinics
- Research facilities
- Corporate and industrial settings
- Student/patient/client's residences

SLPAs differ from other support personnel, such as speech and language aides, instructional aides, communication aides, and so forth, both in the level of training and in the amount of supervision and oversight. According to ASHA (n.d.-a), "Aides have a different, usually narrower, training base and more limited scope of responsibilities than SLPAs."

The use of SLPAs is not new in the field of speech-language pathology. ASHA has had documents addressing support personnel as early as the 1960s. The role of the SLPA in the field of speech-language pathology continues to evolve, however, given changes in health and educational service delivery models, increases in the number of individuals with communication disorders, expansion in the scope of services provided by SLPs, and the rising costs of providing these services.

ASHA (2013) outlines that "some tasks, procedures, or activities used to treat individuals with communication and related disorders can be performed successfully by individuals others than an SLP, if the persons conducting the activity are properly trained and super-

vised by ASHA-certified and/or licensed SLPs" (Executive Summary, para. 1). This chapter outlines recommendations for the training and use of SLPAs. Recommendations for the supervision of SLPAs are summarized in Chapter 2.

ASHA is the national professional organization in the United States in the field of speech-language pathology. For the purpose of this book, recommendations and standards are reviewed applicable to SLPAs in the United States, using ASHA recommendations and practice guidelines. At the writing of this book, ASHA's primary policy document on the training, use, and supervision of SLPAs was *Speech-Language Pathology Assistant Scope of Practice* (ASHA, 2013). This document is available in Appendix 1–A and can also be retrieved at http://www.asha.org/

Internationally, there is variability in professional classification, services provided, and the use of assistants in the field of speech-language pathology. For individuals interested in obtaining information about SLPAs outside the United States, Appendix 1–B contains a summary of related international professional organizations. This information is also available at http://www.asha.org/ (ASHA, n.d.-a.). These organizations are a good starting point in understanding if SLPAs exist at similar levels in other parts of the world. The International Association of Logopedics and Phoniatrics is also a source of information on this topic (http://www.ialp.info/).

In the United States, regulations for the training, use, and supervision of support personnel vary from state to state. The governing bodies that regulate or oversee the use of SLPAs also vary from state to state. In some locations, the state department of education (or applicable educational body) establishes and oversees specific requirements for SLPA training, use, and supervision in a school setting. In some locations, state licensing boards regulate SLPA training, use, and supervision in nonschool settings. In some cases, educational setting-specific requirements overlap with those of noneducation requirements, but in others they differ.

Figure 1–1 contains a map highlighting states with official designation and/or regulation of SLPAs (ASHA, n.d.-a.). States not highlighted in gray are those that either: (a) do not have an official regulating mechanism specifically for SLPAs (although they may recognize that SLPs use assistants, aides, or other types of paraprofessionals) or (b) use paraprofessional designations, other than SLPA, such as communication aides, communication technicians, SLP apprentices, SLP paraprofessionals, and so forth.

As an SLPA, if you are working in a setting with formal licensure, certification, or registration requirements for support personnel, it is imperative that you adhere to any applicable laws, regulations, and procedures. Not doing so could compromise the care of the individuals you serve and place you and your supervisor in legal jeopardy for actions outside the standards of that state. SLPAs should familiarize themselves with the most recent information in their locations. Realize as well that state standards may change on an annual basis or without notice. Hence, it is your responsibility as an SLPA to become familiar with and stay abreast of the most recent regulations in your location.

ASHA's State Advocacy Team maintains a page on ASHA's website that summarizes individual state requirements, including information about support personnel requirements in each state (ASHA, n.d.-a). This is an invaluable resource for SLPAs (available at http://www.asha .org/advocacy/state/). SLPAs should also go directly to the regulating body in their state for information regarding applicable SLPA regulations, laws, and procedures. An Internet search using applicable terms such as *speech-language pathology assistant, support personnel, registration, certification,* or *licensure,* as well as the name of your individual state, will likely yield this contact information.

Last, before a detailed discussion about SLPA training and use is provided, it is helpful to understand what documents and guidelines are available on this (and related topics) from ASHA. Appendix 1–C contains a description of cardinal sources from ASHA relative to SLPAs. ASHA also maintains a "Frequently Asked Questions" section on its website with current and helpful information about SLPAs (ASHA, n.d.-c). (This information is available at http://www .asha.org). Recently, ASHA also created "practice portals" for professionals to access ASHA resources and policies on a given topic. The practice portal on the subject of SLPAs is highly valuable for current information on the topic of SLPAs, support personnel, and related topics. It can be accessed via http://www.asha .org/Practice-Portal/Professional-Issues/ Speech-Language-Pathology-Assistants/ or by searching *practice portal* and *SLPA* on ASHA's website (http://www.asha.org/).

The information discussed in this book applies to documents published by ASHA at the writing of this book. As an SLPA, you should have ASHA's website as a favorite on your home page for ready access. Similar to state regulations, ASHA policies and documents can change over time. As such, it is critical that as an SLPA, you keep abreast of recent information from ASHA applicable to SLPAs.

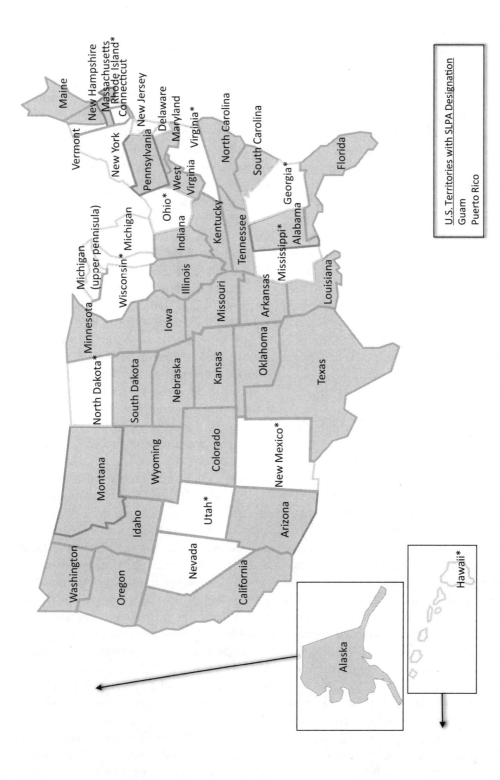

Figure 1–1. States with formal speech–language pathology assistant (SLPA) designations (ASHA, n.d.-b). *Note.* States highlighted in gray formally recognize SLPAs, through registration, certification, licensure, or some other formal mechanism. Asterisks denote states with formal designations in the field of speech–language pathology, other than SLPA, such as communication aide, technican, speech–language pathology paraprofessional, and so forth.

Following a description of SLPA use and training, the final section of this chapter describes ASHA affiliation for SLPAs, which is an additional avenue for keeping connected to ASHA's professional community.

SLPA MINIMUM QUALIFICATIONS

As noted earlier, required training and education will vary by state, but ASHA (2013, Minimal Qualifications of an SLPA, para. 1)[1] recommends the following minimum qualifications for SLPAs:

a. An associate's degree in an SLPA program, or a bachelor's degree in a speech-language pathology or communication disorders program
b. Successful completion of a minimum of one hundred (100) hours of supervised field work experience or its clinical experience equivalent
c. Demonstration of competency in the skills required of an SLPA.

SLPA DUTIES AND RESPONSIBILITIES

ASHA expectations for SLPAs working in the field of speech-language pathology include performing only those tasks that are prescribed by an SLP and adhering to all applicable guidelines and regulations, including state licensure and related rules regarding SLPAs in specific settings. Specifically, ASHA states that SLPAs are expected to do the following (ASHA, 2013, Expectations of an SLPA, para. 1)[1]:

- Seek employment only in settings in which direct and indirect supervision are provided on a regular and systematic basis by an ASHA-certified and/or licensed SLP.
- Adhere to the responsibilities for SLPAs and refrain from performing tasks or activities that are the sole responsibility of the SLP.
- Perform only those tasks prescribed by the supervising SLP.
- Adhere to all applicable state licensure laws and rules regulating the practice of speech-language pathology, such as those requiring licensure or registration of support personnel.
- Conduct oneself ethically within the scope of practice and responsibilities for an SLPA.
- Actively participate with the SLP in the supervisory process.
- Consider securing liability insurance.
- Actively pursue continuing education and professional development activities.

ASHA's (2013) document makes a specific point of highlighting those activities SLPAs should not engage in, as they are specifically outside an SLPA's scope of service (Box 1–1). If you find yourself in a situation during your training or at any point during the course of your employment as an SLPA where you engage in (or are asked to perform) any of these activities, this is a clear warning sign that you should seek immediate assistance in addressing this issue. Chapter 3 discusses ethical dilemmas such as this and recommendations for resolving this ethical conflict.

8 *Speech–Language Pathology Assistants: A Resource Manual*

Box 1–1. Activities Outside an SLPA's Scope of Practice
(ASHA, 2013, Responsibilities Outside the Scope of SLPAs, para. 1[1])

An SLPA must *not*:

a. Represent himself or herself as an SLP.
b. Perform standardized or nonstandardized diagnostic tests, formal or informal evaluations, or swallowing screenings/checklists.
c. Perform procedures that require a high level of clinical acumen and technical skill (e.g., vocal tract prosthesis shaping or fitting, vocal tract imaging and oral pharyngeal swallow therapy with bolus material).
d. Tabulate or interpret results and observations of feeding and swallowing evaluations performed by SLPs.
e. Participate in formal parent conferences, case conferences, or any interdisciplinary team without the presence of the supervising SLP or other designated SLP.
f. Provide interpretative information to the student/patient/client, family, or others regarding the patient/client status or service.
g. Write, develop, or modify a student's, patient's, or client's treatment plan in any way.
h. Assist with students, patients, or clients without following the individualized treatment plan prepared by the certified SLP and/or without access to supervision.
i. Sign any formal documents (e.g., treatment plans, reimbursement forms, or reports).
j. Select students, patients, or clients for service.
k. Discharge a student, patient, or client from services.
l. Make referrals for additional service.
m. Disclose clinical or confidential information either orally or in writing to anyone other than the supervising SLP.
n. Develop or determine the swallowing strategies or precautions for patients, family, or staff.
o. Treat medically fragile students/patients/clients independently.
p. Design or select augmentative and alternative communication systems or devices.

Now that you know what an SLPA must *not* do, ASHA's 2013 scope-of-practice document also outlines activities that are within the scope of responsibilities of an SLPA, including duties in the areas of service delivery, administrative support, and prevention and advocacy (ASHA, 2013).

Service Delivery

In the area of service delivery, ASHA recommends that SLPAs identify themselves to clients, their families, and fellow service providers, both verbally and in writing, and given a name badge (ASHA, 2013). Furthermore, as discussed in Chapter 3, SLPAs are expected to conduct themselves ethically, maintain client confidentiality, and adhere to all federal and state regulations in the provision of services in schools and medical settings. Provided SLPAs are under the direction of a qualified SLP and given adequate training and supervision, Box 1–2 outlines ASHA's recommendations for activities within the scope of an SLPA related to service delivery. SLPAs "may not perform tasks when a supervising SLP

Box 1–2. SLPA Scope of Responsibility: Service Delivery
(ASHA, 2013, Service Delivery, para. 1[1])

a. Assist the SLP with speech, language, and hearing screenings **without** clinical interpretation.
b. Assist the SLP during assessment of students, patients, and clients exclusive of administration and/or interpretation.
c. Assist the SLP with bilingual translation during screening and assessment activities exclusive of interpretation.*
d. Follow documented treatment plans or protocols developed by the supervising SLP.
e. Provide guidance and treatment via telepractice to students, patients, and clients who are selected by the supervising SLP as appropriate for this service delivery model.
f. Document student, patient, and client performance (e.g., tallying data for the SLP to use; preparing charts, records, and graphs) and report this information to the supervising SLP.
g. Program and provide instruction in the use of augmentative and alternative communication devices.
h. Demonstrate or share information with patients, families, and staff regarding feeding strategies developed and directed by the SLP.
i. Serve as interpreter for patients/clients/students and families who do not speak English.*
j. Provide services under SLP supervision in another language for individuals who do not speak English and English-language learners.*

---

*Note: In the area of interpretation and translation, Chapter 5 contains a discussion of the use of SLPAs as interpreters and translators, including ASHA (2004) recommendations for training in this area.

cannot be reached by personal contact, phone, pager, or other immediate or electronic means" (ASHA, 2013, Minimum Requirements in Frequency and Amount of Supervision, para. 1).[1] Furthermore, the purpose of an SLPA is to support the SLP in the provision of services, not to increase the caseload numbers of the SLP. ASHA recommends that SLPAs have liability insurance as protection for malpractice during service provision. Your employer may provide this insurance for you or you may be expected to independently acquire liability insurance. This should be done prior to providing services to clients. ASHA offers discounts on this insurance for SLPAs who are affiliated with ASHA as an associate.

Administrative Support

In addition to providing clinical services, SLPAs may provide administrative support to their supervisor, including the activities listed in Box 1–3.

Prevention and Advocacy

SLPAs may also assist their supervisor in activities related to the prevention of com-municative disorders and advocacy for individuals with communicative disorders and their families. Box 1–4 highlights activities within the scope of responsibilities of an SLPA in this area.

SLPA JOB DESCRIPTION: A DAY IN THE LIFE OF AN SLPA

After reading lists of duties and responsibilities, many SLPAs in training still often ask, "What will my job be like as an SLPA?" This is a valid question to ask but a difficult one to answer. The settings in which SLPAs work are highly variable, as are the populations of individuals for which SLPAs provide services. Equally variable is the nature of tasks SLPAs perform in these different settings. Appendix 1–D contains several stories, collected from SLPAs throughout the United States, which tell of a "Day in the Life" of a specific SLPA. Appendix 1–E contains a narrative from an SLPA, describing her role as an SLPA in a medical setting. Last, Appendices 1–F and 1–G contain examples of sample job descriptions for SLPAs in a medical and educational setting (respectively). Each of these docu-

---

> **Box 1–3. SLPA Scope of Responsibility: Administrative Support** (ASHA, 2013, Administrative Support, para. 1)[1]
>
> a. Assist with clerical duties, such as preparing materials and scheduling activities, as directed by the SLP.
> b. Perform checks and maintenance of equipment.
> c. Assist with departmental operations (scheduling, recordkeeping, safety/maintenance of supplies and equipment).

> **Box 1–4. SLPA Scope of Responsibility: Prevention and Advocacy** (ASHA, 2013, Prevention and Advocacy, para. 1)[1]
>
> a. Present primary prevention information to individuals and groups known to be at risk for communication disorders and other appropriate groups; promote early identification and early intervention activities.
> b. Advocate for individuals and families through community awareness, health literacy, education, and training programs to promote and facilitate access to full participation in communication, including the elimination of societal, cultural, and linguistic barriers.
> c. Provide information to emergency response agencies for individuals who have communication and/or swallowing disorders.
> d. Advocate at the local, state, and national levels for improved public policies affecting access to services and research funding.
> e. Support the supervising SLP in research projects, in-service training, public relations programs, and marketing programs.
> f. Participate actively in professional organizations.

ments sheds a different light on the role of an SLPA. Ultimately, learning firsthand by meeting and speaking directly with SLPAs and SLPs themselves is one of the best ways to learn more about the field of speech-language pathology and the roles of an SLPA.

COMPETENCY ASSESSMENT

Webster's dictionary defines *competent* as "having requisite or adequate ability or qualities" or "having the capacity to function or develop in a particular way" (Merriam-Webster, 2003). Being a competent SLPA requires knowledge and the practical application of this knowledge in the execution of specific tasks (e.g., skill).

In all settings, on-the-job training will be required to develop your knowledge and skills as an SLPA. To be competent in the performance of your SLPA duties in a specific work environment, you will need additional knowledge and skills beyond what you learned in a training program to become an SLPA.

In the field of speech-language pathology, assessment based on competency is often used. As discussed in Chapter 2, it is your supervisor's responsibility to outline what specific competencies are required for you to operate effectively as an SLPA in your unique setting (ASHA, 2013). Your supervisor is also responsible for creating a mechanism for assessing your competency in these areas and for developing ways to improve your knowledge and skills to required levels. As an

SLPA, it is your responsibility to be aware of the knowledge and skills that will be required of you and to strive for competency in all areas.

Appendix 1–H (and the CD of this book) contains an example of a competency-based measurement, given the responsibilities within the scope of an SLPA (ASHA, 2013). You will note it uses a continuum in rating the responsibilities of an SLPA on a scale from *does not meet* (1) to *far exceeds requirements* (5). Table 1–1 contains a description of performance levels for this scale. It is important to remember, however, when descriptions of competency indicate the word *independent*, this does not mean SLPAs are performing any activity without the supervision of an SLP (e.g., operating as an independent clinician). Rather, this designation means that, under a supervising SLP's guidance, an SLPA has obtained a level of competency that allows her or him to operate with proficiency in the task described. Appendix I–L contains additional evaluation tools and forms, recommended by ASHA, for documenting the presence/degree of core proficiency levels for SLPAs.

These competency-based assessments illustrate an important point to consider throughout your career as an SLPA. Competency is reflected in your level of performance at any given point in time, for a specific set of circumstances (task, client, and setting). Your competency will vary in different areas. You will likely not be equally competent across everything you do as an SLPA. That is completely normal. In fact, to expect that you will be perfect and exceed competencies in everything you do misses the potential of this type of assessment.

In every setting, additional, more specific competencies will be required, beyond the basic framework of SLPA responsibilities and job duties outlined by ASHA. For example, there will be specific knowledge and skills needed in working with young children with autism spectrum disorder (ASD). These may be similar in some respects but different from the knowledge and skills needed in working with adults with aphasia. Similarly, if you are working in a school setting, there may be specific competencies needed in that setting that differ from those of a medical or private practice setting. As an SLPA, when you enter a training or employment setting, it is critical that you review all competency assessment tools applicable to you and ask your supervisor about the range of specific knowledge and skills that will be required of you in that unique setting.

Table 1–1. Examples of Competency-Based Assessment Levels (ASHA, 2013)

Does not meet	Requires education and training at the introductory level
Needs improvement	Requires input from supervisor or other resource for routine cases.
Meets requirements	Demonstrates proficiency independently in most cases: independently seeks resources for additional support
Exceeds requirements	Independently demonstrates proficiency for routine to complex cases
Far exceeds requirements	Demonstrates proficiency at all levels of complexity; able to serve as a role model to other staff

Beyond minimal competency, as an SLPA, you should always strive for higher levels of performance in all areas of knowledge and skill applicable to your role as an SLPA. Your goal should be to continue to improve and enhance your knowledge and skills throughout your career. SLPAs who recognize there is always room for improvement and who seek ways to improve their performance are those who reach the highest levels of performance as an SLPA. ASHA also stipulates that SLPAs must "actively pursue continuing education and professional development activities" (ASHA 2013, Expectations of an SLPA, para. 1). Furthermore, many individual state regulating bodies specifically outline the amount and nature of continuing education required for an SLPA to maintain licensure, certification, or registration in that state. You should be familiar with what is required in your individual state.

It is your responsibility to seek out applicable continuing education opportunities. You can work with your supervising SLP in identifying these opportunities, but ultimately you as a professional SLPA are responsible for initiating them. Chapter 4 offers suggestions in the area of self-assessment/reflection as a mechanism for evaluating your own skills and abilities and then, importantly, seeking avenues for improvement. Self-assessment/reflection is also a valuable process in identifying areas of formal continuing education and professional growth.

ASHA AFFILIATION

In 2011, ASHA initiated a new program that offered affiliation status to support personnel, including SLPAs, audiology assistants, and other support personnel in the field of communication sciences and disorders (Robinson, 2010). According to ASHA's president at the time, this new program was created to improve patient care by: (a) providing leadership in reconciling national inconsistencies regarding the training, use, and supervision of support personnel across the United States and (b) offering resources for support personnel and their supervisors (Robinson, 2010). This program is not a certification program. SLPA affiliates are referred to as ASHA associates. They are not full members of ASHA as they are not eligible to vote or hold elected positions. In addition, ASHA does not provide direct oversight or regulation of certification for ASHA associates. This responsibility remains with the applicable state educational and/or statutory/regulatory bodies. ASHA associates, do however, have access to many ASHA member benefits (ASHA, 2011, para. 5), including the following:

- Networking opportunities with other assistants
- Affinity benefits
- Consultation with ASHA professional practices staff
- Listing and search capabilities on ASHA's online member and affiliate directory
- Opportunities to participate in advocacy efforts
- Participation in mentoring programs
- Reduced registration fees for education programs and products
- Access to the online Career Center
- Subscription to *The ASHA Leader* and access to *The ASHA Leader Online* (*ALO*)
- Access to four online scholarly journals

- Subscription to an e-newsletter for assistants
- Access to an assistants' e-group (e-mail discussion list/forum/social network)
- Opportunity to earn professional development hours (PDHs) in training specifically designed for SLPAs and audiology assistants.

You are eligible to apply for ASHA affiliation if:

1. You are employed as an SLPA and are supervised by an ASHA-certified SLP.
2. You have completed your training as an SLPA, but you are not currently employed as an SLPA.

If you are employed as an SLPA, your supervisor must sign, attesting that she or he is supervising you in accordance with ASHA policies and procedures on support personnel and that you are qualified to perform the tasks of an SLPA. If you have completed your SLPA training but are not employed, the director for your SLPA training program must sign, attesting that you have received training to become an SLPA and that you are qualified to perform the tasks of an SLPA.

ASHA associates must agree to the following (ASHA, 2011):

- Adhere to all applicable policies pertaining to the use and supervision of support personnel, including performing only those tasks assigned by a supervising speech-language pathologist or audiologist.
- Work only under the supervision of an ASHA-certified speech-language pathologist or audiologist.

- Adhere to all applicable state (province) laws and rules regulating the professions listed above.
- Pay annual fees to maintain their affiliation.

Additional information about becoming an ASHA associate, including associate program frequently asked questions (McNeilly, 2010), can be found on ASHA's website (http://www.asha.org/associates/).

REFERENCES

American Speech-Language-Hearing Association (ASHA). (n.d.-a.). *Audiology and speech-language pathology associations outside of the United States.* Retrieved from http://www.asha.org/members/international/intl_assoc.htm

American Speech-Language-Hearing Association (ASHA). (n.d.-b.). *ASHA state-by-state.* Retrieved from http://www.asha.org/advocacy/state/

American Speech-Language-Hearing Association (ASHA). (n.d.-c.). *Frequently asked questions: Speech-language pathology assistants (SLPAs).* Retrieved July 19, 2013, from http://www.asha.org/associates/SLPA-FAQs/

American Speech-Language-Hearing Association (ASHA). (2011, July 5). Welcome! ASHA initiates new affiliation category for assistants. *ASHA Leader.* Retrieved from http://www.asha.org/Publications/leader/2011/110705/Welcome--ASHA-Initiates-New-Affiliation-Category-for-Assistants/

American Speech-Language-Hearing Association (ASHA). (2013). *Speech-language pathology assistant scope of practice.* Retrieved from http://www.asha.org/policy

McCrea, E., & Brasseur, J. (2003). *The supervisory process in speech-language pathology and audiology.* Boston, MA: Pearson Education.

McNeilly, L. (2010, November). ASHA will roll out associates program in 2011. *ASHA Leader.* Retrieved from http://www.asha.org/

Publications/leader/2010/101123/ASHA-Will-Roll-Out-Associates-Program-in-2011.htm

Merriam-Webster. (2003). *Merriam-Webster's collegiate dictionary* (11th ed.). Springfield, MA: Author.

Robinson, T. L., Jr. (2010). Associates in ASHA: A new initiative. *ASHA Leader.* Retrieved from http://www.asha.org/Publications/leader/2010/100803/From-President-100803.htm

CHAPTER ENDNOTE

1. American Speech-Language-Hearing Association. (2013). *Speech-language pathology assistant scope of practice.* Retrieved from http://www.asha.org/policy. © Copyright 2013 American Speech-Language-Hearing Association. All rights reserved. Reprinted with permission.

APPENDIX 1–A

ASHA Speech–Language Pathology Assistant Scope of Practice (ASHA, 2013)

TABLE OF CONTENTS

- About This Document
- Dedication
- Executive Summary
- Introduction
- Statement of Purpose
- Qualifications for a Speech-Language Pathology Assistant
  - Minimum Recommended Qualifications for a Speech-Language Pathology Assistant
  - Expectations of a Speech-Language Pathology Assistant
- Responsibilities Within the Scope for Speech-Language Pathology Assistants
  - Service Delivery
  - Administrative Support
  - Prevention and Advocacy
- Responsibilities Outside the Scope for Speech-Language Pathology Assistants
- Practice Settings
- Ethical Considerations
  - Principle of Ethics I
  - Principle of Ethics I, Rule A
  - Principle of Ethics I, Rule D
  - Principle of Ethics I, Rule E
  - Principle of Ethics I, Rule F
  - Principle of Ethics II, Rule B
  - Principle of Ethics II, Rule D
  - Principle of Ethics IV, Rule B
- Liability Issues
- Speech-Language Pathologist's Supervisory Role

- Qualifications for a Supervising Speech-Language Pathologist
- Additional Expectations of the Supervising Speech-Language Pathologist
- Guidelines for SLP Supervision of Speech-Language Pathology Assistants
  - SLP to SLPA Ratio
  - Minimum Requirements for the Frequency and Amount of Supervision
- Conclusion
- Definitions
- References

ABOUT THIS DOCUMENT

This scope of practice for the speech-language pathology assistant (SLPA) was developed by the American Speech-Language-Hearing Association (ASHA) Speech-Language Pathology Assistant Scope of Practice ad hoc committee. It was approved by ASHA's Board of Directors (January 2013). Members of the committee were DeAnne Wellman Owre (chair), Diane L. Eger, Ashley Northam, Mary Jo Schill, Rosemary Scott, Monica Marruffo, and Lemmietta McNeilly (ex officio). Gail J. Richard, vice president for speech-language pathology practice, served as the monitoring vice president. The composition of the ad hoc committee included

ASHA-certified speech-language pathologists with specific knowledge and experience working with support personnel in clinical practice in schools, health care, and/or private practice, as well as two members who have served on the ASHA Board of Ethics (Diane L. Eger and Mary Jo Schill).

The document is intended to provide guidance for SLPAs and their supervisors regarding ethical considerations related to the SLPA practice parameters. The document addresses how SLPAs should be utilized and what specific responsibilities are within and outside their roles of clinical practice. Given that standards, licensure, and practice issues vary from state to state, this document delineates ASHA's policy for the use of SLPAs.

DEDICATION

In loving memory of Lisa Cabiale O'Connor (1937–2012), whose dedication, commitment, and perseverance contributed to ensuring integrity and quality in addressing the topic of SLPAs within the ASHA structure.

EXECUTIVE SUMMARY

This scope of practice presents a model for the training, use, and supervision of support personnel in speech-language pathology. Support personnel in speech-language pathology, or speech-language pathology assistants (SLPAs), perform tasks as prescribed, directed, and supervised by ASHA-certified speech-language pathologists (SLPs). Support personnel

can be used to increase the availability, frequency, and efficiency of services.

Some tasks, procedures, or activities used to treat individuals with communication and related disorders can be performed successfully by individuals other than SLPs if the persons conducting the activity are properly trained and supervised by ASHA-certified and/or licensed SLPs. The decision to shift responsibility for implementation of the more repetitive, mechanical, or routine clinical activities to SLPAs should be made only by qualified professionals and only when the quality of care and level of professionalism will not be compromised. The utilization of evidence and ethical and professional judgment should be at the heart of the selection, management, training, supervision, and use of support personnel.

This scope of practice specifies the qualifications and responsibilities for an SLPA and indicates the tasks that are the exclusive responsibilities of the SLP. Additionally, the document provides guidance regarding ethical considerations when support personnel provide clinical services and outlines the supervisory responsibilities of the supervising SLP.

INTRODUCTION

The SLPA scope of practice provides information regarding the training, use, and supervision of assistants in speech-language pathology that was established by the American-Speech-Language-Hearing Association to be applicable in a variety of work settings. Training for SLPAs should be based on the type of tasks specified in their scope of responsibility. Specific education and on-the-job training may be necessary to prepare assistants for unique roles in professional settings (e.g., hospitals and schools).

ASHA has established an associate affiliation program for support personnel in speech-language pathology and audiology. Individuals who are working in this capacity under the direct supervision of ASHA-certified SLPs or audiologists are eligible for this category of affiliation with ASHA.

ASHA has addressed the topic of support personnel in speech-language pathology since the 1960s. In 1967, the Executive Board of ASHA established the Committee on Supportive Personnel and in 1969 the document *Guidelines on the Role, Training and Supervision of the Communicative Aide* was approved by the Legislative Council (LC). In the 1990s, several entities—including committees, a task force, and a consensus panel—were established, and the LC passed a position statement, technical report, guidelines, and curriculum content for support personnel. In 2002, ASHA developed an approval process for SLPA programs, and in 2003, a registration process for SLPAs was established. Both were discontinued by vote of the LC because of fiscal concerns. In 2004, a position statement on the training, use, and supervision of support personnel in speech-language pathology was passed by the LC. Since then, the number of SLPAs has increased primarily in schools and private practice settings. Specific guidance from ASHA continues to be requested by ASHA members in many states.

This document does not supersede federal legislation and regulation requirements or any existing state licensure laws, nor does it affect the interpretation or implementation of such laws. The document may serve, however, as a guide for the development of new laws or, at the appropriate time, for revising existing licensure laws.

STATEMENT OF PURPOSE

The purpose of this document is to define what is within and outside the scope of responsibilities for SLPAs who work under the supervision of properly credentialed SLPs. The following aspects are addressed:

a. parameters for education and professional development for SLPAs;
b. SLPAs' responsibilities within and outside the scope of practice;
c. examples of practice settings;
d. information for others (e.g., special educators, parents, consumers, health professionals, payers, regulators, members of the general public) regarding services SLPAs perform;
e. information regarding the ethical and liability considerations for the supervising SLP and the SLPA;
f. supervisory requirements for the SLP and the SLPA.

QUALIFICATIONS FOR A SPEECH–LANGUAGE PATHOLOGY ASSISTANT

Minimum Recommended Qualifications for a Speech–Language Pathology Assistant

An SLPA must complete an approved course of academic study, field work under the supervision of an ASHA-certified and/or licensed SLP, and on-the-job training specific to SLPA responsibilities and workplace behaviors.

The academic course of study must include or be equivalent to:

a. an associate's degree in an SLPA program
   or
   a bachelor's degree in a speech-language pathology or communication disorders program
   and
b. successful completion of a minimum of one hundred (100) hours of supervised field work experience or its clinical experience equivalent
   and
c. demonstration of competency in the skills required of an SLPA.

Expectations of a Speech–Language Pathology Assistant

a. Seek employment only in settings in which direct and indirect supervision are provided on a regular and systematic basis by an ASHA-certified and/or licensed SLP.
b. Adhere to the responsibilities for SLPAs specified in this document and refrain from performing tasks or activities that are the sole responsibility of the SLP.
c. Perform only those tasks prescribed by the supervising SLP.
d. Adhere to all applicable state licensure laws and rules regulating the practice of speech-language pathology, such as those requiring licensure or registration of support personnel.

e. Conduct oneself ethically within the scope of practice and responsibilities for an SLPA.
f. Actively participate with the SLP in the supervisory process.
g. Consider securing liability insurance.
h. Actively pursue continuing education and professional development activities.

RESPONSIBILITIES WITHIN THE SCOPE FOR SPEECH–LANGUAGE PATHOLOGY ASSISTANTS

The supervising SLP retains full legal and ethical responsibility for the students, patients, and clients he or she serves but may delegate specific tasks to the SLPA. The SLPA may execute specific components of a speech and language program as specified in treatment plans developed by the SLP. Goals and objectives listed on the treatment plan and implemented by the SLPA are only those within their scope of responsibilities and are tasks the SLP has determined the SLPA has the training and skill to perform. The SLP must provide at least the minimum specified level of supervision to ensure quality of care to all persons served. The amount of supervision may vary and must depend on the complexity of the case and the experience of the assistant. Under no circumstances should use of the ASHA Code of Ethics or the quality of services provided be diluted or circumvented by the use of an SLPA. Again, the use of an SLPA is optional, and an SLPA should be used only when appropriate.

Provided that the training, supervision, and planning are appropriate, tasks in the following areas of focus may be delegated to an SLPA.

Service Delivery

a. Self-identify as SLPAs to families, students, patients, clients, staff, and others. This may be done verbally, in writing, and/or with titles on name badges.
b. Exhibit compliance with The Health Insurance Portability and Accountability Act (HIPAA) and Family Educational Rights and Privacy Act (FERPA) regulations, reimbursement requirements, and SLPAs' responsibilities.
c. Assist the SLP with speech, language, and hearing screenings **without** clinical interpretation.
d. Assist the SLP during assessment of students, patients, and clients exclusive of administration and/or interpretation
e. Assist the SLP with bilingual translation during screening and assessment activities exclusive of interpretation; refer to *Knowledge and Skills Needed by Speech-Language Pathologists and Audiologists to Provide Culturally and Linguistically Appropriate Services* (ASHA, 2004).
f. Follow documented treatment plans or protocols developed by the supervising SLP.
g. Provide guidance and treatment via telepractice to students, patients, and clients who are selected by the supervising SLP as appropriate for this service delivery model.
h. Document student, patient, and client performance (e.g., tallying data for the SLP to use; preparing charts, records, and graphs) and report this information to the supervising SLP.
i. Program and provide instruction in the use of augmentative and alternative communication devices.
j. Demonstrate or share information with patients, families, and staff regarding feeding strategies developed and directed by the SLP.
k. Serve as interpreter for patients/clients/students and families who do not speak English.
l. Provide services under SLP supervision in another language for individuals who do not speak English and English-language learners.

Administrative Support

a. Assist with clerical duties, such as preparing materials and scheduling activities, as directed by the SLP.
b. Perform checks and maintenance of equipment.
c. Assist with departmental operations (scheduling, recordkeeping, safety/maintenance of supplies and equipment).

Prevention and Advocacy

a. Present primary prevention information to individuals and groups known to be at risk for communication disorders and other appropriate groups; promote early identification and early intervention activities.
b. Advocate for individuals and families through community awareness, health literacy, education, and training programs to promote and facilitate access to full participation in communication, including the elimination of societal, cultural, and linguistic barriers.
c. Provide information to emergency response agencies for individuals who have communication and/or swallowing disorders.

d. Advocate at the local, state, and national levels for improved public policies affecting access to services and research funding.
e. Support the supervising SLP in research projects, in-service training, public relations programs, and marketing programs.
f. Participate actively in professional organizations.

RESPONSIBILITIES OUTSIDE THE SCOPE FOR SPEECH–LANGUAGE PATHOLOGY ASSISTANTS

There is potential for misuse of an SLPA, particularly when responsibilities are delegated by administrative or nonclinical staff without the approval of the supervising SLP. It is highly recommended that the *ASHA Scope of Practice in Speech-Language Pathology* (ASHA, 2007) and the *ASHA Code of Ethics* (ASHA, 2010) be reviewed with all personnel involved when employing an SLPA. It should be emphasized that an individual's communication or related disorder and/or other factors may preclude the use of services from anyone other than an ASHA-certified and/or licensed SLP. The SLPA should not perform any task without the approval of the supervising SLP. The student, patient, or client should be informed that he or she is receiving services from an SLPA under the supervision of an SLP.

The SLPA should *not* engage in the following:

a. represent himself or herself as an SLP;
b. perform standardized or nonstandardized diagnostic tests, formal or informal evaluations, or swallowing screenings/checklists;
c. perform procedures that require a high level of clinical acumen and technical skill (e.g., vocal tract prosthesis shaping or fitting, vocal tract imaging and oral pharyngeal swallow therapy with bolus material);
d. tabulate or interpret results and observations of feeding and swallowing evaluations performed by SLPs;
e. participate in formal parent conferences, case conferences, or any interdisciplinary team without the presence of the supervising SLP or other designated SLP;
f. provide interpretative information to the student/patient/client, family, or others regarding the patient/client status or service;
g. write, develop, or modify a student's, patient's, or client's treatment plan in any way;
h. assist with students, patients, or clients without following the individualized treatment plan prepared by the certified SLP and/or without access to supervision;
i. sign any formal documents (e.g., treatment plans, reimbursement forms, or reports; the SLPA **should** sign or initial informal treatment notes for review and co-sign with the supervising SLP as requested);
j. select students, patients, or clients for service;
k. discharge a student, patient, or client from services;
l. make referrals for additional service;
m. disclose clinical or confidential information either orally or in writing to anyone other than the supervising SLP (the SLPA must comply with current HIPPA and FERPA guidelines) unless mandated by law;

n. develop or determine the swallowing strategies or precautions for patients, family, or staff;

o. treat medically fragile students/patients/clients independently;

p. design or select augmentative and alternative communication systems or devices.

PRACTICE SETTINGS

Under the specified guidance and supervision of an ASHA-certified SLP, SLPAs may provide services in a wide variety of settings, which may include, but are not limited to, the following:

a. public, private, and charter elementary and secondary schools;

b. early intervention settings, preschools, and day care settings;

c. hospitals (in- and outpatient);

d. residential health care settings (e.g., long-term care and skilled nursing facilities);

e. nonresidential health care settings (e.g., home health agencies, adult day care settings, clinics);

f. private practice settings;

g. university/college clinics;

h. research facilities;

i. corporate and industrial settings;

j. student/patient/client's residences.

ETHICAL CONSIDERATIONS

ASHA strives to ensure that its members and certificate holders preserve the highest standards of integrity and ethical practice. The *ASHA Code of Ethics* (2010) sets forth the fundamental principles and rules considered essential to this purpose. The code applies to every individual who is: (a) a member of ASHA, whether certified or not, (b) a nonmember holding the ASHA Certificate of Clinical Competence, (c) an applicant for membership or certification, or (d) a Clinical Fellow seeking to fulfill standards for certification.

Although some SLPAs may choose to affiliate with ASHA as associates, the Code of Ethics does not directly apply to associates. However, any individual who is working in a support role (technician, aide, assistant) under the supervision of an SLP or speech scientist must be knowledgeable about the provisions of the code. It is imperative that the supervising professional and the assistant behave in a manner that is consistent with the principles and rules outlined in the ASHA Code of Ethics. Since the ethical responsibility for patient care or for subjects in research studies cannot be delegated, the SLP or speech scientist takes overall responsibility for the actions of the assistants when they are performing assigned duties. If the assistant engages in activities that violate the Code of Ethics, the supervising professional may be found in violation of the code if adequate oversight has not been provided.

The following principles and rules of the ASHA Code of Ethics specifically address issues that are pertinent when an SLP supervises support personnel in the provision of services or when conducting research.

Principle of Ethics I

Individuals shall honor their responsibility to hold paramount the welfare of persons they serve professionally or who are participants in research and scholarly activities and they shall treat animals involved in research in a humane manner.

Guidance

The supervising SLP remains responsible for the care and well-being of the client or research subject. If the supervisor fails to intervene when the assistant's behavior puts the client or subject at risk or when services or procedures are implemented inappropriately, the supervisor could be in violation of the Code of Ethics.

Principle of Ethics I, Rule A

Individuals shall provide all services competently.

Guidance

The supervising SLP must ensure that all services, including those provided directly by the assistant, meet practice standards and are administered competently. If the supervisor fails to intervene or correct the actions of the assistant as needed, this could be a violation of the Code of Ethics.

Principle of Ethics I, Rule D

Individuals shall not misrepresent the credentials of assistants, technicians, support personnel, students, Clinical Fellows, or any others under their supervision, and they shall inform those they serve professionally of the name and professional credentials of persons providing services.

Guidance

The supervising SLP must ensure that clients and subjects are informed of the title and qualifications of the assistant. This is not a passive responsibility; that is, the supervisor must make this information easily available and understandable to the clients or subjects and not rely on the individual to inquire about or ask directly for this information. Any misrepresentation of the assistant's qualifications or role could result in a violation of the Code of Ethics by the supervisor.

Principle of Ethics I, Rule E

Individuals who hold the Certificate of Clinical Competence shall not delegate tasks that require the unique skills, knowledge, and judgment that are within the scope of their profession to assistants, technicians, support personnel, or any nonprofessionals over whom they have supervisory responsibility.

Guidance

The supervising SLP is responsible for monitoring and limiting the role of the assistant as described in these guidelines and in accordance with applicable licensure laws.

Principle of Ethics I, Rule F

Individuals who hold the Certificate of Clinical Competence may delegate tasks related to provision of clinical services to assistants, technicians, support personnel, or any other persons only if those services are appropriately supervised, realizing that the responsibility for client welfare remains with the certified individual.

Guidance

The supervising SLP is responsible for providing appropriate and adequate direct and indirect supervision to ensure that the services provided are appropriate and meet practice standards. The SLP should document supervisory activities and adjust the amount and type of supervision to ensure that the Code of Ethics is not violated.

Principle of Ethics II, Rule B

Individuals shall engage in only those aspects of the professions that are within the scope of their professional practice and competence, considering their level of education, training, and experience.

Guidance

The supervising SLP is responsible for ensuring that he or she has the skills and competencies needed in order to provide appropriate supervision. This may include seeking continuing education in the area of supervision practice.

Principle of Ethics II, Rule D

Individuals shall not require or permit their professional staff to provide services or conduct research activities that exceed the staff member's competence, level of education, training, and experience.

Guidance

The supervising SLP must ensure that the assistant only performs those activities and duties that are defined as appropriate for the level of training and experience and in accordance with applicable licensure laws. If the assistant exceeds the practice role that has been defined for him or her, and the supervisor fails to correct this, the supervisor could be found in violation of the Code of Ethics.

Principle of Ethics IV, Rule B

Individuals shall prohibit anyone under their supervision from engaging in any practice that violates the Code of Ethics.

Guidance

Because the assistant provides services as "an extension" of those provided by the professional, the SLP is responsible for informing the assistant about the Code of Ethics and monitoring the performance of the assistant. Failure to do so could result in the SLP's being found in violation of the Code.

LIABILITY ISSUES

Individuals who engage in the delivery of services to persons with communication disorders are potentially vulnerable to accusations of engaging in unprofessional practices. Therefore, liability insurance is recommended as a protection for malpractice. SLPAs should consider the need for liability coverage. Some employers provide it for all employees. Other employers defer to the employee to independently acquire liability insurance. Some universities provide coverage for students involved in practicum/fieldwork. Checking for liability insurance coverage is the responsibility of the SLPA and needs to be done prior to providing services.

SPEECH-LANGUAGE PATHOLOGIST'S SUPERVISORY ROLE

Qualifications for a Supervising Speech-Language Pathologist

Minimum qualifications for an SLP who will supervise an SLPA include:

a. current ASHA certification and/or state licensure,
b. completion of at least 2 years of practice following ASHA certification,
c. completion of an academic course or at least 10 hours of continuing education credits in the area of supervision, completed prior to or concurrent with the first SLPA supervision experience.

Additional Expectations of the Supervising Speech-Language Pathologist

a. Conduct ongoing competency evaluations of the SLPAs.
b. Provide and encourage ongoing education and training opportunities for the SLPA consistent with competency and skills and needs of the students, patients, or clients served.
c. Develop, review, and modify treatment plans for students, patients, and clients that SLPAs implement under the supervision of the SLP.
d. Make all case management decisions.
e. Adhere to the supervisory responsibilities for SLPs.

f. Retain the legal and ethical responsibility for all students, patients, and clients served.
g. Adhere to the principles and rules of the ASHA Code of Ethics.
h. Adhere to applicable licensure laws and rules regulating the practice of speech-language pathology.

GUIDELINES FOR SLP SUPERVISION OF SPEECH-LANGUAGE PATHOLOGY ASSISTANTS

It is the SLP's responsibility to design and implement a supervision system that protects the students', patients', and clients' care and maintains the highest possible standards of quality. The amount and type of supervision should meet the minimum requirements and be increased as needed based on the needs, competencies, skills, expectations, philosophies, and experience of the SLPA and the supervisor; the needs of students, patients, and clients served; the service setting; the tasks assigned; and other factors. More intense supervision, for example, would be required in such instances as the orientation of a new SLPA; initiation of a new program, equipment, or task; or a change in student, patient, or client status (e.g., medical complications). Functional assessment of the SLPA's skills with assigned tasks should be an ongoing, regular, and integral element of supervision. SLPs and SLPAs should treat each other with respect and interact in a professional manner.

As the supervisory responsibility of the SLP increases, overall responsibilities will change because the SLP is responsible for the students, patients, and clients as well as for supervision of the SLPA.

Therefore, adequate time for direct and indirect supervision of the SLPA(s) and caseload management must be allotted as a critical part of the SLP's workload. The purpose of the assistant level position is not to significantly increase the caseload size for SLPs. Assistants should be used to deliver services to individuals on the SLP's caseload. Under no circumstances should an assistant have his or her own caseload.

Diagnosis and treatment for the students, patients, and clients served remains the legal and ethical responsibility of the supervisor. Therefore, the level of supervision required is considered the minimum level necessary for the supervisor to retain direct contact with the students, patients, and clients. The supervising SLP is responsible for designing and implementing a supervisory plan that protects consumer care, maintains the highest quality of practice, and documents the supervisory activities.

The supervising SLP must:

a. hold a Certificate of Clinical Competence in Speech-Language Pathology from ASHA and/or a state licensure (where applicable),
b. have an active interest in use of and desire to use support personnel,
c. have practiced speech-language pathology for at least 2 years following ASHA certification,
d. have completed or be currently enrolled in at least one course or workshop in supervision for at least 1.0 CEUs (10 clock hours).

The relationship between the supervising SLP and the SLPA is paramount to the welfare of the client. Because the clinical supervision process is a close, interpersonal experience, the supervising SLP should participate in the selection of the SLPA when possible.

SLP to SLPA Ratio

Although more than one SLP may provide supervision of an SLPA, an SLP should **not** supervise or be listed as a supervisor for more than two full-time equivalent (FTE) SLPAs in any setting or combination thereof. The supervising SLP should assist in determining the appropriate number of assistants who can be managed within his or her workload. When multiple supervisors are used, it is critical that the supervisors coordinate and communicate with each other so that minimum supervisory requirements are met and that the quality of services is maintained.

Minimum Requirements for the Frequency and Amount of Supervision

First 90 Workdays

A total of at least 30% supervision, including at least 20% direct and 10% indirect supervision, is required weekly. Direct supervision of student, patient, and client care should be no less than 20% of the actual student, patient, and client contact time weekly for each SLPA. This ensures that the supervisor will have direct contact time with the SLPA as well as with the student, patient, or client. During each week, data on every student, patient, and client seen by the SLPA should be reviewed by the supervisor. In addition, the direct supervision should be scheduled so that all students, patients, and clients seen by the assistant are directly supervised in a timely manner. Supervision days and time of day (morning/afternoon) may be alternated to ensure that all students, patients, and clients receive some direct contact with the SLP **at least once every 2 weeks**.

After First 90 Workdays

The amount of supervision can be adjusted if the supervising SLP determines the SLPA has met appropriate competencies and skill levels with a variety of communication and related disorders.

Minimum ongoing supervision must always include documentation of direct supervision provided by the SLP to each student, patient, or client **at least every 60 calendar days**.

A minimum of 1 hour of direct supervision weekly and as much indirect supervision as needed to facilitate the delivery of quality services must be maintained.

Documentation of all supervisory activities, both direct and indirect, must be accurately recorded.

Furthermore, 100% direct supervision of SLPAs for medically fragile students, patients, or clients is required.

The supervising SLP is responsible for designing and implementing a supervisory plan that ensures the highest standard of quality care can be maintained for students, patients, and clients. The amount and type of supervision required should be consistent with the skills and experience of the SLPA; the needs of the students, patients, and clients; the service setting; the tasks assigned; and the laws and regulations that govern SLPAs. Treatment of the student, patient, or client remains the responsibility of the supervisor.

Direct supervision means on-site, in-view observation and guidance while a clinical activity is performed by the assistant. This can include the supervising SLP viewing and communicating with the SLPA via telecommunication technology as the SLPA provides clinical services, because this allows the SLP to provide ongoing immediate feedback. Direct supervision does not include reviewing a taped session at a later time.

Supervision feedback should provide information about the quality of the SLPA's performance of assigned tasks and should verify that clinical activity is limited to tasks specified in the SLPA's ASHA-approved responsibilities. Information obtained during direct supervision may include, but is not limited to, data relative to: (a) agreement (reliability) between the assistant and the supervisor on correct/incorrect recording of target behavior, (b) accuracy in implementation of assigned treatment procedures, (c) accuracy in recording data, and (d) ability to interact effectively with the patient, client, or student during presentation and application of assigned therapeutic procedures or activities.

Indirect supervision does not require the SLP to be physically present or available via telecommunication in real time while the SLPA is providing services. Indirect supervisory activities may include demonstration tapes, record review, review and evaluation of audio- or videotaped sessions, and/or supervisory conferences that may be conducted by telephone and/or live, secure webcam via the Internet. The SLP will review each treatment plan as needed for timely implementation of modifications.

An SLPA may not perform tasks when a supervising SLP cannot be reached by personal contact, phone, pager, or other immediate or electronic means. If for any reason (i.e., maternity leave, illness, change of jobs) the supervisor is no longer available to provide the level of supervision stipulated, the SLPA may not perform assigned tasks until an ASHA-certified and/or state-licensed SLP with experience and training in supervision has been designated as the new supervising SLP.

Any supervising SLP who will not be able to supervise an SLPA for more than 1 week will need to: (a) inform the SLPA of the planned absence and (b) make other arrangements for the SLPA's supervision of services while the SLP is unavailable or (c) inform the clients/student/patients that services will be rescheduled.

CONCLUSION

It is the intent of this document to provide guidance for the use of speech-language pathology assistants in appropriate settings, thereby increasing access to timely and efficient speech-language services. It is the responsibility of the supervising speech-language pathologists to stay abreast of current guidelines and to ensure the quality of services rendered.

DEFINITIONS

Accountability: Accountability refers to being legally responsible and answerable for actions and inactions of self or others during the performance of a task by the SLPA.

Direct Supervision: Direct supervision means on-site, in-view observation and guidance by an SLP while an assigned activity is performed by support personnel. Direct supervision performed by the supervising SLP may include, but is not limited to, the following: observation of a portion of the screening or treatment procedures performed by the SLPA, coaching the SLPA, and modeling for the SLPA. The supervising SLP must be physically present during all services provided to a medically fragile client by the SLPA (e.g., general and telesupervision). The SLP can view and communicate with the patient and SLPA live via real-time telecommunication technology to supervise the SLPA, giving the SLP the opportunity to provide immediate feedback. This does not include reviewing a taped session later.

Indirect Supervision: Indirect supervision means the supervising SLP is not at the same facility or in close proximity to the SLPA, but is available to provide supervision by electronic means. Indirect supervision activities performed by the supervising SLP may include, but are not limited to, demonstration, record review, review and evaluation of audio- or video-taped sessions, and interactive television and supervisory conferences that may be conducted by telephone, e-mail, or live webcam.

Interpretation: Summarizing, integrating, and using data for the purpose of clinical decision making, which may only be done by SLPs. SLPAs may summarize objective data from a session to the family or team members.

Medically Fragile: A term used to describe an individual who is acutely ill and in an unstable condition. If such an individual is treated by an SLPA, 100% direct supervision by an SLP is required.

Screening: A pass-fail procedure to identify, without interpretation, clients who may require further assessment following specified screening protocols developed by and/or approved by the supervising SLP.

Speech-Language Pathology Aides/Technician: Aides or technicians are individuals who have completed on-the-job training, workshops, and so forth and work under the direct supervision of ASHA-certified SLPs.

Speech-Language Pathology Assistant: Individuals who, following academic coursework, clinical practicum, and credentialing, can perform tasks prescribed, directed, and supervised by ASHA-certified SLPs.

Supervising Speech-Language Pathologist: An SLP who is certified by ASHA and has been practicing for at least 2 years following ASHA certification, has completed not less than ten (10) hours of continuing professional development in supervision training prior to supervision of an SLPA, and who is licensed and/or credentialed by the state (where applicable).

Supervision: The provision of direction and evaluation of the tasks assigned to an SLPA. Methods for providing supervision include direct supervision, indirect supervision, and telesupervision.

Support Personnel: Support personnel in speech-language pathology perform tasks as prescribed, directed, and supervised by ASHA-certified SLPs. There are different levels of support personnel based on training and scope of responsibilities. Support personnel include SLPAs and speech-language pathology aides/technicians. ASHA is operationally defining these terms for ASHA resources. Some states use different terms and definitions for support personnel.

Telepractice: This refers to the application of telecommunications technology to delivery of professional services at a distance by linking clinician to client, or clinician to clinician, for assessment, intervention, and/or consultation.

Telesupervision: The SLP can view and communicate with the patient and SLPA in real time via Skype, webcam, and similar devices and services to supervise the SLPA, providing the opportunity for the SLP to give immediate feedback. This does not include reviewing a taped session later.

REFERENCES

American Speech-Language-Hearing Association. (2004). *Knowledge and skills needed by speech-language pathologists and audiologists to provide culturally and linguistically appropriate services.* Retrieved from http://www.asha.org/policy

American Speech-Language-Hearing Association. (2007). *Scope of practice in speech-language pathology.* Retrieved from http://www.asha.org/policy

American Speech-Language-Hearing Association. (2010). *Code of ethics.* Retrieved from http://www.asha.org/policy

---

Source: American Speech-Language-Hearing Association. (2013). *Speech-language pathology assistant scope of practice.* Available from http://www.asha.org/policy. © Copyright 2013 American Speech-Language-Hearing Association. All rights reserved.

APPENDIX 1–B

Audiology and Speech–Language Pathology Associations Outside of the United States (ASHA, n.d.)

Available at: http://www.asha.org/members/international/intl_assoc.htm

Argentina

Asociacion Argentina de logopedia Foniatria y Audiologia (ASALFA)
http://www.asalfa.org.ar/
E-mail: asalfa@ciudad.com.ar

Australia

Speech Pathology Australia
http://www.speechpathology australia.org.au/
E-mail: office@speechpathology australia.org.au

Austria

Bundesverband Diplomierte Logopadinnen Oesterreich
http://www.logopaedieaustria.at/de/welcome.htm
E-mail: office@logopaedieaustria.at

Oesterreichische Gesellschaft für Sprachheilpädagogik (OGS)
E-mail: office@sprachheilpaedagogik.at

Oesterreichische Gesellschaft für Logopadie, Phoniatrie u.Pädaudiologie
E-mail: gerhard.friedrich@meduni-graz.at

Belgium

International Bureau for AudioPhonology (BIAP)
E-mail: secretariat@biap.org

Vlaamse Vereniging voor Logopedisten Belgium (VVL)
E-mail: pol.demeyere@skynet.be

Brazil

Sociedade Brasileira de Fonoaudiologia
E-mail: diretoria@sbfa.org.br
Official journal: *Revista da Sociedade Brasileira de Fonoaudiologia*

Canada

Canadian Association of Speech-Language Pathologists and Audiologists (CASLPA)
E-mail: execdirector@caslpa.ca

Canadian Hard of Hearing Association
The Canadian Hard of Hearing Association is "Canada's only nation-wide non-profit consumer organization run by and for hard of hearing people."
2415 Holly Lane, Suite 205,
Ottawa, Canada, K1V 7P2
Phone: 613-526-1584
Fax: 613-526-4718

Cyprus

Association of Registered Speech Language Pathologists of Cyprus
E-mail: info@speechtherapy.org.cy

The Czech Republic

The Association of Clinical Logopedics in the Czech Republic
Czech Phoniatric and Paedaudiologic Society

Denmark

Audiologopaedisk Forening—Denmark (ALF)
E-mail: alf@alf.dk

Dansk Selskab for Logopaedi og Foniatri
E-mail: ibthomsen@mail.dk

Egypt

Egyptian Society for Phoniatrics and Logopedics
E-mail: nkotby@cng.com.eg

Finland

Finnish Association of Speech and Language Research
E-mail: matti.lehtihalmes@oulu.fi

France

Association pour la Rééducation de la Parole du Langage Oral et Ecrit et de la Voix (ARPLOEV)
10, rue de l'Arrivée
F-75015 Paris, France

Federation Nationale des Orthophonistes
145, Bd Magenta—75010 Paris, France
Phone: 33/1 4035 6375
Fax: 33/1 4037 4142
E-mail: fno@wanadoo.fr

Société Française de Phoniatrie
Dr. M. A. Faure
Service ORL et Audio
Faculté de médecine
F-25000 Besançon, France

Comité Français d'Audiophonologie
Dr. J. Leman
13, rue Albert Camus
F-595790 Ronchin, France

Germany

Deutsche Gesellschaft für Phoniatrie und Pädaudiologie e.V.
E-mail: martina.hoellrigl@uki.at

Deutsche Gesellschaft für Sprachheilpädagogik e.V.
E-mail: info@dgs-ev.de

Deutscher Bundesverband für Logopadie e.V.
E-mail: info@dbl-ev.de

Greece

Panhellenic Association of Logopedics
E-mail: info@logopedists.gr

Association of Scientists of Speech Pathology—Speech Therapy of Greece
E-mail: info@selle.gr

Hungary

Hungarian Association of Phonetics, Phoniatrics and Logopedics
E-mail: hlia@freE-mail.hu

Iceland

The Icelandic Association of Speech Therapists
E-mail: talmein@talmein.is

India

Indian Speech and Hearing Association
All India Institute of Speech and Hearing
Manasagangothri
Mysore, India 570006
E-mail: director@aiishmysore.in

Indonesia

Indonesian Speech Therapist Association
Kramat VII / 27, Jakarta Pusat 10430, Indonesia
E-mail: munas_ikatwi@mail.com
Phone: 62-0818139926 (Hikmah)
(Hikmatun Sadiah A.Md TW.,S.Pd)

Ireland

The Irish Association of Speech and Language Therapists (IASLT)
E-mail: info@iaslt.com

Israel

The Israeli Speech, Hearing and Language Association (ISHLA)
E-mail: ishla@netvision.net

Italy

Societa Italiana di Foniatria e Logopedia (SIFEL)

Japan

Japan Society of Logopedics and Phoniatrics (JSLP)
E-mail: onsei@jslp.org

The Japanese Association of Communication Disorders
E-mail: jslha@cd.inbox.ne.jp

The Japanese Association of Speech-Language-Hearing Therapists (JAS)
E-mail: kaiingai@jaslht.gr.jp

Korea

The Korean Society of Logopedics and Phoniatrics (KSLP)
E-mail: hschoi@yumc.yonsei.ac.kr

The Korean Academy of Speech-Language Pathology and Audiology
Do-Heung Ko, PhD, President
Okchon-dong
Chunchon 200-702, Korea
Phone: +82-33-254-1561
Fax: +82-33-240-1561
E-mail: dhko@hallym.ac.kr

Lithuania

Lithuanian Logopedic Association
E-mail: lla@su.lt

Malaysia

Malaysian Association of Speech-Language & Hearing (MASH)
P.O. Box 610, Pejabat Pos Jalan Sultan

46770 Petaling Jaya, Selangor
President: Linda Blankenette
E-mail: mash1995@yahoo.com

Malta

Malta Association of Speech and Language Pathologists
E-mail: info@aslpmalta.org

Mexico

Sociedad Mexicana de Audiologia y Foniatria
Apartado Postal 101–06
Col. Insurgentes Cuicuilco
04530 Mexico D.F.

The Netherlands

Nederlandse Vereniging voor Logopedie en Foniatrie (NVLF)
E-mail: p.plokker@nvlf.nl

Nederlandse Vereniging voor Stem-, Spraak- en Taalpathologie (NVSST)
E-mail: egerr@skno.azm.nl

New Zealand

New Zealand Speech Language Therapists Association
E-mail: nzsta@speechtherapy.org.nz

Nigeria

Nigerian Speech and Hearing Association
Dept. of Surgery, ENT Unit
College of Medicine
Idi-Araba, P.M.B.
12003 Lagos, Nigeria

Norway

Norsk Logopedlag
E-mail: ellen-malm.ofte@norsk. logopedlag.no

Philippines

Philippine Association of Speech
   Pathologists (PASP)
E-mail: pasp_secretariat@yahoo.com

Poland

Phoniatric Section of the Polish ENT
   Society
E-mail: bwoznica@ump.edu.pl

Polish Logopaedic Society
E-mail: biuro@logopedia.lublin.pl

Portugal

Associacao Portuguesa de Terapeutas
   da Fala
E-mail: geral@aptf.org
President: Catarina Olim
Avenida Miguel Bombarda, n° 8F Casal
   Minhoto, Santo Amaro de Oeiras,
   2780-343 Oeiras

Russia

The Russian Public Academy of Voice
E-mail: foncentr@mail.ru

Singapore

The Speech-Language Hearing
   Association Singapore
E-mail: secretary@shas.org.sg

Slovenia

Slovenian Logopedics Association (SAL)
President 2012: Nada Zemva
E-mail: nada.zemva@ir-rs.si

South Africa

South African Speech Language Hearing
   Association (SASLHA)
E-mail: admin@saslha.co.za

Spain

Sociedad Medica Espanola de Foniatria
   (SOMEF)

E-mail: info@somef.net

Association Espanola de Logopedia
   Foniatria y Audiologia (AELFA)
E-mail: secretaria@aelfa.org

Sweden

Swedish Association of Phoniatrics and
   Logopedics (SFFL)
E-mail: astrid.frylmark@telia.com

The Swedish Association of Logopedists
   (DIK)
E-mail: ingrid.kongslov@dik.se

Svenska LogopedFörbundet (Swedish
   Association of Speech-Language
   Pathologists)
Box 760, S-13 124
Nacka, Sweden
Phone: 46/8-466 2400
Fax: 46/8-466 2424
E-mail list: slof@dik.se

Swedish Association of Hard of Hearing
   People (HRF)
   The HRF envisions "a society where
   impaired hearing is not a hinder, but a
   natural part of a diverse community;
   a society without discrimination, one
   where all of Sweden's one million
   hard of hearing people can participate
   in studies, work and cultural
   activities, and where good aids are a
   right, not a question of income."
Gävlegatan 16, Box 6605, 113 84
Stockholm, Sweden

Switzerland

Schweizerische Arbeitsgemeinschaft für
   Logopädie (SAL)
E-mail: info@shlr.ch

Deutsche Gesellschaft für Sprach- und
   Stimmheilkunde e.V.
E-mail: office@dgss-ev.org

Societe Romande d'Audiologie
Phoniatrie et Logopedie Switzerland
(SRAPL)
E-mail: secretariat@srapl.ch

Schweizerische Gesellschaft fur
Phoniatrie, Logopädie und Audiologie
(SGPLA)

Taiwan

The Speech-Language-Hearing
Association of the Republic of China
E-mail: slha@slh.org.tw

Turkey

Association of Speech and Language
Pathologists (DKBUD)
Ahmet Rasim Sok. 9/3
Çankaya, Turkey
Phone: +90 532 33194 22
E-mail: info@dkbud.org

Association of Voice, Speech, Swallowing
Society
Büyükdere Cad. Tankaya Apt. No: 18/1
80260, Şişli - İSTANBUL
Phone: +90 (212) 233 11 26

Fax: +90 (212) 233 11 27
E-mail: info@skybd.org

United Kingdom

The British Voice Association (BVA)
E-mail: bva@dircon.co.uk

The Royal College of Speech & Language
Therapists United Kingdom (RCSLT)
E-mail: info@rcslt.org

Venezuela

Federacion Latino-Americana de
Sociedades de Foniatria
Logopedia y Audiologia (FLASFLA)
Dr. Oscar Ferrer Roo
Apartado de Chacao 60.209
Caracas 1060, Venezuela

Vietnam

Liaison Office of the Socialist Republic of
Vietnam
1233 20th Street, NW, Suite 400
Washington, DC 20036
Phone: 202-861–0737
Fax: 202-861–0917

APPENDIX 1–C

Relevant ASHA Documents

SLPA Scope of Practice

American Speech-Language-Hearing Association. (2013). *Speech-language pathology assistant scope of practice*. Available from http://www.asha.org/policy

Code of Ethics (Chapter 3, Appendix A)

American Speech-Language-Hearing Association. (2010). *Code of ethics*. Available from http://www.asha.org/policy

Confidentiality (Chapter 3, Appendix D)

American Speech-Language-Hearing Association. (2013). *Confidentiality*. Available from http://www.asha.org/policy

Ethical Issues Concerning the Use of Support Personnel

American Speech-Language-Hearing Association. (2004). *Support personnel*. Available from http://www.asha.org/policy

SLP Scope of Practice

American Speech-Language-Hearing Association. (2007). *Scope of practice in speech-language pathology*. Available from http://www.asha.org/policy

Clinical Supervision in SLP (in General)

American Speech-Language-Hearing Association. (2008). *Clinical supervision in speech-language pathology* [Technical report]. Available from http://www.asha.org/policy

APPENDIX 1–D

A Day in the Life of an SLPA: Interviews/Advice From SLPAs

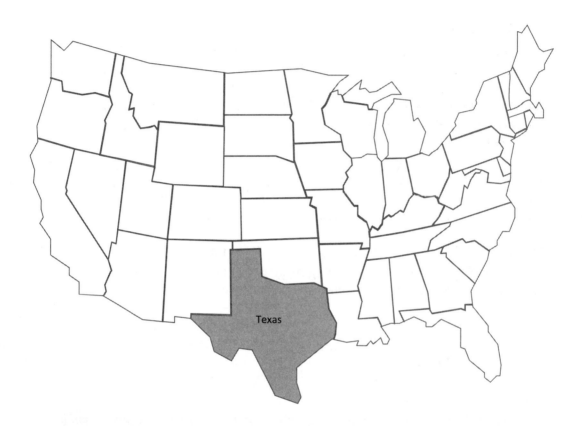

A DAY IN THE LIFE OF SARA

A Traveling SLPA

Sara is a licensed speech-language pathology assistant (SLPA) in the state of Texas. According to the American Speech-Language-Hearing Association (ASHA) (n.d., Statutory and Regulatory Requirements, para. 1), obtaining an SLPA license in Texas requires the following:

(a) a baccalaureate degree with an emphasis in communicative sciences and disorders,

(b) proof of completion of no fewer than 24 semester hours in speech-language pathology/audiology, and

(c) no fewer than 25 hours of clinical observation in the area of speech-language pathology *and* 25 hours of clinical assisting experience in speech-language pathology.

SLPAs in Texas must be supervised by a licensed speech-language pathologist (SLP) at least 2 hours per week, of which at least 1 hour must be face-to-face supervision at the location where the SLPA is employed.

Sara earned a bachelor's degree in communicative disorders. She feels fortunate to have attended a bachelor's program that also offered her the opportunity to obtain 100 hours of clinical practicum as an SLPA.

Sara is currently employed as an SLPA for a company that provides services to individuals in home settings, head start programs, and daycares. A typical day for Sara consists of traveling to these different locations to provide treatment services. Sara typically sees clients for 30-minute treatment sessions and makes about 125 to 200 visits per month. Her clients are very diverse, many of whom come from low-income households. They range in age from as young as 18 months to as old as 17 years. They have a wide spectrum of disorders, including a variety of speech and language impairments.

Rewards

Sara enjoys building rapport with her clients and their families. She finds the most rewarding aspect of her job the positive impact that she can make on her clients' lives and in seeing the joy of the children she works with when she travels to their homes to provide services. She reports that in some cases, her clients and their families tell her that her services are the highlight of their day/week.

Challenges

Sara has found that one of the challenges of her job is moving from home to home, hauling her equipment in and out of her car. She feels, though, that being in a client's home is also a big advantage, as she is able to get to know the parents and families of her clients.

Words of Wisdom

Sara reports that being an SLPA is "highly rewarding." To individuals interested in pursuing a career as an SLPA, Sara recommends you attend a school that offers an opportunity to complete your degree in communicative disorders, as well as obtain the needed observation and clinical hours required to become an SLPA.

Reference

American Speech-Language-Hearing Association (ASHA). (n.d.). *ASHA state-by-state.* Retrieved from http://www.asha.org/Advocacy/state/info/TX/Texas-Support-Personnel-Requirements/

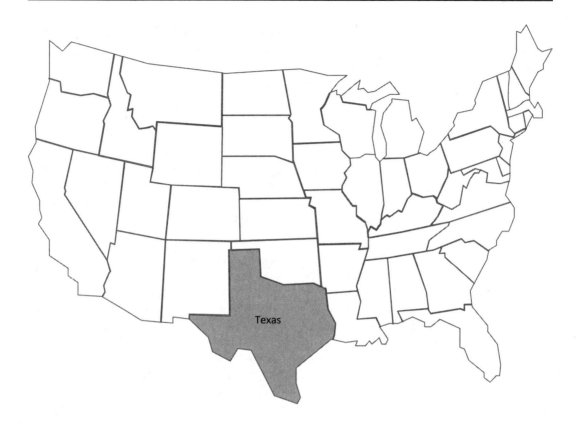

A DAY IN THE LIFE OF STEPHANIE

Never Give Up!

Stephanie is a licensed SLPA in the state of Texas. She has a bachelor's degree in communicative disorders and completed 50 hours of clinical practicum as part of her training to become an SLPA. She has been an SLPA for 5 years.

Stephanie currently works in a private practice, providing treatment services to individuals who range in age from 2 to 11 years, including individuals with autism spectrum disorder (ASD), speech sound disorder (SSD), stuttering, Down syndrome, and cleft lip/palate.

A typical day for Stephanie starts at 8:30 a.m. First, she retrieves the speech folders for each client on her treatment schedule. These folders contain an initial evaluation, testing, monthly summary reports, a calendar, and speech notes (which include each client's individual goals). Next, Stephanie plans her sessions, writing out the goals developed by her supervising SLP and possible activities for each. She then decides which activities work best for each client's goals and collects her materials.

Stephanie sees three to five clients every morning and then an additional three to four clients in the afternoon. Treatment is provided on a one-to-one basis, although sometimes social skills are targeted in group sessions. During her sessions, she tallies the client's responses on a blank sheet of paper, where she has written each client's goals for that session.

After her sessions, Stephanie writes a formal Subjective Objective Assessment and Plan (SOAP) note. Her supervising SLP reviews these notes at the end of each day.

Stephanie is also charged with keeping the treatment rooms orderly, which includes cleaning and sanitizing materials. She also assists with administrative duties, such as auditing therapy folders quarterly, to ensure all needed information is present and up to date. Stephanie participates twice weekly in team meetings, one with the entire staff and the other with her fellow SLPAs and SLP supervisor.

Rewards

Stephanie's greatest reward as an SLPA is watching her clients make progress.

Challenges

Stephanie's biggest challenge is working with children who have behavioral issues, such as children who are not compliant with requests during the session. She also has clients who can exhibit aggressive behavior during treatment sessions when they become frustrated or are asked to complete nondesired tasks.

Words of Wisdom

Stephanie's words of wisdom to new SLPAs are: (a) take the time to do research about different diagnoses/disabilities and (b) "don't give up!" When she first started working as an SLPA, Stephanie worked primarily with individuals with ASD. She recalls this was very challenging because many of her clients did not interact with her. As Stephanie put it, they seemed to be "in their own world." She also recalls they often cried, screamed, hit, or bit themselves.

In these early days of her career, Stephanie remembers sitting in her car during lunch one day, crying and thinking, "I can't do this. I don't know what I am doing!" Her supervising SLP told her, once you understand autism, working with clients will not be so hard. For Stephanie, this advice was absolutely correct. With perseverance, research, and a knowledgeable supervising SLP, Stephanie now has the techniques needed to help her clients succeed (both those with ASD and all her clients). Now, she remembers to take it one day at a time, and she realizes, "I can do this!"

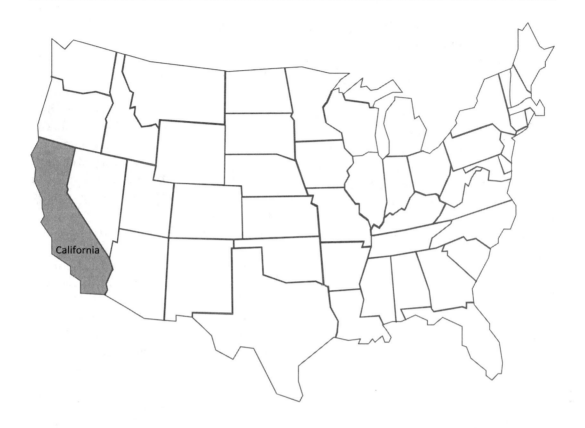

A DAY IN THE LIFE OF MIKA

Training to be an SLP

Mika is a licensed SLPA in the state of California. According to ASHA (n.d., Statutory and Regulatory Requirements, para. 1), to obtain an SLPA license in California requires at least one of the following qualifications:

- an associate of arts or sciences degree from an SLPA-accredited and board-approved program, or
- a bachelor's degree in speech-language pathology or communicative disorders from an accredited and board-approved program, *and* completion of 70 hours of fieldwork/clinical experience.

Mika has a bachelor's degree in communicative disorders and completed 100 hours of clinical practicum as an SLPA.

Mika currently works as an SLPA in a private practice, providing treatment services to children, mostly ages 2 to 5 years, who have a variety of impairments, including expressive/receptive language delay and ASD. She also provides treatment to older children, as part of a social skills group, focused on pragmatic skills, such as problem solving, perspective taking, appropriate/inappropriate conversation topics, understanding nonverbal cues, and so forth. These groups comprise three to five children, with similar ages and abilities, all who have been diagnosed with ASD.

Mika's typical day is roughly 8 hours. She arrives 30 minutes early to review each client's file and any notes from her supervising SLP. In the mornings, she also gathers the toys and materials needed for each session. She carries out treatment goals, mostly through play-based intervention. Her treatment sessions occur throughout the course of her day and are generally 50-minute sessions, provided on a one-on-one basis with each client. In the afternoons, Mika prepares files and lesson plans for the next day. She also answers phones and helps with administrative duties, as needed.

Mika is currently enrolled in a graduate program in speech-language pathology and plans to obtain her master's degree. Her long-term goal is to become a fully licensed and ASHA-certified SLP. She plans to continue working as an SLPA while attending graduate school. She feels that her experience as an SLPA will allow her to incorporate what she has learned in the therapy room with what she learns in the classroom. She is very eager to learn more, including procedures for assessment/diagnosis and an expanded range of treatment procedures. She is particularly excited to participate in internships and clinical practicum with individuals she has not yet worked with as an SLPA, such as individuals with swallowing disorders, aphasia, and so forth.

Rewards

Mika feels extremely lucky to be working with a supervising SLP and fellow clinicians who view her as a full member of a team. Her greatest reward is in having an opportunity to provide services to clients on a one-on-one basis for 1-hour sessions. She believes this provides truly individualized treatment, which leads to dramatic progression over time. She says that "watching her clients inch closer and closer to their goals is an amazing feeling." As an SLPA, she has been able to make a connection with her clients and share in their feeling of excitement when they progress, make changes, and overcome challenges.

Challenges

Mika finds controlling the environment, addressing behavior, and building rapport among the most challenging aspects of her role as an SLPA. She believes that to be truly effective as an SLPA, she must be able to multitask, simultaneously implementing treatment goals (as developed by her supervising SLP), collecting data, and modifying the environment. This must be done while taking into consideration each client's behavior/performance/needs, such as the following:

- Will this client cry?
- Is this the first time away from mom or dad?
- How do I keep the client on task while I take notes?
- What encourages good behavior?
- How do I make therapy fun but still task driven?

Words of Wisdom

First and foremost, Mika recommends that all SLPAs thoroughly understand their scope of practice. Mika also stresses that as an SLPA, you must be knowledgeable and passionate about what you do.

Mika has learned that it is important to know pertinent information in the field, but it is equally important to deliver what you know in a motivating and fun environment that is geared to each client's individual needs. She recommends that SLPAs take advantage of their environment and be willing to learn. She has found it very helpful to observe other clinicians and brainstorm additional ways she can improve her performance as an SLPA.

Reference

American Speech-Language-Hearing Association (ASHA). (n.d.). *ASHA state-by-state.* Retrieved from http://www.asha.org/Advocacy/state/info/CA/California-Support-Personnel-Requirements/

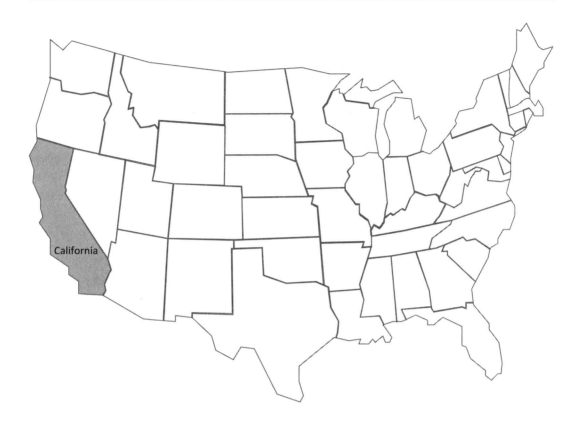

A DAY IN THE LIFE OF JACKIE

Set Yourself Apart

Jackie is a licensed SLPA in the state of California. Jackie became an SLPA by completing an associate's degree in speech-language pathology assisting. Jackie currently works in a public school setting, with children in kindergarten through eighth grade. She works at two separate elementary school campuses, providing treatment to students with a variety of impairments, including individuals with SSD and ASD. Between her two campuses, Jackie works in self-contained, functional skills classrooms and ASD-specific classrooms.

A typical day for Jackie consists of language and articulation "pull-out" treatment, when she works with students on a one-on-one basis or in small groups, and "push-in" treatment, provided to students in self-contained classrooms. A big part of Jackie's job includes collaborating with teachers for scheduling treatment sessions and data collection and recordkeeping. She also plays an active role in assisting her supervising SLP, when needed, in performing in-class observations and screenings.

Rewards

For Jackie, her greatest reward as an SLPA is in developing relationships with students and in observing their progress. She believes this comes from providing ongoing services and keeping accurate records.

Challenges

Jackie finds scheduling treatment for students in multiple grade levels, each with individual needs, to be one of the most challenging aspects of her job.

Words of Wisdom

Jackie's words of wisdom for a new SLPA are to "set yourself apart by having an area of specialty (autism, AAC, sign language)." She believes to be a successful SLPA, you must learn as much as you can during and after your training to become an SLPA. Jackie attends professional development workshops on a regular basis to enhance her skills. In California, SLPA are required to complete 12 hours of continuing professional development (CPD) every 2 years (ASHA, n.d.). Jackie accrues well over this minimum and feels it has been the secret to her success. She also believes being a team player is critical and recommends that new SLPAs be open to completing any and all tasks within their scope of practice.

Reference

American Speech-Language-Hearing Association (ASHA). (n.d.). *ASHA state-by-state.* Retrieved from http://www.asha.org/Advocacy/state/info/CA/California-Support-Personnel-Requirements/

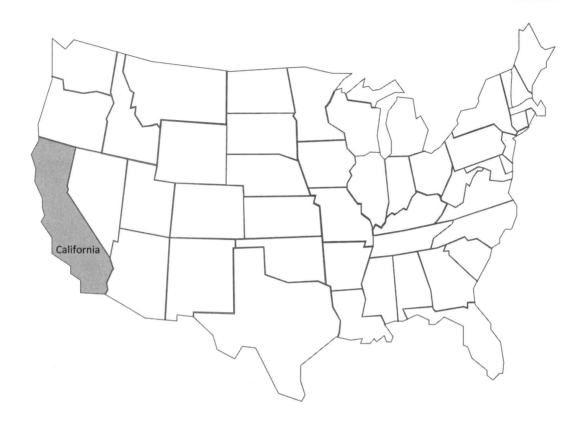

A DAY IN THE LIFE OF SUSAN

A Bilingual SLPA

Susan is a licensed SLPA in the state of California. Susan has an associate's degree in speech-language pathology assisting and completed 216 hours of clinical practicum with both children and adults as part of her training to become an SLPA.

Susan works in a public school setting in California with children ages 3 to 12 years, many of whom have articulation problems, language delays, or both. She also works with individuals with Down syndrome, ASD, and other disabilities. The students at her school have diverse cultural and linguistic backgrounds. Many come from low-income households.

Susan works an 8-hour day. She spends 2 hours per day completing paperwork, preparing materials for therapy sessions, performing recordkeeping, and working with the office manager to contact parents, teachers, and representatives from other disciplines to schedule individualized educational plan (IEP) meetings, including preparing notices and documents for IEP meetings. She also assists her supervisor in preparing material to share with parents. Often these materials go beyond solely speech and language domains, such as resources for affordable clothing, low-cost medical and dental services, and activities for parents to do with their children outside of school. The remainder of her day is spent providing therapy to students, in small groups or on a one-on-one basis. She also assists her supervising SLPs in screenings and assessment of new and current Spanish-speaking students.

Susan is a bilingual SLPA (Spanish). According to ASHA's (2013) scope-of-practice document, bilingual SLPAs who have been provided with adequate training, planning, and supervision may perform the following tasks (Service Delivery, para. 1):

1. Assist the SLP with bilingual translation during screening and assessment activities exclusive of interpretation
2. Serve as interpreter for patients/clients/students and families who do not speak English
3. Provide services under SLP supervision in another language for individuals who do not speak English and English-language learners.

Susan performs each of these tasks, at her school sites, on a regular basis. She is also called to assist with bilingual assessment at the eight schools within her district. She received training both as an interpreter and in conducting bilingual assessments alongside district SLPs. She has hands-on experience through her work as an SLPA and received training as a district translator. She has learned to be flexible in her role as a bilingual SLPA and notes that "one size does fit all." She has noticed in working as a bilingual SLPA that often materials are not available in other languages, and in these cases, she works with her supervising SLP to translate information for her clients and their families. She feels that is critical in providing a connection with her client's families and granting them equal access to resources. She also conducts the majority of treatment in Spanish.

Rewards

According to Susan, the most rewarding part of her job as an SLPA is seeing the growth in the students she works with and having them actually exit the speech program. She looks forward to hearing about their achievements as they transition to junior high and high school settings.

Challenges

Susan's greatest challenge is not always having the right or current tools to work with her students, such as computer programs, iPads, or material in general. She has at times spent her own money on materials, supplies, and reinforcements for her students, as her school district does not consistently provide these items.

Words of Wisdom

Susan thinks those training to be an SLPA should have a realistic picture of what it means to be an SLPA. She says it is not always like textbooks and classes can make it seem. There are real challenges in working as an SLPA, such as when you may not have the resources or tools you need to do your job effectively. Susan's advice is not to become an SLPA for the money but because you love working with children, especially those with disabilities and behavioral challenges. She has also found it very valuable to get to know as much as she can about the clients she works with as an SLPA. She reads their reports carefully and tries to get a sense of their family life and circumstances, such as who they are living with, whether they are immigrants and which country they are from, their economic background, whether multiple families are living in the home, and whether they live in a house, apartment, motel, and so forth. She finds this helps her to understand her clients better and to find ways to motivate them to do their best and be successful.

Reference

American Speech-Language-Hearing Association (ASHA). (2013). *Speech-language pathology assistant scope of practice*. Retrieved from http://www.asha.org/policy/SP2013-00337/

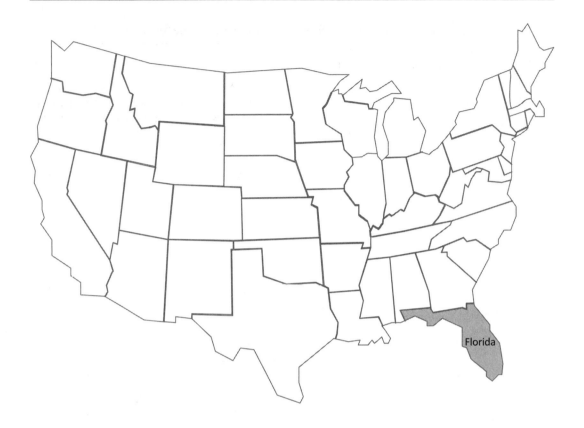

A DAY IN THE LIFE OF LAURE

An Amazing Field

Laure is a licensed SLPA in Florida. In Florida, to be certified as an SLPA, one must complete the following:

> A bachelor's degree from a regionally accredited college or university, including completion of 24 semester hours as specified by the board from a Council for Higher Education–accredited institution

SLPAs also receive on-the-job training by a licensed SLP, who maintains responsibility for all services performed by the SLPA (ASHA, n.d.). SLPAs in Florida must also complete 20 continuing education (CE) units per biennium certificate renewal (2 of these hours must be in an approved course related to the prevention of medical errors) (ASHA, n.d., para. 1).

Laure has a bachelor's degree in management information systems. She also completed more than 200 hours of practicum (24 semester hours) to obtain her license as an SLPA. Laure is currently enrolled in a master's program in communication science and disorders. She has three semesters left in completing her master's degree.

She currently works in a private practice setting with children ranging in age from 3 to 13 years. Half her caseload in this setting consists of individuals with SSD and specifically those with articulation goals. She also works with individuals with delays in receptive and/or expressive language skills. A typical day for Laure consists of providing therapy services, as directed by her supervising SLP, often using play-based, child-directed approaches. For the most part, Laure sees clients individually, but there are times when she also works with small groups of students.

Rewards

Laure really enjoys the relationship she has been developing with her supervising SLP. She has also been able to develop an excellent rapport with her clients, their parents, and school personnel. She loves seeing her clients' progress and watching them grow and develop both personally and academically.

Challenges

Laure finds the most challenging aspect of her job is that of managing client behavior, especially for students with severe developmental delays, who may exhibit high levels of frustration, and for younger children, who need consistent structure and redirection. She has noticed that sometimes helping a client to participate and remain on task may be as simple as

discovering the client's likes and dislikes and determining what learning modality works best. For example, she has found that some children do not respond well to auditory-visual stimulation, and in that case, they may need a more kinesthetic approach where they are allowed to touch and do things themselves. Other children may just need positive, visual reinforcement, which gives them instant reward for small successes.

Words of Wisdom

Laure's advice to new SLPAs is to "hang in there because this is an amazing field." Laure recalls that when she first started, she was "so green," with little experience. However, after doing this for the past year, she has found it to be truly rewarding and cannot help but say to others who are considering going into this field, especially those who may be struggling to get through their training, that it is well worth it!

Reference

American Speech-Language-Hearing Association (ASHA). (n.d.). *ASHA state-by-state.* Retrieved from http://www.asha.org/Advocacy/state/info/FL/Florida-Support-Personnel-Requirements/

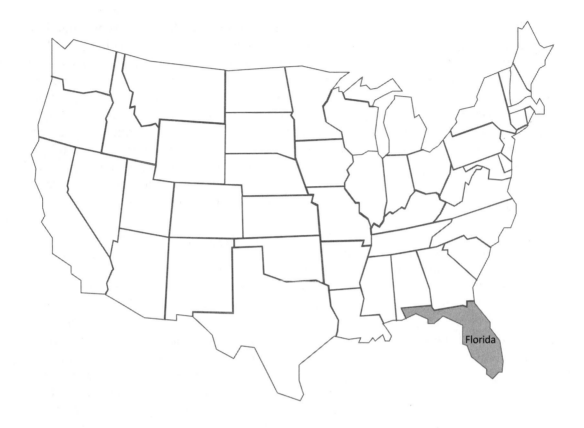

A DAY IN THE LIFE OF ALYSON

There Are No Wrong Questions

Alyson is a licensed SLPA in the state of Florida. She has a bachelor's degree in communicative disorders and completed 20 hours of clinical practicum as part of her training to become an SLPA. Alyson works part-time for a private practice, providing services to individuals ages 3 to 12 years with primarily SSD and language impairments. She is currently working and applying to graduate schools as she hopes to complete her master's degree and become a fully certified SLP.

Rewards

Alyson says the most rewarding aspect of her job as an SLPA is seeing the progress her clients make, whether it be little or big gains.

Challenges

For Alyson, the most challenging aspects of working as an SLPA are finding the right activities/materials to work effectively with each client. She feels that without the clinical and educational background that comes with a master's degree, she does not always know where to begin.

Words of Wisdom

Alyson recommends that SLPAs, regardless of their experience, should "ask lots of questions." She often faces problems/situations that she is not sure how to address, but she feels fortunate to work in a friendly and safe environment where everyone is willing to help one another. She regularly seeks the guidance of her supervising SLP. She feels there are no wrong questions, but the important thing is to ask.

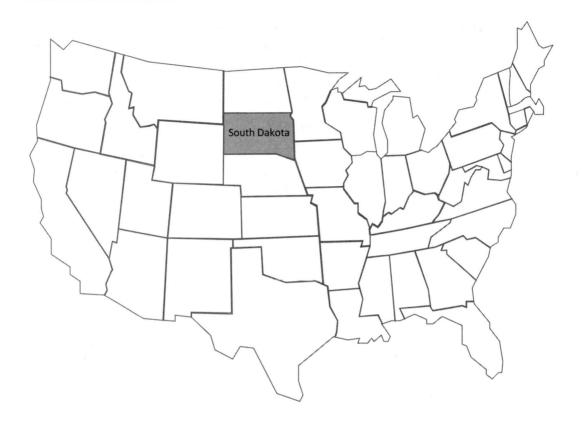

A DAY IN THE LIFE OF JENNIFER

Two Sites and Two Supervisors

Jennifer is a licensed SLPA in the state of South Dakota. To obtain a license in South Dakota, individuals must (ASHA, n.d.):

1. hold an associate's degree in SLPA or a bachelor's degree, with major emphasis in speech-language pathology or communication disorders, from an accredited academic institution;
2. complete a minimum of 100 clock hours of supervised clinical practicum as an SLPA, while either on the job or during academic preparation; and
3. have committed no act for which disciplinary action is justified.

SLPAs in South Dakota must be supervised by a licensed SLP with at least 3 years of experience (ASHA, n.d.). Jennifer has an associate's degree in speech language pathology assisting, which included both observation and 100 hours of fieldwork experience as an SLPA.

Jennifer works in an elementary school setting, with grades kindergarten through third grade. She primarily works with individuals with SSD and in particular students with goals targeting articulation. She also provides services to students with fluency and language disorders. Jennifer's time is split between two different school sites, each with a designated supervising SLP. Her supervising SLPs see the clients she treats once per week. She also meets with both her supervisors once per week to discuss students, materials, and anything else that might come up for the week.

Most days, Jennifer provides treatment to students back to back, with a short break in her day for lunch and to travel between sites. She plans for her treatment sessions after school or one afternoon a week designated for related paperwork and planning. Her treatment is usually provided to small groups of students with similar goals.

Rewards

For Jennifer, the most rewarding aspect of being an SLPA is getting to see the progress students make from one year to the next. She also feels fortunate to have supervisors who have different styles, so she is able to learn from both.

Challenges

Jennifer finds the most challenging aspect of her job as an SLPA is working with students who have challenging behaviors. She says you never know what type of day a student is having and need to be prepared.

Words of Wisdom

Jennifer's words of wisdom for new SLPAs are to remember that each student is unique. Jennifer believes you can find the right way to help each student if you keep in mind that every little thing is a learning experience for that student. If you do not feel like they accomplished enough during a specific session, Jennifer encourages new SLPAs to remember that more sessions are ahead (and to try again).

Reference

American Speech-Language-Hearing Association (ASHA). (n.d.). *ASHA state-by-state.* Retrieved from http://www.asha.org/Advocacy/state/info/SD/South-Dakota-Support-Personnel-Requirements/

APPENDIX 1-E

A Glimpse Into the World of Speech-Language Pathology Assistants (SLPAs) in the Health Care Setting

Jeneane Douglas

I hear the following question often from my physical therapy and occupational therapy coworkers (and even a few speech-language pathologists) in the hospital where I work: "Just what is a speech-language pathology assistant (SLPA), anyway?" As a licensed physical therapist assistant (LPTA) for 22 years and an SLPA (with Oregon state certification) for 4, I answer with the comparison of the certified occupational therapist assistant (COTA) and LPTA.

The American Speech-Language-Hearing Association (ASHA) describes SLPAs as "support personnel with academic and/or on the job training who carry out tasks prescribed, directed, and supervised by ASHA certified speech-language pathologists." However, unlike assistants in occupational and physical therapy, education and training requirements, certification/licensure, and scope and complexity of practice for SLPAs vary greatly across the United States. ASHA's new associates program may be instrumental in providing national advocacy and awareness of the SLPA as a distinct and valuable occupation.

The first recipients of associates' degrees in occupational therapy graduated in 1956; physical therapy assistants followed suit in 1969. SLPA-specific educational programs with practical and thorough coursework did not graduate its first class until 2002 from Pasadena City College. Today, there are approximately 21 training programs in the United States and 7 in Canada.

Each state has its own licensure or certification requirements. In 2006, for example, Oregon mandated a curriculum for SLPAs, who require certification by the state Board of Examiners for Speech-Language Pathology and Audiology. Oregon's 2-year program culminates in either a certificate or associate's degree in speech-language pathology. Individuals with a bachelor's degree in communication sciences and disorders may also apply for certification if they complete coursework commensurate with an SLPA program and a 100-hour practicum with 100% direct (line of sight or sound) supervision provided by an ASHA-certified speech-language pathologist (SLP). Oregon also requires certification renewal every 2 years and continuing education.

In the medical rehabilitation setting, SLPAs carry out a variety of duties. At Providence Neurodevelopmental Center and Center for Medically Fragile Children, a long-term pediatric skilled nursing facility in Portland, Oregon, the day begins with consultation with nursing, medical, and therapy staff. The supervising SLP outlines which patients may require direct treatment time and provides recommendations for those sessions. Plans may include augmentative and alternative communication (AAC) instruction (for patients and center staff) as well as joint treatment sessions with occupational and physical therapy staff. Each child in the facility has a communication and medical need to be addressed. Patients range in age from infancy to 21 years and have complex diagnoses, including genetic syndromes, epilepsy, and cerebral palsy that can lead to significant disabilities and communication needs. Elin Bishop, a state-certified SLPA, is one of many SLPAs in Oregon and other states who provide medically based speech-language services under the guidance of their supervising SLPs. Bishop has chosen medical speech-language pathology because of its many rewards. The most enjoyable part of her job, she says, is "being with the children. It is so rewarding and inspiring to see how far some of these kids have come."

At my facility—the Easter Seals Children's Therapy Center in Salem, Oregon —children with complex medical diagnoses are at the forefront of concern and care. Some of these diagnoses are the subjects of investigations at the Centers for Disease Control and Prevention's Undiagnosed Diseases Program.

In the course of my day, I might be with children climbing up the outdoor play structure (and discussing locative basic concepts and working on gross motor skills); discussing types of snacks during imaginative play; working on stance activities at the toy kitchen; using augmentative and alternative communication during play with wind-up cars, a doll house, or many other toys in a speech-treatment room; selecting books from the book nook; or even playing cotton-ball hockey and having a kazoo and whistle jam session with a client working on oral motor skills.

My two fellow SLPAs at the children's therapy center also confer with supervising SLPs, attend meetings with other medical discipline staff and AAC support providers, and take multiple continuing education courses to keep up on the many diagnoses of center patients. Children may present with articulation, phonology, fluency, or other communication disorders as well as needs related to cleft lip and palate, and pragmatic and other communication concerns related to autism, Down syndrome, epilepsy, Rett syndrome, and other diagnoses.

Medical SLPAs may require medically based continuing education. They also maintain consistent communication with the supervising SLP as well as with other members of the multidisciplinary rehabilitation team, service providers in school settings, and primary physicians and specialists. They also consult with AAC providers on acquiring equipment and follow-through. We also communicate with parents, who often attend outpatient visits and are eager to comply with home program recommendations.

My SLPA responsibilities are quite different, in that all of my documentation requires input from my supervising SLP; assessments and plans are to be completed solely by the SLP, who also attends meetings and confers with other providers and parents/caregivers. Supervision requirements are also vastly different; the SLPA requires line-of-sight or sound supervision for 10% of all client interaction and 10% indirect (assistance with home programs, case conferences, etc.). Supervision records must be stored for 3 years in case of an audit.

SLPAs are assets to clinicians in health care and in schools. Revonda Miller, an SLPA in North Carolina, explains that "we are a great addition to an SLP's practice by extending the amount of treatment (and billables) provided. We can provide all services except swallowing. Our training is directly in service provision, not theory and diagnosis, which are the responsibility of the supervising SLP."

Despite the similarities in education and treatment abilities for SLPAs and LPTAs, the occupational outlook, employment opportunities, and salaries for SLPAs lag behind their LPTA counterparts. Mary Pitt, an SLPA in Texas, moved away from family and friends in Florida because of the dearth of job opportunities in her home state. It is my hope that the ASHA Associate Membership program will assist with advocacy so that one day, my fellow acute-care medical rehabilitation staffers in occupational and physical therapy will no longer ask, "What is an SLPA anyway?" but instead say, "Welcome to the PT/OT/SLP team, SLPAs!"

REFERENCE

Douglas, J. (n.d.). *A glimpse into the world of speech-language pathology assistants (SLPAs) in the health care setting*. Retrieved from http://www.asha.org/associates/slpas-in-health-care/ © Copyright American Speech-Language-Hearing Association. All rights reserved.

APPENDIX 1–F

Sample Job Description—Medical Setting

SLPA JOB DESCRIPTION

Medical Facility Example

General Summary

The speech-language pathology assistant, as a member of an interdisciplinary team, works under the supervision of a certified speech-language pathologist in implementation of services for the rehabilitation of patients with speech, language, cognitive, swallowing, oral muscular, augmentative alternative communication disorders, and hearing impairments.

Essential Duties and Responsibilities

1. Prepares patients for treatment.
2. Prepares treatment areas and equipment for use.
3. Implements documented treatment plans developed by speech-language pathologist.
4. Accurately collects and records subjective and objective data.
5. Records patient status with regard to established objectives as stated in the treatment plan and reports this information to the supervising speech-language pathologist.
6. Assists the speech-language pathologist in the assessment of patients.
7. Orders supplies and equipment.
8. Engages in various clerical tasks including entry of orders for patient care, filing, billing, and ordering of equipment and supplies.

9. Maintains and cleans equipment, adhering to infection control protocol.
10. Maintains the confidentiality of information pertaining to patients and their families.
11. Behaves in accordance with the mission and values of the organization.
12. Participates in quality improvement initiatives as directed by the speech-language pathologist.
13. Respects and appropriately considers age, gender, cultural background, and related factors when providing services.

Supplemental Duties and Responsibilities

1. Participates in educational activities for patients, families, and other health professionals.
2. Participates in organizational committees as time, interest, and necessity dictate.

Required Education, Experience, and Licensure

1. The SLPA must meet state requirements for health.
2. The SLPA must have one of the following:
   - Associate's degree from a speech-language pathology assistant program;
   - Bachelor's degree in speech-language pathology;
   - Completion of a college-based speech-language pathology assistant certificate program;

- Required education as designated by the state licensing board or other regulatory agency.

Required Skills and Abilities

1. Knowledge of speech-language pathology treatment and equipment.
2. Ability to follow oral and written directions, including treatment plans.
3. Ability to work under direct and indirect supervision.
4. Ability to show excellent judgment for continuation or discontinuation of a patient's treatment under conditions of pain or discomfort.
5. Analytical skills necessary to identify and report changes in the patient and equipment.
6. Flexibility and adaptability, as the job combines patient care, clinic/equipment maintenance, and clerical responsibilities.
7. Ability to pay close attention to visual and auditory detail.
8. Ability to use a variety of computer programs for documentation and patient treatment.
9. Ability to push wheelchair-bound patients and assist ambulatory patients.
10. Ability to walk and stand up for 90% of the work day.

Working Conditions

1. Work is a combination of sedentary and physical activities completed in a normal patient care and office environment.
2. Travel in a company or personal vehicle may be required.
3. Exposure to body fluids is frequent. Exposure to blood-borne pathogens and other infectious material is possible.
4. Exposure to verbally and/or physically aggressive patients is possible.

Reporting Relationships

The SLPA is directly and indirectly supervised by a certified speech-language pathologist. The supervising SLP maintains legal and moral responsibility for all services provided by the SLPA and ensures that such services are in compliance with the ASHA Code of Ethics, ASHA Guidelines for Speech-Language Pathology Assistants, and state licensure laws.

Source: Reprinted with permission from *Practical Tools and Forms for Supervising Speech-Language Pathology Assistants.* © 2013. American Speech-Language-Hearing Association. All rights reserved.

APPENDIX 1–G

Sample Job Description—Educational Setting

SLPA JOB DESCRIPTION

Educational Facility Example

General Summary

The speech-language pathology assistant, as a member of an educational team, works under the supervision of a certified speech-language pathologist in implementation of services for children/students with speech, language, cognitive, voice, swallowing, oral muscular, augmentative/alternative communication disorders, and hearing impairments.

Essential Duties and Responsibilities

1. Prepares work area and materials for use.
2. Accompanies the student from the classroom to the service area or prepares classroom for service delivery.
3. Implements documented treatment/intervention plans developed by the speech-language pathologist.
4. Accurately collects and records subjective and objective data.
5. Records student's status with regard to established objectives as stated in the treatment plan and reports this information to the supervising speech-language pathologist.
6. Assists the speech-language pathologist in the assessment of students.
7. Orders supplies and equipment.
8. Engages in various clerical tasks, including filing and copying.

9. Maintains and cleans equipment, adhering to infection control protocol.
10. Maintains the confidentiality of information pertaining to students and their families.
11. Behaves in accordance with the educational facility guidelines.
12. Respects and appropriately considers age, gender, cultural/linguistic background, and related factors when providing services.

Supplemental Duties and Responsibilities

1. Participates in educational facility activities and committees as requested by the speech-language pathologist.
2. Participates in classroom activities as requested by the speech-language pathologist.
3. Participates in conferences as requested by the speech-language pathologist.

Required Education, Experience, and Licensure

1. The SLPA must meet state and facility requirements for health.
2. The SLPA must have one of the following:
   - Associate's degree from a speech-language pathology assistant program;
   - Bachelor's degree in speech-language pathology;
   - Completion of a college-based speech-language pathology assistant certificate program;

- Required education as designated by the state licensing board or other regulatory agency.

Required Skills and Abilities

1. Knowledge of speech-language pathology equipment, materials, and procedures.
2. Ability to follow oral and written directions, including intervention plans.
3. Ability to work with students individually and in groups.
4. Ability to interact appropriately with others involved in the student's program, including the teacher, parent, and other personnel.
5. Analytical skills necessary to identify and report changes in the student or equipment.
6. Flexibility and adaptability, as the job combines direct intervention, classroom work, equipment/materials maintenance, and clerical responsibilities.
7. Ability to pay close attention to visual and auditory detail.
8. Ability to use a variety of computer programs for intervention and documentation.

9. Ability to walk and stand up for 90% of the work day.

Working Conditions

1. Work is a combination of sedentary and physical activities completed in a normal educational environment.
2. Travel between educational facilities in a personal vehicle may be required.
3. Exposure to body fluids and other infectious material is possible.
4. Exposure to verbally and/or physically aggressive students is possible.

Reporting Relationships

The SLPA is directly and indirectly supervised by a certified speech-language pathologist. The supervising SLP maintains legal and moral responsibility for all services provided by the SLPA, and ensures that such services are in compliance with the ASHA Code of Ethics, ASHA Guidelines for Speech-Language Pathology Assistants, state regulatory/licensure laws, and educational facility guidelines.

Source: Reprinted with permission from *Practical Tools and Forms for Supervising Speech-Language Pathology Assistants.* © 2013. American Speech-Language-Hearing Association. All rights reserved.

Example of Competency–Based Assessment

*SLPA Scope of Responsibilities Competency Assessment**

PROFESSIONAL CONDUCT						
	Does Not Meet	*Needs Improvement*	*Meets Requirements*	*Exceeds Requirements*	*Far Exceeds Requirements*	*COMMENTS*
Refrains from performing tasks or activities that are the sole responsibility of the SLP; performs only those tasks prescribed by the supervising SLP.						
Adheres to all applicable state licensure laws and rules regulating the practice of speech-language pathology, such as those requiring licensure or registration of support personnel.						
Conducts oneself ethically, within the scope of practice and responsibilities for an SLPA.						
Actively participates with the SLP in the supervisory process.						
Actively pursues continuing education and professional development activities.						

continues

Appendix 1–H. *continued*

SERVICE DELIVERY

	Does Not Meet	Needs Improvement	Meets Requirements	Exceeds Requirements	Far Exceeds Requirements	COMMENTS
Identifies self as an SLPA to families, students, patients, clients, staff, and others.						
Maintains client confidentiality; exhibits compliance with the Health Insurance Portability and Accountability Act (HIPAA) and Family Educational Rights and Privacy Act (FERPA) regulations, reimbursement requirements, and SLPAs' responsibilities.						
Assists with speech, language, and hearing screenings without clinical interpretation.						
Assists during assessment of students, patients, and clients exclusive of administration and/or interpretation.						
Assists with bilingual translation during screening and assessment activities exclusive of interpretation.						
Follows documented treatment plans or protocols developed by the supervising SLP.						

	Does Not Meet	Needs Improvement	Meets Requirements	Exceeds Requirements	Far Exceeds Requirements	COMMENTS
Provides guidance and treatment via telepractice to students, patients, and clients, as directed by the supervising SLP.						
Documents student, patient, and client performance (e.g., tallying data for the SLP to use; preparing charts, records, and graphs) and reports this information to the supervising SLP.						
Programs and provides instruction in the use of augmentative and alternative communication (AAC) devices.						
Demonstrates or shares information with patients, families, and staff regarding feeding strategies developed and directed by the supervising SLP.						
As applicable, serves as interpreter for patients/clients/students and families who do not speak English.						
As applicable, provides services under SLP supervision in another language for individuals who do not speak English and English-language learners.						

continues

Appendix 1–H. *continued*

ADMINISTRATIVE SUPPORT						
	Does Not Meet	*Needs Improvement*	*Meets Requirements*	*Exceeds Requirements*	*Far Exceeds Requirements*	*COMMENTS*
Assists with clerical duties, such as preparing materials and scheduling activities.						
Performs checks and maintenance of equipment.						
Assists with departmental operations (scheduling, recordkeeping, safety/maintenance of supplies and equipment).						
PREVENTION AND ADVOCACY						
	Does Not Meet	*Needs Improvement*	*Meets Requirements*	*Exceeds Requirements*	*Far Exceeds Requirements*	*COMMENTS*
Presents primary prevention information to individuals and groups known to be at risk for communication disorders and other appropriate groups; promotes early identification and early intervention activities.						

	Does Not Meet	Needs Improvement	Meets Requirements	Exceeds Requirements	Far Exceeds Requirements	COMMENTS
Advocates for individuals and families through community awareness, health literacy, education, and training programs to promote and facilitates access to full participation in communication, including the elimination of societal, cultural, and linguistic barriers.						
Provides information to emergency response agencies for individuals who have communication and/or swallowing disorders.						
Advocates at the local, state, and national levels for improved public policies affecting access to services and research funding.						
Supports the supervising SLP in research projects, in-service training, public relations programs, and marketing programs.						
Participates actively in professional organizations.						

Note: Competencies based on ASHA (2013). *Speech-language pathology assistant scope of practice*. Retrieved from http://www.asha.org/policy

Recommendations for additional training/education: _____

_____

_____

APPENDIX 1–I

Technical Proficiency Checklist

Verification of Technical Proficiency of a Speech-Language Pathology Assistant

Speech-Language Pathology Assistant Name: _____

Supervisor(s) Name: _____

Program/Facility Name: _____

Skills	Achievement of Skill	
	Yes	No
Clerical/Administrative Skills		
Assists with clerical skills and departmental operations (e.g., preparing materials, scheduling activities, keeping records)		
Participates in in-service training		
Performs checks, maintenance, and calibration of equipment		
Supports supervising SLP in research projects and public relations programs		
Collects data for quality improvement		
Prepares and maintains patient/client charts, records, graphs for displaying data		
Interpersonal Skills		
Uses appropriate forms of address with patient/client, family, caregivers, and professionals (e.g., Dr., Mr., Mrs., Ms.)		
Greets patient/client, family, and caregiver and identifies self as a speech-language pathology assistant		
Restates information/concerns to supervising SLP as expressed by patient/client, family, and caregivers as appropriate		
Directs patient/client, family, and caregivers to supervisor for clinical information		
Is courteous and respectful in various communication situations		
Uses language appropriate to a patient/client, family, or caregiver's education level, communication style, developmental age, communication disorder, and emotional state		
Demonstrates awareness of patient/client needs and cultural values		
Conduct in Work Setting		
Recognizes own limitations within the ASHA SLP Assistant Scope of Practice		
Upholds ethical behavior and maintains confidentiality as described in the ASHA SLP Assistant Scope of Practice		

Skills	Achievement of Skill	
	Yes	No
Maintains client records in accordance with confidentiality regulations/laws as prescribed by supervising SLP		
Discusses confidential patient/client information only at the direction of supervising SLP		
Identifies self as an assistant in all written and oral communication with the client/patient, family, caregivers, and staff		
Demonstrates ability to explain to supervising SLP the scope of information that should be discussed with the patient/client, family, caregivers, and professionals		
Arrives punctually and prepared for work-related activities		
Completes documentation and other tasks in a timely manner		
Maintains personal appearance and language expected for the specific work setting		
Evaluates own performance		
Uses screening instruments and implements treatment protocols only after appropriate training and only as prescribed by supervising SLP		
Seeks clarification from supervising SLP as needed to follow the prescribed treatment or screening protocols		
Actively participates in interaction with supervisor demonstrating use of supervisor's feedback		
Maintains accurate records representing assigned work time with patients/clients		
Implements appropriate infection control procedures and universal precautions consistent with the employer's standards and guidelines		
Implements injury prevention strategies consistent with employer's standards and guidelines		
Uses appropriate procedures for physical management of clients according to employer's standards and guidelines and state regulations		
Technical Skills as Prescribed by Supervising SLP		
Accurately administers screening instruments, calculates and reports the results of screening procedures to supervising SLP		
Provides instructions that are clear, concise, and appropriate to the client's developmental age, level of understanding, language use, and communication style		
Follows treatment protocol as developed and prescribed by supervising SLP		
Provides appropriate feedback to patients/clients as to accuracy of their responses		
Identifies and describes relevant patient/client responses to supervising SLP		
Identifies and describes relevant patient/client, family, and caregiver behaviors to supervising SLP		
Uses appropriate stimuli, cues/prompts with the patient/client to elicit target behaviors as defined in the treatment protocol		

continues

Appendix 1–I. *continued*

Skills	Achievement of Skill	
	Yes	No
Maintains on-task or redirects off-task behavior of patients/clients in individual or group treatment, consistent with the patient/client's developmental age, communication style, and disorder		
Provides culturally appropriate behavioral reinforcement consistent with the patient/client's developmental age and communication disorder		
Accurately reviews and summarizes patient/client performance		
Uses treatment materials that are appropriate to the developmental age and communication disorder of the patient/client and the culture of the patient/client/family		
Starts and ends the treatment session on time		
Obtains co-signature of supervising SLP on documentation		
Accurately records target behaviors as prescribed by supervising SLP		
Accurately calculates chronological age of the patient/client		
Correctly calculates and determines percentages, frequencies, averages, and standard scores		
Uses professional terminology correctly in communication with supervising SLP		
Maintains eligible records, log notes, and written communication		
Appropriately paces treatment session to ensure maximum patient/client response		
Implements designated treatment objectives/goals in specific appropriate sequence		

Source: Reprinted with permission from *Practical Tools and Forms for Supervising Speech-Language Pathology Assistants.* © 2013. American Speech-Language-Hearing Association. All rights reserved.

APPENDIX 1–J

Direct Observation Skills Brief Checklist—Medical Setting

Speech-Language Pathology Assistant: _____

Supervising SLP: _____

Patient/Client Observed: _____

Date/Time of Observation: _____

Rate the following on a scale of 1 (disagree) to 5 (agree).

Interpersonal Skills

1. Maintains appropriate patient/client relationship.	○1 ○2 ○3 ○4 ○5
2. Demonstrates appropriate level of self-confidence.	○1 ○2 ○3 ○4 ○5
3. Considers patient's needs.	○1 ○2 ○3 ○4 ○5
4. Considers patient's cultural values.	○1 ○2 ○3 ○4 ○5
5. Uses language appropriate for patient's age and education.	○1 ○2 ○3 ○4 ○5
6. Is courteous and respectful at all times.	○1 ○2 ○3 ○4 ○5

Personal Qualities

1. Arrives punctually for the treatment session.	○1 ○2 ○3 ○4 ○5
2. Arrives prepared for the treatment session.	○1 ○2 ○3 ○4 ○5
3. Appearance is appropriate for the treatment session.	○1 ○2 ○3 ○4 ○5
4. Recognizes professional boundaries during treatment session.	○1 ○2 ○3 ○4 ○5
5. Stays within professional boundaries during treatment session.	○1 ○2 ○3 ○4 ○5

Technical and Treatment Skills

1. Completes assigned tasks within designated treatment session.	○1 ○2 ○3 ○4 ○5
2. Uses appropriate materials based on treatment plan.	○1 ○2 ○3 ○4 ○5
3. Uses materials that are age and culturally appropriate.	○1 ○2 ○3 ○4 ○5
4. Uses materials that are motivating.	○1 ○2 ○3 ○4 ○5
5. Prepares the treatment/intervention settings to meet the needs of the patient/client.	○1 ○2 ○3 ○4 ○5
6. Accurately determines correct vs. incorrect responses.	○1 ○2 ○3 ○4 ○5
7. Provides appropriate feedback as to the response accuracy.	○1 ○2 ○3 ○4 ○5
8. Verbally reports the session.	○1 ○2 ○3 ○4 ○5
9. Provides appropriate documentation of the session.	○1 ○2 ○3 ○4 ○5

Comments:

Source: Reprinted with permission from *Practical Tools and Forms for Supervising Speech-Language Pathology Assistants.* © 2013. American Speech-Language-Hearing Association. All rights reserved.

APPENDIX 1–K

Direct Observation Skills Brief Checklist—Educational Setting

Speech-Language Pathology Assistant: _____

Supervising SLP: _____

Student Observed: _____

Date/Time of Observation: _____

Rate the following on a scale of 1 (disagree) to 5 (agree).

Interpersonal Skills
1. Maintains appropriate relationship with student   ○1 ○2 ○3 ○4 ○5
2. Demonstrates appropriate level of self-confidence.   ○1 ○2 ○3 ○4 ○5
3. Considers the student's cultural/linguistic needs.   ○1 ○2 ○3 ○4 ○5
4. Uses language appropriate for student's age and education.   ○1 ○2 ○3 ○4 ○5
5. Is courteous and respectful at all times.   ○1 ○2 ○3 ○4 ○5

Personal Qualities
1. Arrives punctually for the intervention session.   ○1 ○2 ○3 ○4 ○5
2. Arrives prepared for the intervention session.   ○1 ○2 ○3 ○4 ○5
3. Appearance is appropriate for the intervention session.   ○1 ○2 ○3 ○4 ○5
4. Recognizes professional boundaries during the intervention session.   ○1 ○2 ○3 ○4 ○5
5. Stays within professional boundaries during the intervention session.   ○1 ○2 ○3 ○4 ○5

Technical and Intervention Skills
1. Completes assigned tasks within the designated session.   ○1 ○2 ○3 ○4 ○5
2. Uses appropriate materials based on treatment plan.   ○1 ○2 ○3 ○4 ○5
3. Uses materials that are age and culturally appropriate.   ○1 ○2 ○3 ○4 ○5
4. Uses materials that are motivating.   ○1 ○2 ○3 ○4 ○5
5. Prepares the intervention setting to meet the needs of the student.   ○1 ○2 ○3 ○4 ○5
6. Accurately determines correct vs. incorrect responses.   ○1 ○2 ○3 ○4 ○5
7. Provides appropriate feedback as to the response accuracy.   ○1 ○2 ○3 ○4 ○5
8. Verbally reports the session.   ○1 ○2 ○3 ○4 ○5
9. Provides appropriate documentation of the session.   ○1 ○2 ○3 ○4 ○5

Comments:

Source: Reprinted with permission from *Practical Tools and Forms for Supervising Speech-Language Pathology Assistants.* © 2013. American Speech-Language-Hearing Association. All rights reserved.

Skills Proficiency Checklist

SLPA: _____ Supervising SLP: _____

Skills or Proficiency	Self-Rating		Supervising SLP Rating			
	Date	Proficiency Level	Date	Proficiency Level	How Learned	Demonstrated

Competence Levels
1. *Little or no experience*
2. *Some experience, requires practice/assist.*
3. *Proficient with occasional supervision*
4. *Proficient with independent performance*

How Learned
Observation
On-the-job training
Class
Video
Policy/procedure

Demonstrated
Direct observation
Test (written/verbal)
Certificate/license
Discussion
Other

CHAPTER 2

Defining Roles: Supervision and Mentoring

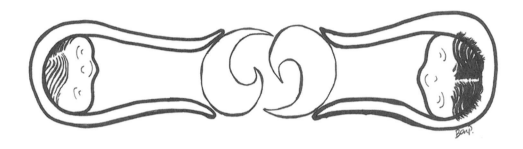

People seldom improve when they have no other model but themselves to copy.
Oliver Goldsmith (Irish poet and playwright)

SUPERVISION

Role of Your Supervisor

Speech-language pathology assistants (SLPAs) operate under the supervision of a qualified speech-language pathologist (SLP). As an SLPA, an important question to ask is, "What is the role of my supervisor?" Understanding the role of your supervisor allows you to practice as an SLPA given prescribed regulations. The American Speech-Language-Hearing Association (ASHA) has recommended guidelines relative to the supervision of SLPAs and the roles and responsibilities of those who supervise SLPAs (ASHA, 2013). The overarching theme in these recommendations casts the primary role of the supervisor as one of decision maker in directing the nature of services provided and as the individual responsible for providing oversight in protecting the patient/client's safety and in ensuring the highest quality of care. The SLPA's goal is also one of maintaining the highest quality care for the individuals she or he serves.

In this context, as the image at the start of the chapter suggests, the supervisor and SLPA are partners in bringing excellent care to individuals with communicative disorders. Ultimately, though, "diagnosis and treatment for the students, patients, and clients served remains the legal and ethical responsibility of the supervisor" (ASHA, 2013, Guidelines for SLP Supervision of SLPAs, para. 1). The responsibility for patient care cannot be delegated to an SLPA. The SLPA's services should be viewed as an extension of the SLP, not an alternative to services provided by the SLP. The purpose of SLPA services should not be to significantly increase the caseload size of the SLP (ASHA, 2013). This means that SLPAs should be used to deliver services only to those individuals on the supervising SLP's caseload. Importantly, as discussed in Chapter 1, ASHA details that "under no circumstances should an assistant have his or her own caseload" (ASHA, 2013, Guidelines for SLP Supervision of SLPAs, para. 2).

Just as you are expected to be very familiar with your roles and responsibilities, you should also be familiar with those of your supervisor. ASHA expects that SLPA supervisors will do the following (ASHA, 2013, Qualifications of an SLPA, para. 2)[1]:

1. Conduct ongoing competency evaluations of the SLPA.
2. Provide and encourage ongoing education and training opportunities for the SLPA consistent with competency and skills and needs of the students, patients, or clients served.
3. Develop, review, and modify treatment plans for students, patients, and clients that SLPAs implement under the supervision of the SLP.

4. Make all case management decisions.
5. Adhere to the supervisory responsibilities for SLPs.
6. Retain the legal and ethical responsibility for all students, patients, and clients served.
7. Adhere to the principles and rules of the ASHA Code of Ethics.
8. Adhere to applicable licensure laws and rules regulating the practice of speech-language pathology.

Amount and Type of Supervision

A question also asked is, "How much will I be supervised?" or "How much supervision is required?" ASHA also provides detailed recommendations in this area (Box 2–1; ASHA, 2013). ASHA categorizes the type of supervision, including *direct supervision*, which is onsite, in-view observation and guidance, and *indirect supervision*, which is conducted without direct in-view observation and guidance, such as during record review, review and evaluation of audio- or videotaped sessions, and so forth (ASHA, 2013). As outlined in Box 2–1, within the first 90 days, ASHA recommends that SLPAs receive a total of at least 30% direct and indirect supervision weekly (with no less than 20% supervision for direct patient/client contact activities). After the first 90 days, ASHA recommends no less than 20% supervision weekly (with no less than 10% direct supervision).

ASHA states that the supervisor must make herself or himself available to the SLPA for immediate contact while the SLPA is performing her or his duties. SLPAs may not perform tasks when "a supervising SLP cannot be reached by

Box 2–1. Minimum Frequency and Amount of Supervision
(ASHA, 2013, Minimum Requirements for Frequency and Amount of Supervision, para. 1)[1]

- *First 90 workdays:* A total of at least 30% supervision, including at least 20% direct and 10% indirect supervision, is required weekly. Direct supervision of student, patient, and client care should be no less than 20% of the actual student, patient, and client contact time weekly for each SLPA.
- Direct supervision should be scheduled so that all students, patients, and clients seen by the assistant are directly supervised in a timely manner. Supervision days and time of day (morning/afternoon) may be alternated to ensure that all students, patients, and clients receive some direct contact with the SLP at least once every 2 weeks.
- *After first 90 workdays:* The amount of supervision can be adjusted if the supervising SLP determines the SLPA has met appropriate competencies and skill levels with a variety of communication and related disorders.
- A minimum of 1 hour of direct supervision weekly and as much indirect supervision as needed to facilitate the delivery of quality services must be maintained.
- One hundred percent direct supervision of SLPAs for medically fragile students, patients, or clients is required.

personal contact, phone, pager, or other immediate or electronic means" (ASHA, 2013, Minimal Requirements for the Frequency and Amount of Supervision, para. 11). This means that if your supervising SLP is not available, your service provision to clients must be discontinued until adequate supervision can be obtained, including things like extended absences due to maternity leave, illness, or if your supervisor leaves that site to accept employment elsewhere (ASHA, 2013).

ASHA guidelines detail the *minimal* level of supervision recommended. Each supervisor will be responsible for determining the actual amount and nature of supervision an SLPA receives, taking into consideration things such as an SLPA's experience, the clients served, the setting, and the tasks assigned. It is anticipated that more supervision will be needed when you begin a position or when you perform tasks that are new to you. ASHA recommends that supervisors establish a schedule, which allows them to review the data collected on every client seen by the SLPA on a weekly basis (ASHA, 2013). Furthermore, to ensure adequate supervision, ASHA recommends that the supervisor provide direct contact to every client seen by the SLPA at least every 2 weeks and that SLPs not supervise more than three SLPAs at a time (ASHA, 2013). Remember, too, that individual state regulating agencies may differ in the minimal levels of supervision required. As discussed in Chapter 1, you should familiarize yourself with all applicable regulations in your individual state relative to minimal levels of supervision. Chapter 1 contains details on how to obtain this information.

Supervisor Training and Credentials

ASHA guidelines also contain recommendations in the area of supervisor qualifications (Box 2–2). As can be seen, ASHA recommends that supervisors have an ASHA Certificate of Clinical Competence (CCC) and applicable state licensure, as well as at least 2 years' experience as an SLP, following certification. Preservice training and continuing education in supervision are also recommended, including at least 10 hours of continuing education on the topic of supervision. It is also important that a supervisor has a desire to supervise

an SLPA and that she or he has the time and resources needed to do so. These are important questions to ask when interviewing for an SLPA position and when you consider employment as an SLPA.

Documenting Supervision

ASHA recommends that supervisors document the actual amount and nature of supervision an SLPA receives and that the supervisor participate in performance appraisals of the SLPA (ASHA, 2013). Documentation of supervision includes:

- Documentation of *all* supervisory activities, both direct and indirect
- Documentation of specific services provided to the client, as well as documentation that direct supervision was provided by the SLP, at least every 60 calendar days for each client served

The manner in which your supervision is documented will vary across settings and supervisors. Examples of forms used for recording supervision are located in Appendices 2–A to 2–C. Chapter 1 con-

---

Box 2–2. Qualifications of a Supervising SLP
(ASHA, 2013, Qualifications for Supervising SLP, para. 1)[1]

- Hold a Certificate of Clinical Competence in Speech-Language Pathology from ASHA and/or state licensure (where applicable)
- Have an active interest in use of and desire to use support personnel
- Have pràcticed speech-language pathology for at least 2 years following ASHA certification
- Have completed or be currently enrolled in at least one course or workshop in supervision for at least 1.0 CEUs (10 clock hours)

tains additional details on common evaluation practices, including a discussion of competency-based assessment and samples of ASHA-recommended proficiency checklists and observation forms.

Supervisory Relationship

When discussing rules and regulations applicable to supervision, often missed is the importance of the relationship between you and your supervisor. Remember that both you and your supervisor are responsible for establishing a good working relationship. It is a two-way street. The level of service you are able to provide will depend heavily on the nature of the supervisory relationship you are able to develop *together*. Ideally, the relationship you develop is one of reciprocity or, as McCready (2007) described, a relationship in which both the SLPA and the supervisor give and take mutually and complement one another professionally. The use of active listening and good conflict resolution will be at the heart of this relationship (McCready, 2007). The sections that follow address expectations, supervisory conferences, and feedback, each of which is important to fostering a good working relationship with your supervisor.

Expectations

Expectations set the stage for all workplace behaviors. Your supervisor will have expectations for you in the performance of your duties as an SLPA. You will also have expectations of your supervising SLP in the execution of her or his duties as your supervisor. These expectations will likely be at multiple levels, changing given specific circumstances. It is impossible to list everything that will be expected of you or what you can expect of your supervisor. As such, it is critical that you have an ongoing dialogue about these expectations. Many work place conflicts occur between a supervisor and a supervisee when there is a misunderstanding about what is expected of each person. A good rule of thumb is to never assume you know what is expected. Rather, directly clarifying expectations is the best course of action.

Supervisory Conferences

Supervisory conferences are a critical part of supervision. A fair amount of research has been conducted on the nature of supervisory conferences in the field of speech-language pathology, most of it directed at the supervisor in terms of her role in these conferences (e.g., supervisor training, communication, style, etc.) (McCrea & Brasseur, 2003). From a supervisee's perspective, though, it is important that you also look closely at your role in shaping supervisory conferences. First, realize that a supervisory conference is not a static, once per year event, like a performance review for employment purposes. Rather, they are an ongoing dialogue between you and your supervisor. These interactions can take many forms, depending on your setting, such as formal weekly or daily meetings (or "conferences"), or more informal discussions with your supervisor. These conferences are an opportunity to receive feedback, share/clarify expectations, address clinical issues/concerns, develop goals, seek avenues of skill development, and further shape the nature of the relationship between you and your supervisor. Some ways you can contribute to this process are as follows:

1. *Work with your supervisor to establish a routine schedule for conferences.* It is most effective to establish a routine schedule for conferences versus, for example, meeting as available or as needed (Dowling, 2001).
2. *Help to develop the agenda for your conferences by providing questions and suggested items to discuss, in advance of the next conference.* Make a list of any pressing questions you may have for your supervisor. If possible, providing this to your supervisor in advance of the conference time will be helpful. As time is often limited, select your questions carefully to maximize your conference time.
3. *Take notes about items discussed and things that require your follow-up.* Keep a journal of conferences, recording questions, answers, to-do lists, and any other important aspects of this process; however, you should not record any personal information about

your clients in this journal. If you want to make clinical notes, use initial or client pseudonyms.
4. *Contribute actively to the discussion during the conference.* Use this opportunity to ask questions and clarify information presented. This is also an opportunity for you to share your perspectives on related issues.
5. *Employ good interpersonal communication and good listening skills.*
6. *After the conference, take time to reflect on the content as well as your contributions and ways to enhance conferences in future.* Use your notes to reflect back on the discussion and any additional observations, questions, comments, or concerns. These can be addressed at the next conference.

Feedback

As may be evident at this point, feedback is a key component of the supervisory process (McCrea & Brasseur, 2003; Nelson, 2009). Box 2–3 highlights characteristics of effective feedback. Supervisees across all levels of training generally

---

Box 2–3. Characteristics of Effective Feedback
(ASHA, n.d.-a, pp. 26–27)[2]

Effective feedback is:

1. Given for a good reason
2. Specific and descriptive
3. Relevant
4. About behavior that can be changed
5. Given at appropriate time (usually right after observation but in an appropriate setting)
6. Open to discussion
7. A balance of positive and negative

recognize the value of *effective* feedback (Moss, 2007). In two recent studies conducted by this author, feedback was specifically highlighted by SLPAs and SLPAs in training as important to both clinical success and satisfaction with training and supervision (Ostergren, 2012; Ostergren & Aguilar, 2012).

As an SLPA, you will receive feedback from your supervisor in a variety of ways. As discussed above, these may include formal feedback through competency assessments and performance evaluation tools. You will also receive feedback via informal methods, including verbal comments and discussion during supervisory conferences and/or informal written notes from your supervisor (McCrea & Brasseur, 2003). Feedback may occur after task completion or during, as would be the case if a supervisor participated in a therapy session with you, commenting and guiding your behavior. As an SLPA, you should seek both formal and informal feedback from your supervisor. Both will be important in helping develop your skills and thereby providing the highest quality of care for the clients you serve.

It is critical that you receive this feedback in a way that is productive in shaping your skills but also in a manner that shapes the nature of future feedback. Providing and receiving feedback, especially negative feedback, is not always easy, particularly if this feedback involves aspects of the supervisory relationship and/or personal issues (Nelson, 2009). Some suggestions for ways you can enhance this process are the following:

- *Don't take it personally!* SLPAs who develop exceptional skills are those who realize, no matter what the task, there is always

room for improvement, and *effective* feedback will help you to improve. If your supervisor suggests areas to improve, view this as an opportunity to change and grow in your skills as an SLPA.

- *Keep an open mind and to try to see your supervisor's perspective in the feedback provided.*

- *Use reflection when you receive feedback.* First listen or read (in the case of written feedback) and attempt to understand *before* you react or respond.

- *Know yourself and let your supervisor know your preference for the method of feedback.* Do you prefer verbal, written, a combination of feedback? It is okay to let your supervisor know your preference, but be careful to take into consideration the demands on the supervisor in this respect. For example, receiving extensive written feedback on every task performed is not realistic, but working with your supervisor to identify tasks where specific written feedback may be helpful to you is.

- *Seek modifications to feedback, as needed.* If you are receiving feedback that is overly critical or overly positive, discuss this with your supervisor. Similarly, if the feedback is not specific or descriptive, ask for clarification. If the feedback is not given in time for you to implement changes, problem solve with your supervisor ways to change the timing of feedback in the future. Remember, though, to employ good interpersonal communication skills and tact when requesting modifications to feedback.

Supervisory conferences are an excellent time to discuss the nature of the feedback you receive. As an SLPA, you will receive feedback, but you can also offer feedback to your supervisor about the supervisory process. In preparation for discussions about the feedback, it is helpful to reflect back on the nature of effective feedback. That is, are you receiving positive and negative feedback, is it given about behaviors that you can change and at an appropriate time so that you can incorporate change into future performance, and is it specific, descriptive, and relevant? These are all areas that can be discussed with your supervisor in optimizing feedback.

MENTORING

Mentoring is defined as "a developmental partnership through which one person shares knowledge, skills, information, and perspective to foster the personal and professional growth of someone else" (ASHA, n.d.-a, p. 3). SLPAs often view their supervisor as a mentor, but it is important to remember that these roles are not synonymous (ASHA, 2008). The primary role of a supervisor, as discussed above, is in ensuring client safety and the highest quality of care. This is done by providing oversight and accountability to the process, including, for example, by "providing grades or conducting performance evaluations or documenting professional behavior and clinical performance" (ASHA, 2008, Mentoring

in Supervision, para. 1). Mentors, on the other hand, are individuals who are not necessarily charged with this oversight but take an active role in fostering the development of your professional and/or personal growth. Having a professional mentor is important and has been shown to be related to increases in work satisfaction and career-related motivation/ involvement, as well as a more positive self-image of the mentee and more positive attitudes toward workplace interpersonal relationships (Eby, Allen, Evans, Ng, & DuBois, 2008).

It may be that your supervisor also views herself or himself as a mentor to you. If so, this is excellent. You can foster this relationship by taking into consideration the roles of a mentee (Box 2–4), as well as the roles of a mentor (Box 2–5). If your supervisor does not view her or his role as a mentor to you, this is okay, too. In that case, this is an opportunity for you to develop a mentoring relationship with another individual. Ideally, as an SLPA, it is highly valuable to develop relationships with multiple mentors who each have a vested interest in shaping your professional and personal growth. Remember, too, that a mentor is not necessarily *all purpose*. Mentors can serve different roles, both personal and professional, depending on your goals.

Finding a mentor can seem like an intimidating and mysterious task. The truth is that some mentoring relationships will develop naturally and others will require work on your part in identifying and cultivating a suitable mentoring relationship. It is also true that a certain amount of chemistry, in terms of connecting personally with that person, will be an important part of this process (ASHA, n.d.-a). There may also be failed attempts where a mentor-mentee relationship looks

Box 2–4. Roles of a Mentee (ASHA, n.d.-a, pp. 7–8)[2]

- **Driver of Relationship**
  Identify the skills, knowledge, and/or goals that you want to achieve and communicate them to your mentor. Bring up new topics that are important to you at any point and give feedback to your mentor.
- **Development Planner**
  Maintain a mentoring plan and work with your mentor to set up goals, developmental activities, and time frames.
- **Resource Partner**
  Work with your mentor to seek resources for learning; identify people and information that might be helpful.
- **Teacher**
  Look for opportunities to give back to your mentor; share any information that you think might be valuable.
- **Continuous Learner**
  Take full advantage of this opportunity to learn.

Box 2–5. Roles of a Mentor (ASHA, n.d.-a, pp. 8–9)[2]

- **Coach/Adviser**
  Give advice and guidance, share ideas, and provide feedback. Share information on "unwritten rules for success" within the environment/organization.
- **Source of Encouragement/Support**
  Act as a sounding board for ideas/concerns about school/career choices, providing insights into possible opportunities. Provide support on personal issues if appropriate.
- **Resource Person**
  Identify resources to help the mentee enhance personal development and career growth. Expand the mentee's network of contacts.
- **Champion**
  Serve as an advocate for the mentee whenever the opportunity presents itself. Seek opportunities for increased visibility for the mentee.
- **Devil's Advocate**
  When appropriate, play devil's advocate to help the mentee think through important decisions and strategies.

promising but does not expand to its fullest potential for a variety of reasons. Do not let this discourage you from seeking mentors.

The mentee is the driver of a mentoring relationship. As such, the first step in this process is for you to identify your personal and professional goals. That is, "What do you hope to accomplish from a mentoring relationship?" or "What skills or knowledge do you hope to gain?" Next, you can explore formal and informal channels for identifying individuals who may have an interest in helping you to accomplish these goals.

Professional organizations, such as ASHA, are often a good place to explore more formal channels of mentoring. At the writing of this text, ASHA had mentoring programs for student members and also for professional SLP and audiology members but not yet for ASHA associates. It may be that these programs are now available, so check ASHA's website for additional information. Even if formal programs are not specifically structured for ASHA associates, ASHA's resources in this area can be helpful. Another avenue in identifying formal mentoring programs is through state speech, language, and hearing associations. You can explore their websites or contact your regional representative to see if formal mentoring programs are available to you. Similarly, if you are employed in a large company or school district, check with your human resources department to see if there are any formal mentoring programs offered to employees.

You can also seek mentors through more informal channels. Start by making a list of individuals in your professional and personal environments or those you have met at various points in your career or education who may be potential mentors. Compare this list to your personal and professional goals and see if there are any potential matches. If someone listed has not already reached out to you as a mentor, you will need to make first contact in initiating this relationship. Try first to develop an open line of communication and personal contact with that person before jumping into questions about mentoring (Hannon, n.d.). Getting to know each other's personal styles will allow you and your potential mentor to see if your personalities are a good fit. The next step will be to share your interests and related professional or personal goals with that person. Starting out with a, "Will you be my mentor?" question can be too formal and may seem like a big commitment. You can begin instead by asking for advice on a single issue or problem and then build from there (Hannon, n.d.). If that person seems receptive to answering your questions and offering insight, keep the relationship going. Acknowledge that person's assistance and look for ways you can in turn offer support or information to your mentor. Try to establish regular contact with that person, keeping in mind the roles of the mentor and mentee as you continue to foster this relationship.

Regardless of how you identify a mentor (formally or informally), be active in growing this relationship. Box 2–6 contains a few additional suggestions for maintaining a successful mentoring relationship.

Last, once you have a mentor and have established a positive working relationship, it is important to set goals that you and your mentor can work to accomplish (ASHA, n.d.-b). You should write them down and keep track of your prog-

Defining Roles: Supervision and Mentoring **83**

> ## Box 2–6. Guidelines for Mentoring Success
> ### (ASHA, n.d.-a, pp. 12–13)[2]
>
> - Be sure you are clear on how often you will communicate; whether it will be by phone, e-mail, or both; how quickly you will respond; and confidentiality.
> - Make contact frequently, especially during the first few weeks, to build a trusting relationship.
> - Respect your mentee/mentor's experience and views even if you don't agree.
> - Follow up when you make a commitment to get information or take action.
> - Don't ever leave your mentor hanging. If you don't respond, the mentor will feel that he or she wasn't helpful. You never want to leave someone who has volunteered to help with this kind of impression.
> - Be appreciative of whatever you get from your mentee/mentor; learn his or her strengths and seek or offer advice in these areas.
> - Work hard to make the relationship a two-way street. This means you should always be on the lookout for information/ resources that might be of interest to your mentee/mentor (e.g., articles you read or information you come across).
> - Be flexible and enjoy the experience!

ress in achieving your goals in a journal or calendar. ASHA (n.d.-b)[2] recommends the following tips for successful goal writing:

1. Be specific in your goals.
2. Set a goal for something you really want to accomplish.
3. Break up your goals into manageable subgoals.
4. Give yourself credit when you accomplish a goal.
5. Categorize your goals by the areas of your life that you would like to improve (e.g., financial, career, educational, social, etc.).
6. Review your goals daily.
7. Involve family, friends, and colleagues for support, motivation, and resources.

REFERENCES

American Speech-Language-Hearing Association (ASHA). (n.d.-a). *The power of passionate* mentoring: *The ASHA gathering place mentoring manual*. Rockville, MD: Author. Retrieved February 2, 2013, from http://www.asha.org/uploadedFiles/students/gatheringplace/MentoringManual.pdf

American Speech-Language-Hearing Association (ASHA). (n.d.-b). *Writing mentoring goals and objectives*. Retrieved February 2, 2013, from http://www.asha.org/students/gatheringplace/step/goals/

American Speech-Language-Hearing Association (ASHA). (2008). *Clinical supervision in speech-language pathology* [Technical report]. Retrieved from http://www.asha.org/policy

American Speech-Language-Hearing Association (ASHA). (2013). *Speech-language pathology assistant scope of practice*. Retrieved from http://www.asha.org/policy

Dowling, S. (2001). *Supervision: Strategies for successful outcomes and productivity*. Boston, MA: Allyn & Bacon.

Eby, L. T., Allen, T. D., Evans, S. C., Ng, T., & DuBois, D. L. (2008). Does mentoring matter? A multidisciplinary meta-analysis comparing mentored and non-mentored individuals. *Journal of Vocational Behavior, 72*(2), 254–267.

Hannon, K. (n.d.). How to find a mentor. *Forbes*. Retrieved February 2, 2013, from http://www.forbes.com/sites/kerryhannon/2011/10/31/how-to-find-a-mentor

McCrea, E., & Brasseur, J. (2003). *The supervisory process in speech-language pathology and audiology*. Boston, MA: Pearson Education.

McCready, V. (2007, May 8). Supervision of speech-language pathology assistants: A reciprocal relationship. *ASHA Leader*. Retrieved from http://www.asha.org/Publications/leader/2007/070508/f070508b/

Moss, L. B. (2007). Supervisory feedback: A review of the literature. *Perspectives on Administration and Supervision, 17*(1), 10–12.

Nelson, L. (2009). Feedback in supervision. *Perspectives on Administration and Supervision, 19*(1), 19–24.

Ostergren, J. (2012). Bachelor's level speech-language pathology assistants (SLPAs) in California: A bachelor's level clinical practicum course. *Contemporary Issues in Communication Sciences and Disorders, 39*, 1–11.

Ostergren, J., & Aguilar, S. (2012). A survey of speech-language pathology assistants in California: Current trends in demographics, employment, supervision, and training. *Contemporary Issues in Communication Sciences and Disorders, 39*, 121–136.

CHAPTER ENDNOTES

1. American Speech-Language-Hearing Association. (2013). *Speech-language pathology assistant scope of practice*. Retrieved from http://www.asha.org/policy. © Copyright 2013 American Speech-Language-Hearing Association. All rights reserved. Reprinted with permission.

2. American Speech-Language-Hearing Association. (n.d.-a). *The power of passionate mentoring: The ASHA gathering place mentoring manual*. Rockville, MD: Author. Retrieved February 2, 2013, from © Copyright American Speech-Language-Hearing Association. All rights reserved. Reprinted with permission.

APPENDIX 2–A

Supervisor Log of Direct and Indirect Observations

Week ending: _____

SLPA: _____

Supervising SLP: _____

Patient	Mon.	Tues.	Wed.	Thurs.	Fri.	Sat./Sun.
Other Activities						
Billing						
Equipment Maintenance						
Documentation						
Conferences/Inservices						
Other clerical						

Indicate DO for direct observation + time
Indicate IDO for indirect observation + time

Comments:

Source: Reprinted with permission from _Practical Tools and Forms for Supervising Speech-Language Pathology Assistants._ © 2013. American Speech-Language-Hearing Association. All rights reserved.

APPENDIX 2–B

SLPA Weekly Activity Log

Week ending: _____

SLPA: _____

Supervising SLP: _____

Patient	Mon.	Tues.	Wed.	Thur.	Fri.	Sat./Sun.
Total treatment time						
Total direct supervision						

	Mon.	Tues.	Wed.	Thur.	Fri.	Sat./Sun.
Documentation time						
Meeting with supervisor						
Other meetings/ conferences						
Observation of sessions						
Equipment maintenance						
Clerical tasks						

S indicates supervised session.

Source: Reprinted with permission from *Practical Tools and Forms for Supervising Speech-Language Pathology Assistants.* © 2013. American Speech-Language-Hearing Association. All rights reserved.

APPENDIX 2–C

SLPA Weekly Activity Record

SLPA: _____

Supervising SLP: _____

Week ending: _____

Total hours week: _____

Activity	Time Spent
1. Direct patient treatment/intervention	_____
2. Observation of other sessions	_____
3. Meeting with supervising SLP	_____
4. Other meetings/conferences (list)	_____

_____

_____

_____

_____

5. Equipment/materials maintenance	_____
6. Documentation	_____
7. Clerical activities	_____
A. Total time directly observed by the SLP	_____
B. Total treatment time provided this week	_____

Percent of time directly observed by the SLP (A/B)   _____

Source: Reprinted with permission from *Practical Tools and Forms for Supervising Speech-Language Pathology Assistants.* © 2013. American Speech-Language-Hearing Association. All rights reserved.

CHAPTER 3

Ethical Conduct

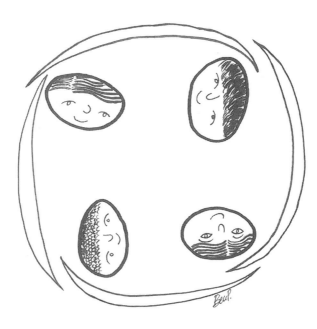

Action indeed is the sole medium of expression for ethics.
Jane Addams (first American woman to receive the Nobel Peace Prize)

ETHICS, MORALS, AND LAW

Webster's dictionary defines *ethics* as "the discipline dealing with what is good and bad and with moral duty and obligation" (Merriam-Webster, 2003). Hence, at its very core, ethics is *the study of* morality, or what is good/bad and right/wrong. *Morals* form the ground rules for society's laws. In contrast, *laws* are enforceable, written rules based on the concepts of justice and equality (Horner, 2003). In the simplest terms, laws dictate what we must do, whereas morals (and thereby ethics) address what we should do (Horner, 2003). A related term, *integrity*, refers to an adherence to high moral standards. As such, a person with professional integrity is someone who adheres to ethical principles in the execution of his or her professional duties.

Often, when students (and professionals) hear that what follows is a discussion of ethics, they brace themselves for a long, difficult discussion of these complex and intertwined terms. However, as Chabon and Morris (2004) highlight, "Ethics is really about helping one to make good decisions" (para. 2). In this light, the study of ethics and an understanding of ethical conduct can be used as a compass in navigating your professional obligations as a speech-language pathology assistant (SLPA).

ASHA CODE OF ETHICS

The concept of professional ethics refers to the "principles of conduct governing an individual or a group" (Merriam-Webster, 2003). The American Speech-Language-Hearing Association (ASHA) has a professional Code of Ethics (ASHA, 2010). According to ASHA, the purpose of this code is to "ensure the highest standards of integrity and ethical principles" (Preamble, para. 1). The code consists of four ethical principles and related rules of ethics that form the basic moral foundation of this code and are meant to be "aspirational and inspirational in nature" (Preamble, para. 5). ASHA's complete Code of Ethics is listed in Appendix 3–A. The four ethical principles of this code are listed in Box 3–1.

ASHA's Code of Ethics states that members, nonmember certificate holders, and individuals who are applying for membership or certification shall observe these principles as "affirmative obligations under all conditions of professional activity," such that "any violation of the spirit and purpose of this Code shall be considered unethical" (ASHA, 2010, Preamble, para. 2). ASHA maintains a Board of Ethics (BOE), charged with the responsibility of reviewing, publishing, and amending ASHA's Code of Ethics and

developing educational programs and materials applicable to ethical conduct (ASHA, 2012).

As discussed in Chapter 1, SLPAs are able to apply to become an ASHA associate. This is an optional designation for qualified support personnel in audiology or speech-language pathology. Individuals with this designation must agree to follow all ASHA policies regarding supporting personnel, working only under the supervision of a qualified CCC-SLP or CCC-A. ASHA associates can access ASHA resources and many ASHA benefits but are not fully designated ASHA "members" or "certificate holders." Hence, although the spirit and moral foundation of ASHA's Code of Ethics are applicable to SLPAs, the exact language of many of the rules of ethics is not consistent with the scope of an SLPA (ASHA, 2013b). As such, a question asked is, "How does ASHA's Code of Ethics apply to SLPAs?" ASHA in its recent revision of the SLPA Scope of Practice (ASHA, 2013b, Ethical Considerations, para. 2) addressed this issue, stating,

> Although some SLPAs may choose to affiliate with ASHA as associates, the Code of Ethics does not directly apply to affiliates. However, any individual who is working in a support role (technician, aide, assistant) under the supervision of an SLP or speech scientist must be knowledgeable about the provisions of the code. It is imperative that the supervising professional and the assistant behave in a manner that is consistent with the principles and rules outlined in the ASHA Code of Ethics.

This newly revised document also reiterates that the ethical responsibility for patient care cannot be delegated to the

> ## Box 3–1. ASHA's Four Ethical Principles (ASHA, 2010)[1]
>
> ### Principle 1 (Responsibility to Clients Served and Research Participants)
> *Individuals shall honor their responsibility to hold paramount the welfare of persons they serve professionally or who are participants in research and scholarly activities, and they shall treat animals involved in research in a humane manner.*
>
> ### Principle 2 (Responsibility of Maintaining Professional Competence)
> *Individuals shall honor their responsibility to achieve and maintain the highest level of professional competence and performance.*
>
> ### Principle 3 (Responsibility to the Public)
> *Individuals shall honor their responsibility to the public by promoting public understanding of the professions, by supporting the development of services designed to fulfill the unmet needs of the public, and by providing accurate information in all communications involving any aspect of the professions, including the dissemination of research findings and scholarly activities, and the promotion, marketing, and advertising of products and services.*
>
> ### Principle 4 (Responsibility to Other Members, Students, and Other Professions and Disciplines)
> *Individuals shall honor their responsibilities to the professions and their relationships with colleagues, students, and members of other professions and disciplines.*

SLPA, and as such, the actions of the assistant in service provision are the responsibility of the supervising SLP. Furthermore, this document specifically states that "if the assistant engages in activities that violate the Code of Ethics, the supervising professional may be found in violation of the code if adequate oversight has not been provided" (ASHA, 2013b, Ethical Consideration, para. 2).

As is likely evident at this point, any discussion of ethics and ethical conduct of an SLPA is intertwined with a discussion of ethical conduct of the supervising SLP.

Appendix 3–B contains a list of ASHA's ethical principles and rules, which are applicable for those who supervise an SLPA. However, for the purpose of this book, ASHA's Code of Ethics is discussed next in relation to SLPAs. Even though not specifically written for SLPAs, analysis of this code *as it applies to the conduct of SLPAs* is highly valuable. Box 3–2 contains a list of key ethical principles and rules that have language that is consistent with the service provision of an assistant. This is not an exhaustive list of all applicable ASHA ethical principles or rules.

Box 3–2. Examples of ASHA's Ethical Principles Potentially Applicable to SLPAs[1]

Principle of Ethics I

A. Individuals shall provide all services competently.

C. Individuals shall not discriminate in the delivery of professional services or the conduct of research and scholarly activities on the basis of race or ethnicity, gender, gender identity/gender expression, age, religion, national origin, sexual orientation, or disability.

M. Individuals shall adequately maintain and appropriately secure records of professional services rendered, research and scholarly activities conducted, and products dispensed, and they shall allow access to these records only when authorized or when required by law.

N. Individuals shall not reveal, without authorization, any professional or personal information about identified persons served professionally or identified participants involved in research and scholarly activities unless doing so is necessary to protect the welfare of the person or of the community or is otherwise required by law.

O. Individuals shall not charge for services not rendered, nor shall they misrepresent services rendered, products dispensed, or research and scholarly activities conducted.

Q. Individuals whose professional services are adversely affected by substance abuse or other health-related conditions shall seek professional assistance and, where appropriate, withdraw from the affected areas of practice.

Principle of Ethics II

B. Individuals shall engage in only those aspects of the professions that are within the scope of their professional practice and competence, considering their level of education, training, and experience.

C. Individuals shall engage in lifelong learning to maintain and enhance professional competence and performance.

E. Individuals shall ensure that all equipment used to provide services or to conduct research and scholarly activities is in proper working order and is properly calibrated.

Principles of Ethics III:

A. Individuals shall not misrepresent their credentials, competence, education, training, experience, or scholarly or research contributions.

B. Individuals shall not participate in professional activities that constitute a conflict of interest.

D. Individuals shall not misrepresent research, diagnostic information, services rendered, results of services rendered, products dispensed, or the effects of products dispensed.

E. Individuals shall not defraud or engage in any scheme to defraud in connection with obtaining payment, reimbursement, or grants for services rendered, research conducted, or products dispensed.

F. Individuals' statements to the public shall provide accurate information about the nature and management of communication disorders, about the professions, about professional services, about products for sale, and about research and scholarly activities.

G. Individuals' statements to the public when advertising, announcing, and marketing their professional services; reporting research results; and promoting products shall adhere to professional standards and shall not contain misrepresentations.

Principle of Ethics IV

A. Individuals shall uphold the dignity and autonomy of the professions, maintain harmonious interprofessional and intraprofessional relationships, and accept the professions' self-imposed standards.

C. Individuals shall not engage in dishonesty, fraud, deceit, or misrepresentation.

D. Individuals shall not engage in any form of unlawful harassment, including sexual harassment or power abuse.

E. Individuals shall not engage in any other form of conduct that adversely reflects on the professions or on the individual's fitness to serve persons professionally.

F. Individuals shall assign credit only to those who have contributed to a publication, presentation, or product. Credit shall be assigned in proportion to the contribution and only with the contributor's consent.

H. Individuals shall reference the source when using other persons' ideas, research, presentations, or products in written, oral, or any other media presentation or summary.

I. Individuals' statements to colleagues about professional services, research results, and products shall adhere to prevailing professional standards and shall contain no misrepresentations.

K. Individuals shall not discriminate in their relationships with colleagues, students, and members of other professions and disciplines on the basis of race or ethnicity, gender, gender identity/

> gender expression, age, religion, national origin, sexual orientation, or disability.
> L. Individuals shall not file or encourage others to file complaints that disregard or ignore facts that would disprove the allegation, nor should the Code of Ethics be used for personal reprisal, as a means of addressing personal animosity, or as a vehicle for retaliation.
> M. Individuals who have reason to believe that the Code of Ethics has been violated shall inform the Board of Ethics.
> N. Individuals shall comply fully with the policies of the Board of Ethics in its consideration and adjudication of complaints of violations of the Code of Ethics.

Any principles that refer to determining the nature of services provided were not included. This was intentional, given that SLPAs do not determine if, when, or how services are provided, nor can they engage in any service provision without the explicit direction and supervision of an SLP (ASHA, 2013b). Those listed in Box 3–2 were deemed core concepts important to any level of service provision, such as confidentiality, competence, nondiscrimination, patient safety, support of the profession and other professionals, and accuracy in public statements. The section that follows will provide a framework for how to view this information in making ethical decisions in your work as an SLPA.

ETHICAL DECISION MAKING

Armed with a discussion of ethics in general and a review of ASHA's Code of Ethics, we now revisit the concept of ethics as a compass in helping you navigate decisions about what you should do in the execution of your daily duties as an SLPA. Rarely do threats to ethical conduct in our professional (or personal) lives present themselves in conveniently identified and easily resolved scenarios. Careful and thoughtful reflection is often required, both in identifying the parameters of a conflict and in suggesting a potential course of action.

Several authors in the field of speech-language pathology have suggested ways of approaching this task using frameworks for ethical decision making (Body & McAllister, 2009; Chabon & Morris, 2004; Irwin, Pannbacker, Powell, & Vekovius, 2007). One framework that appears particularly applicable is Chabon and Morris's (2004) discussion of consensus building in ethical decision making. These concepts have been applied to represent the unique elements of service provision as an SLPA and are represented in Figure 3–1. A worksheet with these principles is available on the CD of this textbook. The sample scenario described in Box 3–3 is a hypothetical one that will be used in describing the use of this framework. The worksheet has been completed for this particular case and is located in Appendix 3–C so you can follow along as you read the description below.

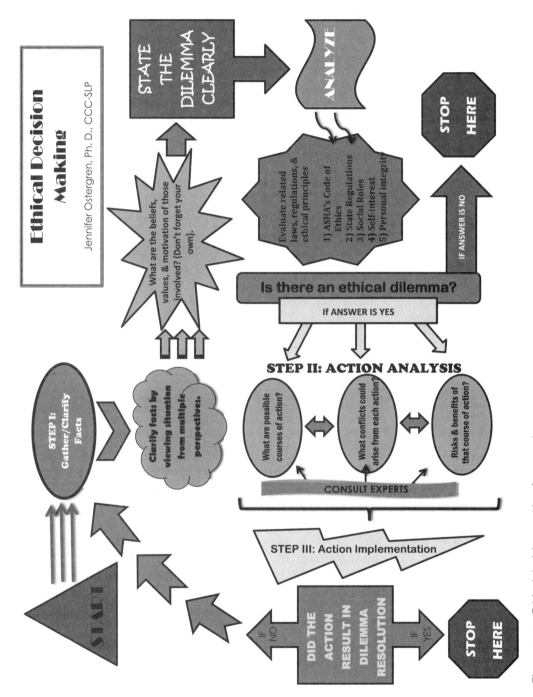

Figure 3–1. Ethical decision-making framework.

Box 3–3. Sample Scenario

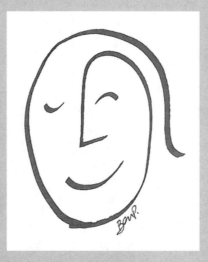

Amber is an SLPA employed in a large, urban elementary school setting. She has worked in this setting for more than a year. She is currently supervised by an experienced SLP who has an ASHA Certificate of Clinical Competence (CCC). Amber herself is an ASHA associate. Amber's supervisor has one of the highest caseloads in their district. Next week, her supervisor has several individualized educational plan (IEP) meetings scheduled. She has expressed to Amber that she is behind schedule in writing documentation for these meetings and in performing follow-up assessments. Amber's supervisor just asked her to perform a diagnostic assessment on a client in preparation for an upcoming IEP meeting. Amber has observed her supervisor administering assessments and has frequently taken part in assisting her supervisor during assessments, such as preparing materials and helping to record data during the assessment; however, consistent with her scope of duties, Amber has not administered these tests independently, nor has she interpreted or summarized the results. Amber and her supervisor have a good working relationship. Amber wants to help her supervisor, but Amber is concerned that this request violates her licensing regulations and ASHA's Code of Ethics. She is unsure how to address this situation.

The initial phase of ethical decision making is the gather/clarify information phase (see Figure 3–1). You can start by making sure that you actually understand the circumstances of a situation accurately and gather any additional facts needed to understand the situation fully. In our sample scenario, it will be important to clarify if in fact the supervisor meant for Amber to perform the assessment on her own (e.g., collecting, summarizing, and interpreting the data). Alternatively, perhaps there had been some form of miscommunication and Amber's supervisor only meant to request that Amber help in administering and/or preparing for this testing (as she has done previously).

As Figure 3–1 indicates, in this phase, it is also important to view the circumstances from all perspectives, considering carefully your own motives and role, as well as those of others involved. In the sample scenario, it will be important to think about why the supervisor made this request and what are the extenuating circumstances surrounding this request. It appears from the details that time and several impending IEP meetings and reports may be a factor. Amber having assisted with tests previously may also bring something relevant to this situation. Amber's role as the assistant and her relationship with her supervisor are also facts to consider further. Amber and her supervisor appear to have a good working relationship, and as such, Amber likely has a desire to help her supervisor, but Amber may also be concerned about how telling her supervisor that she cannot do something may affect her job or this relationship. The sample scenario indicates that Amber is sensitive to that and wants to help her supervisor, if she can. Of course, none of these factors necessarily makes the situation ethical, but they are nonetheless important to consider and may play a role in helping to identify a possible course of action.

Also in this phase, it is important to review any relevant rules, laws, or ethical principles (see Figure 3–1). As a general rule, some important documents for SLPAs to consider in this respect are ASHA's Scope of Practice for SLPAs (ASHA, 2013b, Appendix 1–A, Chap. 1), ASHA's Code of Ethics (ASHA, 2010, Appendix 3–A), and any applicable state regulations or laws governing SLPAs and their supervisors or any other relevant documents. Documents regarding the policies and procedures of your employer may be relevant as well. In the sample scenario, the supervisor is an ASHA CCC-SLP. As such, ASHA's Code of Ethics will be important to consider and will directly relate to the supervisor's actions in this matter. Several of the principles and rules highlighted in Appendix 3–B (Ethical Principles, Rules, and Guidance Pertinent to the Supervision of Support Personnel) appear relevant to this situation, but in particular, the following three seem most applicable.[1]

- **Principle of Ethics I, Rule E:** Individuals who hold the Certificate of Clinical Competence shall not delegate tasks that require the unique skills, knowledge, and judgment that are within the scope of their profession to assistants, technicians, support personnel, or any nonprofessionals over whom they have supervisory responsibility.
- **Principle of Ethics II, Rule D:** Individuals shall not require or permit their professional staff to provide services or conduct research activities that exceed the staff member's competence, level of education, training, and experience.
- **Principle of Ethics IV, Rule B:** Individuals shall prohibit anyone under their supervision from engaging in any practice that violates the Code of Ethics.

In Amber's case, she is an ASHA associate and therefore has agreed to abide by ASHA rules and regulations regarding SLPA use. ASHA's Scope of Practice for SLPAs specifically states that SLPAs should not "perform standardized or nonstandardized diagnostic tests, formal or informal evaluations, or swallowing screenings/checklists" (ASHA, 2013b, Responsibilities Outside the Scope for SLPAs, para. 2). From Amber's perspective as an SLPA, the following two ethical principles seem most related to this situation.[1]

- **Principle of Ethics I, Rule A:** Individuals shall provide all services competently.
- **Principle of Ethics II, Rule B:** Individuals shall engage in only those aspects of the professions that are within the scope of their professional practice and competence, considering their level of education, training, and experience.

Furthermore, Amber is registered as an SLPA in her state, and her state regulations prohibit SLPAs from performing diagnostic assessments.

At the end of the gather/clarify information phase, the next step is to ask yourself, "Is this an ethical dilemma?" (see Figure 3–1). If the answer is no, then you do not appear to be facing an ethical dilemma. If the answer is yes, then the next step is to identify a plausible course of action within the action analysis phase. In the action analysis phase, the first step is to list plausible courses of action. Ask yourself, "What actions can I take?" For each course of action, think about the following:

1. What does that course of action entail? Is it feasible?
2. Who will be affected by that course of action (either negatively or positively)?
3. What are the risks and benefits of that course of action?
4. Will that action result in an ethical resolution to the dilemma at hand?

Obviously, the final consideration in this phase (whether action will result in an ethical resolution) is the most important; however, sometimes it is helpful to start with listing all courses of action.

Ideally, the action analysis phase reveals a course of action which can resolve the ethical dilemma (see Figure 3–1). If not, then an additional branching step may be required. This branching step involves consulting with experts, supervisors, or colleagues. This in fact can occur at any step in the process, when additional assistance or insight is needed, but it is important to remember that self-analysis is key. You are likely the person closest to this situation as it is affecting you personally or professionally. As such, you are the first expert to analyze the situation, bringing in additional insight from outside perspectives, as needed.

A word of caution as well in seeking additional opinions: SLPAs must maintain confidentiality, particularly when discussing any situation that involves your clients or their families. Federal regulations prohibit you from discussing personal information about the clients you serve (Annett, 2001). ASHA's Code of Ethics (2010) also specifically addresses the matter of client confidentiality and confidentiality in relationships with colleagues (Box 3–4). Appendix 3–D contains a copy of ASHA's statement on confidentiality. This topic is also given additional consideration at the end of this chapter.

> ## Box 3–4. Ethical Principles and Rules Involving Confidentiality
> ### (ASHA, 2010)[1]
>
> *Confidentiality of Client Information*
>
> **Principle of Ethics I, Rule K:**
> Individuals shall adequately maintain and appropriately secure records of professional services rendered, research and scholarly activities conducted, and products dispensed and shall allow access to these records only when authorized or when required by law.
>
> **Principle of Ethics I, Rule L:**
> Individuals shall not reveal, without authorization, any professional or personal information about identified persons served professionally or identified participants involved in research and scholarly activities unless required by law to do so, or unless doing so is necessary to protect the welfare of the person or of the community or otherwise required by law.
>
> *Confidentiality in Relationships With Colleagues*
>
> **Principle of Ethics IV, Rule B:**
> Individuals shall not engage in dishonesty, fraud, deceit, misrepresentation, sexual harassment, or any other form of conduct that adversely reflects on the professions or on the individual's fitness to serve persons professionally.
>
> **Principle of Ethics IV, Rule F:**
> Individuals' statements to colleagues about professional services, research results, and products shall adhere to prevailing professional standards and shall contain no misrepresentations.
>
> **Principle of Ethics IV, Rule I:**
> Individuals who have reason to believe that the Code of Ethics has been violated shall inform the Board of Ethics.
>
> **Principle of Ethics IV, Rule J:**
> Individuals shall comply fully with policies of the Board of Ethics in its consideration and adjudication of complaints of violation of the Code of Ethics.

In the sample scenario, as highlighted in Table 3–1, there are several potential courses of action.

The final stage in this process is the action implementation phase (see Figure 3–1). In this stage, you implement the

Table 3–1. Potential Courses of Action for Sample Scenario

Possible Course of Action	Benefits	Risks	Ethical Resolution? (Yes/No)
Amber could assess the client (as requested) but not tell anyone and allow her supervisor to sign the report as if the speech-language pathologist (SLP) was the one who conducted this assessment.	• Amber avoids conflict with her supervisor by not having to tell the supervisor that assessment is outside Amber's scope of responsibilities.	• Violation in ethical principles, for both Amber and her supervisor. • Negative impact in quality of care for the client. • Potential for sanctions from state licensing board, for both Amber and her supervisor. • Potential for sanctions from the American Speech-Language-Hearing Association's (ASHA's) Board of Ethics for Amber's supervisor	No
Amber can tell her supervisor that assessment is not within her scope of responsibilities and as such she is not able to assess the client (as requested). She can, however, offer to assist in the assessment and in any other duties within Amber's scope of responsibilities so that the supervisor has additional time to assess the client.	• No violation in ethical principles. • Quality in client care is maintained, as Amber has reduced the supervisor's workload in other ways so that the client can be assessed by the SLP, who is qualified to do so.	• Amber's supervisor may disagree or may be upset that Amber has refused to do something requested. If good interpersonal skills are used in addressing this situation, this risk may be mitigated.	Yes
Amber could assess the client (as requested) but report her supervisor's conduct to the state licensing board, ASHA's Board of Ethics, and their employer.	• Amber avoids direct conflict with her supervisor by not having to tell the supervisor that assessment is outside Amber's scope of responsibilities.	• Violation in ethical principles, for both Amber and her supervisor.* • Negative impact on quality of care for the client. • Potential for sanctions from state licensing board, for both Amber and her supervisor. *NOTE: Although Amber reported her supervisor to ASHA's Board of Ethics, Amber would still be engaging in unethical conduct as she performed the assessment, which was not in the best interest of the client.	No

Table 3–1. *continued*

Possible Course of Action	Benefits	Risks	Ethical Resolution? (Yes/No)
Amber could not mention this conflict to her supervisor but call in sick the day the assessment is scheduled, so she does not have to assess the client.	• Amber avoids direct conflict with her supervisor by not having to tell her supervisor that assessment is outside Amber's scope of responsibilities. • No sanctions from state licensing board for either Amber or her supervisor as the assessment is not performed by Amber.	• Potential negative impact on quality of care as the assessment may not be performed as needed, which isn't in the best interest of the client. Alternatively, the supervisor may simply reschedule the assessment for another day when Amber is available and in that case the issue has not been resolved and will resurface when Amber returns.	No

course of action decided on in the action analysis phase. At the end of the action implementation phase, hopefully the situation is resolved and the ethical dilemma eliminated. If not, this process starts over again, as you reenter the gather/clarify facts, action analysis, and action implementation phases until a satisfactory conclusion is met. In the sample scenario, the action selected for implementation is that highlighted in bold in Table 3–1. Amber plans to speak directly with her supervisor about her concerns in performing assessments, highlighting that this activity is outside ASHA and state regulations for the scope of responsibilities as an SLPA. Related to this, Amber will offer to stay late to prepare test materials and to rearrange her schedule so that she can assist her supervisor during administration of this assessment. Furthermore, Amber has identified a few clerical tasks she can perform, which will help decrease the demands on her supervisor's sched-ule so that the supervisor has time to complete the assessment.

As this case illustrates, ethical decision making requires careful consideration from multiple perspectives. Making decisions based on ethics takes practice. Using a structured framework like the one discussed above is a first step in developing your skills in this area. Appendix 3–E contains additional sample ethical scenarios applicable to an SLPA. Use the worksheet and framework provided to practice your skills in this area. Taking it a step further by discussing your conclusions with others in the profession is also an excellent way to hone your skills in this area.

Finally, a discussion of ethical conduct would not be complete without highlighting the role of good interpersonal skills and conflict resolution in resolving ethical dilemmas professionally. Chapter 4 addresses this topic in greater detail, including several guiding principles for resolving conflict effectively.

CONFIDENTIALITY

Before we close the chapter on ethics, let's take a closer look at the topic of confidentiality. As highlighted above, when discussing ethical matters, you should maintain confidentiality of client information and confidentiality in your relationships with colleagues. This issue of confidentiality, however, goes beyond discussing an ethical dilemma (Annett, 2001; ASHA, 2013a, O'Neil-Pirozzi, 2001). As is evident in ASHA's confidentiality statement (Appendix 3–D), confidentiality extends to every aspect of your role as an SLPA, including confidentiality of client information and confidentiality in your relationships with other professionals.

Confidentiality of Client Information

As highlighted in Box 3–4, confidentiality of client information encompasses both verbal and written information. In addition, beyond ASHA's Code of Ethics, the privacy and security of documentation are governed by federal regulations outlined in the Health Insurance Portability and Accountability Act (HIPAA) and Family Educational Rights and Privacy Act (FERPA) (U.S. Department of Education, n.d.; U.S. Department of Health and Human Services, n.d.-a, n.d.-b). HIPAA regulations outline rules pertaining to health care providers and health-related information. FERPA regulations outline rules applicable to school personnel and educational records. Both require specific and explicit consent for providers to use and disclose protected information. They also stipulate that individuals have a right to review and correct their official records, be notified of disclosure history, and receive notice of policies regarding disclosure of protected information. As such, as an SLPA, it is critical that you maintain confidentiality of all client information. This confidentiality includes all aspects of a client's care. This means that you must not share the details about any aspect of your services with anyone other than your supervising SLP, those specifically granted access to this information by your client (in writing), or as expressly required by law. This confidentiality includes verbal information, written materials, and audio and video recordings. Written documents and audio and visual recordings must be kept in a secure location and may not be stored, electronically or in hard copy form, in locations where those without specific permission are able to view this information. It is crucial that you take confidentiality seriously. Some reminders to ensure your client's confidentiality include the following:

1. Do not share information about your client with anyone not specifically granted access to this information. This includes sharing information about your client with your family or friends. As they are not specifically authorized service providers, information about your clients should not be shared with them.
2. Do not speak in public locations about your client.
3. Do not remove any documents (written, audio, or visual) from clinical/educational locations.
4. Get specific permission to forward or copy any information about your client.
5. If you are given passwords or access codes to confidential information, do not share this information with others and do not store this information in a public location.

6. Do not dispose of client information without first adequately destroying or removing all confidential information. Your employer should have specific procedures for doing so.

Confidentiality in Relationships With Peers and Colleagues

Confidentiality in relationships with colleagues, peers, and other professionals takes on several meanings (ASHA, 2010, Box 3–4; ASHA, 2013a). First, you should be careful to not misrepresent yourself or others in your verbal or written communications. In addition, when conflicts arise, you should limit discussion of these matters to those involved. This means you should not discuss conflict with colleagues and peers in public locations. If you must seek additional guidance, do so with discretion and confidentiality. Chapter 4 provides additional details about confidentiality in written communications as well.

REFERENCES

American Speech-Language-Hearing Association (ASHA). (2010). *Code of ethics*. Retrieved from http://www.asha.org/policy

American Speech-Language-Hearing Association (ASHA). (2012). *Practices and procedures of the board of ethics*. Retrieved from http://www.asha.org/policy

American Speech-Language-Hearing Association (ASHA). (2013a). *Confidentiality*. Retrieved from http://www.asha.org/policy

American Speech-Language-Hearing Association (ASHA). (2013b). *Speech-language pathol-*ogy assistant scope of practice. Retrieved from http://www.asha.org/policy

Annett, M. M. (2001, February 20). Law concerns privacy, transfer of patient data: New regulations will affect SLPs, audiologists across settings. *ASHA Leader*. Retrieved from http://www.asha.org/Publications/leader/2001/010220/privacy.htm

Body, R., & McAllister, L. (2009). *Ethics in speech and language therapy*. Somerset, NJ: John Wiley.

Chabon, S. S., & Morris, J. F. (2004, February 17). A consensus model for making ethical decisions in a less-than-ideal world. *ASHA Leader*. Retrieved from http://www.asha.org/Publications/leader/2004/040217/040217e.htm

Horner, J. (2003). Mortality, ethics, and law: Introductory concepts. *Seminars in Speech and Language, 24*, 263–274.

Irwin, D., Pannbacker, M., Powell, W., & Vekovius, G. (2007). *Ethics for speech-language pathologists and audiologists: An illustrative casebook*. Clifton Park, NY: Thomson Delmar Learning.

Merriam-Webster. (2003). *Merriam-Webster's collegiate dictionary* (11th ed.). Springfield, MA: Author.

O'Neil-Pirozzi, T. M. (2001). Please respect patient confidentiality. *Contemporary Issues in Communication Sciences and Disorders, 28*, 48–51.

U.S. Department of Education. (n.d.). *Family Educational Rights and Privacy Act (FERPA): General information*. Retrieved February 2, 2013, from http://www2.ed.gov/policy/gen/guid/fpco/ferpa/index.html

U.S. Department of Health and Human Services. (n.d.). *Summary of HIPPA security rules*. Retrieved February 2, 2013, from http://www.hhs.gov/ocr/privacy/hipaa/understanding/summary/index.html

CHAPTER ENDNOTE

1. American Speech-Language-Hearing Association. (2010). *Code of ethics*. Retrieved from http://www.asha.org/policy. © Copyright 2010 American Speech-Language-Hearing Association. Reprinted with permission.

APPENDIX 3–A

ASHA Code of Ethics

TABLE OF CONTENTS

- Preamble
- Principle of Ethics I
- Rules of Ethics
- Principle of Ethics II
- Rules of Ethics
- Principle of Ethics III
- Rules of Ethics
- Principle of Ethics IV
- Rules of Ethics

PREAMBLE

The preservation of the highest standards of integrity and ethical principles is vital to the responsible discharge of obligations by speech-language pathologists, audiologists, and speech, language, and hearing scientists. This Code of Ethics sets forth the fundamental principles and rules considered essential to this purpose.

Every individual who is (a) a member of the American Speech-Language-Hearing Association, whether certified or not, (b) a nonmember holding the Certificate of Clinical Competence from the Association, (c) an applicant for membership or certification, or (d) a Clinical Fellow seeking to fulfill standards for certification shall abide by this Code of Ethics.

Any violation of the spirit and purpose of this Code shall be considered unethical. Failure to specify any particular responsibility or practice in this Code of Ethics shall not be construed as denial of the existence of such responsibilities or practices.

The fundamentals of ethical conduct are described by Principles of Ethics and by Rules of Ethics as they relate to the responsibility to persons served, the public, speech-language pathologists, audiologists, and speech, language, and hearing scientists, and to the conduct of research and scholarly activities.

Principles of Ethics, aspirational and inspirational in nature, form the underlying moral basis for the Code of Ethics. Individuals shall observe these principles as affirmative obligations under all conditions of professional activity.

Rules of Ethics are specific statements of minimally acceptable professional conduct or of prohibitions and are applicable to all individuals.

PRINCIPLE OF ETHICS I

Individuals shall honor their responsibility to hold paramount the welfare of persons they serve professionally or who are participants in research and scholarly activities, and they shall treat animals involved in research in a humane manner.

Rules of Ethics

A. Individuals shall provide all services competently.
B. Individuals shall use every resource, including referral when appropriate,

to ensure that high-quality service is provided.

C. Individuals shall not discriminate in the delivery of professional services or the conduct of research and scholarly activities on the basis of race or ethnicity, gender, gender identity/gender expression, age, religion, national origin, sexual orientation, or disability.

D. Individuals shall not misrepresent the credentials of assistants, technicians, support personnel, students, Clinical Fellows, or any others under their supervision, and they shall inform those they serve professionally of the name and professional credentials of persons providing services.

E. Individuals who hold the Certificate of Clinical Competence shall not delegate tasks that require the unique skills, knowledge, and judgment that are within the scope of their profession to assistants, technicians, support personnel, or any nonprofessionals over whom they have supervisory responsibility.

F. Individuals who hold the Certificate of Clinical Competence may delegate tasks related to provision of clinical services to assistants, technicians, support personnel, or any other persons only if those services are appropriately supervised, realizing that the responsibility for client welfare remains with the certified individual.

G. Individuals who hold the Certificate of Clinical Competence may delegate tasks related to provision of clinical services that require the unique skills, knowledge, and judgment that are within the scope of practice of their profession to students only if those services are appropriately supervised. The responsibility for client welfare remains with the certified individual.

H. Individuals shall fully inform the persons they serve of the nature and possible effects of services rendered and products dispensed, and they shall inform participants in research about the possible effects of their participation in research conducted.

I. Individuals shall evaluate the effectiveness of services rendered and of products dispensed, and they shall provide services or dispense products only when benefit can reasonably be expected.

J. Individuals shall not guarantee the results of any treatment or procedure, directly or by implication; however, they may make a reasonable statement of prognosis.

K. Individuals shall not provide clinical services solely by correspondence.

L. Individuals may practice by telecommunication (e.g., telehealth/e-health), where not prohibited by law.

M. Individuals shall adequately maintain and appropriately secure records of professional services rendered, research and scholarly activities conducted, and products dispensed, and they shall allow access to these records only when authorized or when required by law.

N. Individuals shall not reveal, without authorization, any professional or personal information about identified persons served professionally or identified participants involved in research and scholarly activities unless doing so is necessary to protect the welfare of the person or of the community or is otherwise required by law.

O. Individuals shall not charge for services not rendered, nor shall they misrepresent services rendered, products dispensed, or research and scholarly activities conducted.

P. Individuals shall enroll and include persons as participants in research or teaching demonstrations only if their participation is voluntary, without coercion, and with their informed consent.

Q. Individuals whose professional services are adversely affected by substance abuse or other health-related conditions shall seek professional assistance and, where appropriate, withdraw from the affected areas of practice.

R. Individuals shall not discontinue service to those they are serving without providing reasonable notice.

PRINCIPLE OF ETHICS II

Individuals shall honor their responsibility to achieve and maintain the highest level of professional competence and performance.

Rules of Ethics

A. Individuals shall engage in the provision of clinical services only when they hold the appropriate Certificate of Clinical Competence or when they are in the certification process and are supervised by an individual who holds the appropriate Certificate of Clinical Competence.

B. Individuals shall engage in only those aspects of the professions that are within the scope of their professional practice and competence, considering their level of education, training, and experience.

C. Individuals shall engage in lifelong learning to maintain and enhance professional competence and performance.

D. Individuals shall not require or permit their professional staff to provide services or conduct research activities that exceed the staff member's competence, level of education, training, and experience.

E. Individuals shall ensure that all equipment used to provide services or to conduct research and scholarly activities is in proper working order and is properly calibrated.

PRINCIPLE OF ETHICS III

Individuals shall honor their responsibility to the public by promoting public understanding of the professions, by supporting the development of services designed to fulfill the unmet needs of the public, and by providing accurate information in all communications involving any aspect of the professions, including the dissemination of research findings and scholarly activities, and the promotion, marketing, and advertising of products and services.

Rules of Ethics

A. Individuals shall not misrepresent their credentials, competence, education, training, experience, or scholarly or research contributions.

B. Individuals shall not participate in professional activities that constitute a conflict of interest.

C. Individuals shall refer those served professionally solely on the basis of the interest of those being referred and not on any personal interest, financial or otherwise.

D. Individuals shall not misrepresent research, diagnostic information, services rendered, results of services rendered, products dispensed, or the effects of products dispensed.

E. Individuals shall not defraud or engage in any scheme to defraud in connection with obtaining payment, reimbursement, or grants for services rendered, research conducted, or products dispensed.

F. Individuals' statements to the public shall provide accurate information about the nature and management of communication disorders, about the professions, about professional services, about products for sale, and about research and scholarly activities.

G. Individuals' statements to the public when advertising, announcing, and marketing their professional services; reporting research results; and promoting products shall adhere to professional standards and shall not contain misrepresentations.

PRINCIPLE OF ETHICS IV

Individuals shall honor their responsibilities to the professions and their relationships with colleagues, students, and members of other professions and disciplines.

Rules of Ethics

A. Individuals shall uphold the dignity and autonomy of the professions, maintain harmonious interprofessional and intraprofessional relationships, and accept the professions' self-imposed standards.

B. Individuals shall prohibit anyone under their supervision from engaging in any practice that violates the Code of Ethics.

C. Individuals shall not engage in dishonesty, fraud, deceit, or misrepresentation.

D. Individuals shall not engage in any form of unlawful harassment, including sexual harassment or power abuse.

E. Individuals shall not engage in any other form of conduct that adversely reflects on the professions or on the individual's fitness to serve persons professionally.

F. Individuals shall not engage in sexual activities with clients, students, or research participants over whom they exercise professional authority or power.

G. Individuals shall assign credit only to those who have contributed to a publication, presentation, or product. Credit shall be assigned in proportion to the contribution and only with the contributor's consent.

H. Individuals shall reference the source when using other persons' ideas, research, presentations, or products in written, oral, or any other media presentation or summary.

I. Individuals' statements to colleagues about professional services, research results, and products shall adhere to prevailing professional standards and shall contain no misrepresentations.

J. Individuals shall not provide professional services without exercising independent professional judgment, regardless of referral source or prescription.

K. Individuals shall not discriminate in their relationships with colleagues, students, and members of other professions and disciplines on the basis of race or ethnicity, gender, gender identity/gender expression, age, religion, national origin, sexual orientation, or disability.

L. Individuals shall not file or encourage others to file complaints that disregard or ignore facts that would disprove the allegation, nor should the Code of Ethics be used for personal reprisal, as a means of addressing personal animosity, or as a vehicle for retaliation.

M. Individuals who have reason to believe that the Code of Ethics has been violated shall inform the Board of Ethics.

N. Individuals shall comply fully with the policies of the Board of Ethics in its consideration and adjudication of complaints of violations of the Code of Ethics.

Source: American Speech-Language-Hearing Association. (2010). *Code of ethics.* Available from http://www.asha.org/policy. © Copyright 2010 American Speech-Language-Hearing Association. Reprinted with permission.

APPENDIX 3–B

Ethical Principles, Rules, and Guidance Pertinent to the Supervision of Support Personnel (ASHA, 2013)

ASHA strives to ensure that its members and certificate holders preserve the highest standards of integrity and ethical practice. The *ASHA Code of Ethics* (2010) sets forth the fundamental principles and rules considered essential to this purpose. The code applies to every individual who is (a) a member of ASHA, whether certified or not, (b) a nonmember holding the ASHA Certificate of Clinical Competence, (c) an applicant for membership or certification, or (d) a Clinical Fellow seeking to fulfill standards for certification.

Although some SLPAs may choose to affiliate with ASHA as associates, the Code of Ethics does not directly apply to associates. However, any individual who is working in a support role (technician, aide, assistant) under the supervision of an SLP or speech scientist must be knowledgeable about the provisions of the code. It is imperative that the supervising professional and the assistant behave in a manner that is consistent with the principles and rules outlined in the ASHA Code of Ethics. Since the ethical responsibility for patient care or for subjects in research studies cannot be delegated, the SLP or speech scientist takes overall responsibility for the actions of the assistants when they are performing assigned duties. If the assistant engages in activities that violate the Code of Ethics, the supervising professional may be found in violation of the code if adequate oversight has not been provided.

The following principles and rules of the ASHA Code of Ethics specifically address issues that are pertinent when an SLP supervises support personnel in the provision of services or when conducting research.

Principle of Ethics I

Individuals shall honor their responsibility to hold paramount the welfare of persons they serve professionally or who are participants in research and scholarly activities and they shall treat animals involved in research in a humane manner.

Guidance

The supervising SLP remains responsible for the care and well-being of the client or research subject. If the supervisor fails to intervene when the assistant's behavior puts the client or subject at risk or when services or procedures are implemented inappropriately, the supervisor could be in violation of the Code of Ethics.

Principle of Ethics I, Rule A

Individuals shall provide all services competently.

Guidance

The supervising SLP must ensure that all services, including those provided directly by the assistant, meet practice standards and are administered competently. If the supervisor fails to intervene or correct the actions of the assistant as needed, this could be a violation of the Code of Ethics.

Principle of Ethics I, Rule D

Individuals shall not misrepresent the credentials of assistants, technicians, support personnel, students, Clinical Fellows, or any others under their supervision, and they shall inform those they serve professionally of the name and professional credentials of persons providing services.

Guidance

The supervising SLP must ensure that clients and subjects are informed of the title and qualifications of the assistant. This is not a passive responsibility; that is, the supervisor must make this information easily available and understandable to the clients or subjects and not rely on the individual to inquire about or ask directly for this information. Any misrepresentation of the assistant's qualifications or role could result in a violation of the Code of Ethics by the supervisor.

Principle of Ethics I, Rule E

Individuals who hold the Certificate of Clinical Competence shall not delegate tasks that require the unique skills, knowledge, and judgment that are within the scope of their profession to assistants, technicians, support personnel, or any nonprofessionals over whom they have supervisory responsibility.

Guidance

The supervising SLP is responsible for monitoring and limiting the role of the assistant as described in these guidelines and in accordance with applicable licensure laws.

Principle of Ethics I, Rule F

Individuals who hold the Certificate of Clinical Competence may delegate tasks related to provision of clinical services to assistants, technicians, support personnel, or any other persons only if those services are appropriately supervised, realizing that the responsibility for client welfare remains with the certified individual.

Guidance

The supervising SLP is responsible for providing appropriate and adequate direct and indirect supervision to ensure that the services provided are appropriate and meet practice standards. The SLP should document supervisory activities and adjust the amount and type of supervision to ensure that the Code of Ethics is not violated.

Principle of Ethics II, Rule B

Individuals shall engage in only those aspects of the professions that are within the scope of their professional practice and competence, considering their level of education, training, and experience.

Guidance

The supervising SLP is responsible for ensuring that he or she has the skills and competencies needed in order to provide appropriate supervision. This may include seeking continuing education in the area of supervision practice.

Principle of Ethics II, Rule D

Individuals shall not require or permit their professional staff to provide services or conduct research activities that exceed the staff member's competence, level of education, training, and experience.

Guidance

The supervising SLP must ensure that the assistant only performs those activities and duties that are defined as appropriate for the level of training and experience and in accordance with applicable licensure laws. If the assistant exceeds the practice role that has been defined for him or her, and the supervisor fails to correct this, the supervisor could be found in violation of the Code of Ethics.

Principle of Ethics IV, Rule B

Individuals shall prohibit anyone under their supervision from engaging in any practice that violates the Code of Ethics.

Guidance

Because the assistant provides services as "an extension" of those provided by the professional, the SLP is responsible for informing the assistant about the Code of Ethics and monitoring the performance of the assistant. Failure to do so could result in the SLP's being found in violation of the Code.

REFERENCE

American Speech-Language-Hearing Association. (2010). *Code of ethics*. Retrieved from http://www.asha.org/policy

Note: A full copy of this document is available in Appendix 1–A.

Source: American Speech-Language-Hearing Association. (2013). *Speech-language pathology assistant scope of practice.* Available from http://www.asha.org/policy. © Copyright 2013 American Speech-Language-Hearing Association. All rights reserved. Reprinted with permission.

APPENDIX 3–C

Sample SLPA Ethical Decision-Making Worksheet

STEP 1: GATHER/CLARIFY FACTS*

■ Who is involved in this situation?
Amber and her supervisor.

■ Who is affected by this situation?
Amber, her supervisor, and the client and his or her family (if Amber performs the assessment).

■ What are the motives and roles of others involved in this situation?
Amber's supervisor appears to be motivated by currently pressing issues in terms of a large number of reports and assessments that need to be done soon. Additional clarification may be needed as to why this particular client was highlighted as a person Amber should be involved in assessing. Perhaps Amber and this client have a positive relationship or there is some input Amber's supervisor feels will be valuable from Amber in terms of assessment or the client's progress report. Related to this, Amber can also clarify her supervisor's intent with this request. Was the request that Amber assist in this assessment or that Amber perform this assessment independently? The role of Amber's supervisor is that of Amber's superior, which is a position of power in terms of Amber's employment and performance evaluation, as well as potential future supervision.

■ What is *your own* motive (role) in the situation?
Amber's role is that of an assistant, who works under the direction of her supervisor. Amber may be concerned how her supervisor will react if she tells her she cannot do something, both personally because they appear to have a good relationship but also from an employment and supervision standpoint. Amber may be concerned she will lose her job or be rated poorly on evaluations if she tells her supervisor that assessment is outside of her scope of practice.

■ Describe applicable state regulations/laws (if any).
Regulations for Amber's state licensure specifically state she may not independently assess a client. They do state she can assist with assessment. Similarly, state regulations governing Amber's supervisor also specifically state that she may not delegate tasks such as assessment to support personnel.

Describe applicable employer policies and/or procedures (if any).
No specific employer-related policies or procedures available on this matter were identified.

List applicable ASHA ethical principles and rules of ethics (if any):

Ethical Principle	Ethical Rule
Applicable to Amber	
Principle of Ethics I	*Rule A: Individuals shall provide all services competently.*
Principle of Ethics II	*Rule B: Individuals shall engage in only those aspects of the professions that are within the scope of their professional practice and competence, considering their level of education, training, and experience.*
Applicable to Amber's Supervisor	
Principle of Ethics I	*Rule E: Individuals who hold the Certificate of Clinical Competence shall not delegate tasks that require the unique skills, knowledge, and judgment that are within the scope of their profession to assistants, technicians, support personnel, or any nonprofessionals over whom they have supervisory responsibility.*
Principle of Ethics II	*Rule D: Individuals shall not require or permit their professional staff to provide services or conduct research activities that exceed the staff member's competence, level of education, training, and experience.*
Principle of Ethics IV	*Rule B: Individuals shall prohibit anyone under their supervision from engaging in any practice that violates the Code of Ethics.*

Note: At the end of Step 1 (gather/clarify facts), you should be able to describe the nature of the problem accurately and in depth, factoring in each of the facts in Step 1. If not, continue to gather additional information. If by clarifying the facts, the ethical dilemma no longer exists, stop here. If not, proceed to Step 2 (action analysis).

STEP 2: ACTION ANALYSIS

Possible Course of Action	Benefits	Risks
Amber could assess the client (as requested) but not tell anyone and allow her supervisor to sign the report as if the speech-language pathologist (SLP) was the one who conducted this assessment.	■ Amber avoids conflict with her supervisor by not having to tell the supervisor that assessment is outside Amber's scope of responsibilities.	■ Violation in ethical principles, for both Amber and her supervisor. ■ Negative impact in quality of care for the client. ■ Potential for sanctions from state licensing board, for both Amber and her supervisor. ■ Potential for sanctions from the American Speech-Language-Hearing Association (ASHA's) Board of Ethics for Amber's supervisor.
Amber can tell her supervisor that assessment is not within her scope of responsibilities, and as such, she is not able to assess the client (as requested). She can offer to assist in the assessment and in any other duties within Amber's scope of responsibilities so that the supervisor has additional time to assess the client.	■ No violation in ethical principles. ■ Quality in client care is maintained, as Amber has reduced the supervisor's workload in other ways so that the client can be assessed by the SLP, who is qualified to do so.	■ Amber's supervisor may disagree or may be upset that Amber has refused to do something requested. If good interpersonal skills are utilized in addressing this situation, this risk may be mitigated.

Amber could assess the client (as requested) but report her supervisor's conduct to the state licensing board, ASHA's Board of Ethics, and their employer.	■ Amber avoids direct conflict with her supervisor by not having to tell the supervisor that assessment is outside Amber's scope of responsibilities.	■ Violation in ethical principles, for both Amber and her supervisor.* ■ Negative impact on quality of care for the client. ■ Potential for sanctions from state licensing board, for both Amber and her supervisor. *Note:* Although Amber reported her supervisor to ASHA's Board of Ethics, Amber would still be engaging in unethical conduct as she performed the assessment, which was not in the best interest of the client.
Amber could not mention this conflict to her supervisor but call in sick the day the assessment is scheduled, so she does not have to assess the client.	■ Amber avoids direct conflict with her supervisor by not having to tell her supervisor that assessment is outside Amber's scope of responsibilities. ■ No sanctions from the state licensing board for either Amber or her supervisor as the assessment is not performed by Amber.	■ Potential negative impact on quality of care as the assessment may not be performed as needed, which isn't in the best interest of the client. Alternatively, the supervisor may simply reschedule the assessment for another day when Amber is available. and in that case, the issue has not been resolved and will resurface when Amber returns.

Consult Experts**

- Who are sources of assistance in problem solving this matter (e.g., supervisor, employer, coworker, etc.)?
  Amber has another SLP she has worked closely with in the same district. She may be an additional resource on the matter, given of course that Amber discusses this issue in confidence.

- What are the opinions of experts on your course(s) of action?
  After evaluating the possible course of actions, Amber decided there was only one that resulted in an ethical resolution. She decided not to involve her former supervisor in this matter at this time. For this particular issue, Amber felt she could resolve it without consulting others.

Note: In consulting with others about the situation, you must do so with discretion and complete confidentiality. This is particularly true when the conflict involves a client. Federal law prohibits you from discussing any personal information about your client with anyone other than the SLP responsible for that client's care and those specifically authorized (typically in writing). If so, you should use only generic descriptions, without any names or personal information specifically identifying the individuals involved. You should also have this discussion in a private location where others cannot overhear your conversation.

STEP 3: ACTION IMPLEMENTATION***

- What action did you implement?
  Amber expressed to her supervisor that assessment was not within her scope of responsibilities, and as such, she was not able to assess the client, as requested. She offered to assist in the assessment by preparing the materials. Amber also indicated that she would be willing to stay late to assist with other scheduling and clerical duties needed in preparation for the upcoming individualized educational plans (IEPs).

- What was the outcome of your action?
  Amber's supervisor assessed the client and, with the additional help that Amber provided, was able to meet all her obligations in terms of upcoming IEPs. Amber's professional approach and good interpersonal skills preserved their relationship and helped Amber to feel confident in addressing conflict in the future ethically.

***Note:** The outcome of your action should resolve the ethical dilemma. If not, restart this process over again at Step 1 (gather/clarify facts) and proceed to Step 2 (action analysis) and Step 3 (action implementation) until an ethical resolution is achieved.

APPENDIX 3–D

ASHA Confidentiality Statement (ASHA, 2013)

TABLE OF CONTENTS

- About This Document
- Issues in Ethics Statements: Definition
- Introduction
- Confidentiality Issues in Research
  - Discussion
  - Guidance
- Confidentiality of Client Information
  - Discussion
  - Guidance With Respect to Verbal Communication
  - Guidance With Respect to Written Records
- Student Privacy Issues
  - Discussion
  - Guidance With Respect to Students in Classes
  - Guidance With Respect to Student Clinicians
- Confidentiality in Relation to Peers and Colleagues
  - Discussion
  - Guidance

ABOUT THIS DOCUMENT

This Issues in Ethics statement is a revision of *Confidentiality* (originally published in 2001 and revised in 2004). The Board of Ethics reviews Issues in Ethics statements periodically to ensure that they meet the needs of the professions and are consistent with ASHA policies.

ISSUES IN ETHICS STATEMENTS: DEFINITION

From time to time, the Board of Ethics determines that members and certificate holders can benefit from additional analysis and instruction concerning a specific issue of ethical conduct. Issues in Ethics statements are intended to heighten sensitivity and increase awareness. They are illustrative of the Code of Ethics and intended to promote thoughtful consideration of ethical issues. They may assist members and certificate holders in engaging in self-guided ethical decision making. These statements do not absolutely prohibit or require specified activity. The facts and circumstances surrounding a matter of concern will determine whether the activity is ethical.

INTRODUCTION

Professional persons in health care delivery fields (including those working in the public schools) have legal and ethical responsibilities to safeguard the confidentiality of information regarding the clients in their care. Scholars and those involved in human research have legal and ethical obligations to protect the privacy of persons who agree to participate in clinical studies and other research projects. Children and adults who are legally incompetent have the same right to privacy enjoyed by adults who are competent, though their rights will be mediated by a designated family member or a legal guardian.

There are federal statutes binding on all ASHA members who treat clients or patients, whether they work in health care facilities (where the HIPAA privacy and security rules apply), schools (which operate under the Family Education Rights and Privacy Act, as well as HIPAA), or private practice. There are also stringent federal statutes governing the treatment of human subjects in medical and other forms of scientific research. Individual states also have statutes governing the confidentiality of patient and client information, the protection of data gathered in research, and the privacy of students. It is the responsibility of all members of the speech-language pathology and audiology professions to know these laws and to honor them. Because state laws may vary, professionals moving from one state to another should take special care to familiarize themselves with the legal requirements of the new place of practice or residence. Educational institutions preparing professionals in this field should give significant attention to informing all those entering the field about these legal requirements and should model good practice in their handling of confidential information concerning the students enrolled in their programs. Owners of businesses and managers of facilities should regularly review these legal requirements with the professionals and the staff whom they employ.

Institutions and facilities within which professionals see clients or pursue research may have their own policies concerning safeguarding privacy and maintaining confidential records. It is incumbent on the professionals in such settings to familiarize themselves with such workplace policies and regulations and to perform their work in conformity with these requirements. Owners and managers should make sure that such policies are readily available to their employees. Workplace training is desirable, and periodic reviews are recommended.

The ASHA Code of Ethics (2010) identifies the confidentiality of information pertaining to clients, patients, students, and research subjects as a matter of ethical obligation, not just a matter of legal or workplace requirements. Respect for privacy is implicitly addressed in Principle of Ethics I because to hold paramount the welfare of persons served is to honor and respect their privacy and the confidential nature of the information with which they entrust members of the professions. This broad, general obligation is further specified in both Rules M and N.

Principle I, Rule M: Individuals shall adequately maintain and appropriately secure records of professional services rendered, research and scholarly activities conducted, and products dispensed and they shall allow access to these records only when authorized or when required by law.

Principle I, Rule N: Individuals shall not reveal, without authorization, any professional or personal information about identified persons served professionally or identified participants involved in research and scholarly activities unless doing so is necessary to protect the welfare of the person or of the community or is otherwise required by law.

If there is variation among the different sources of rules on privacy, the professional should follow the most restrictive rule; for example, if the law seems to allow an action that the Code of Ethics seems to prohibit, follow the Code of Ethics. If there is conflict between sources, do what the law requires; for example, if workplace policies conflict on some point with legal requirements for confidential handling of records, the law takes precedence.

CONFIDENTIALITY ISSUES IN RESEARCH

Discussion

Attention to the protection of privacy begins with the planning of a research project, is crucial to the way research on human subjects is conducted, and extends through the review of research results (on both human and animal subjects) for publication and the sharing of data sets. Everyone involved—researchers, human subjects, support personnel, editors, reviewers, and data managers—should be aware of the ethical and legal requirements regarding privacy and should not compromise confidentiality for any reason.

Institutional review boards must be consulted about any research involving human subjects, and informed consent forms must be obtained and honored. Human subjects have a right to expect that their personal information will not be divulged when the results of a study are published or when data sets from a research project are shared with other investigators. Protecting the privacy of research subjects is an obligation for all those who are involved in the research.

Guidance

Data and the personal identities of individual participants in research studies must be kept confidential. There should be careful supervision of staff to make sure that they, too, are adhering to best practices in protecting the confidentiality of all participant data. Some reasonable precautions to protect and respect the confidentiality of participants include:

- disseminating research findings without disclosing personal identifying information;
- storing research records securely and limiting access to authorized personnel only;
- removing, disguising, or coding personal identifying information;
- obtaining written informed consent from the participant (or, in the case of a child, the parent or guardian) to disseminate findings that include photographic/video images or audio voice recordings that might reveal personal identifying information.

Because legal requirements in this area are very strict and because institutions monitor research on human subjects very carefully, professionals should seek further guidance directly from the appropriate personnel in their home institutions.

During the peer review of submitted manuscripts, all findings, information, and graphics in the manuscripts must be treated as highly confidential, and reviewers and editors alike have an obligation to protect findings from any form of premature disclosure. In a blind-review process, the identities of the researchers must be protected. In a double-blind review process, the anonymity of authors and reviewers alike must be scrupulously preserved. Editors and reviewers should make no prepublication use of information they learn from submitted manuscripts.

CONFIDENTIALITY OF CLIENT INFORMATION

Discussion

Clients must be assured that all aspects of their communication with a speech-language pathologist or audiologist regarding themselves or their family members will be held in the strictest confidence. Clients who cannot trust professionals to treat information as confidential may withhold information that is important to assessment and treatment. When professionals disregard the privacy of their clients, the clients are injured in obvious and/or subtle ways. Evaluations, treatment plans and therapy, discussions with the client or the client's relatives, consultations with the family or with other professionals, treatment records, and payment negotiations should all be treated as confidential. All persons who come into possession of client information are equally bound by this requirement. Therapists, supervisors, assistants, and support staff in schools, facilities, and firms overseeing billing services are all prohibited from revealing client information to unauthorized third parties. ASHA members have a responsibility not only for monitoring their own conversations, securing of records, and sharing of client information, but also for ensuring that supervisees and support staff are adhering to ethical requirements regarding privacy. ASHA members who oversee facilities delivering services should have in place policies

and sanctions regarding violations of confidentiality by their employees or by students working under supervision.

Guidance With Respect to Verbal Communication

In the case of a competent adult, no one other than the client herself or himself has the right to authorize the release of information. In the case of a child, only the parent of record or guardian ad litem has this right. It should be noted that there will be cases (e.g., in custody disputes or under custody agreements) in which a biological or adoptive parent has neither the right to know client information nor the right to authorize disclosures. In the case of an incompetent adult, only the designated family member(s) or legal guardian has the right to authorize disclosure. Good practice suggests:

- In all treatment situations, a written form specifying disclosure of information should be provided to, and signed by, the client or client representative at the beginning of treatment.
- Every client record should contain a clear, specific, up-to-date, and easily located statement of who has the right of access to client information and who may authorize the release of such information to other parties.

For any release of information other than that specified in the preliminary privacy agreement or as required by law (e.g., a subpoena), speech-language pathologists and audiologists must obtain a release of information agreement from clients or their designated representatives. This includes obtaining permission to share information with another professional. It is prudent to obtain this permission in writing rather than relying on verbal assent.

In rare cases, courts or administrative bodies with subpoena power may legitimately require the disclosure of confidential information. When a court serves an organization or individual with a subpoena requiring records or other information as evidence in a legal proceeding, typically the professional complies with the request; however, it is often prudent for professionals to seek legal advice in such situations.

Professionals are prohibited from discussing clients in public places—such as elevators, cafeterias, staff lounges, or clinical/business sites—with others, specifically including the practitioner's family members and friends. Practitioners sometimes think that if they do not use the client's name such discussions are acceptable, but this is not true. Any description of, or comment about, a client who is being served constitutes disclosure of confidential information.

The same restrictions that apply to face-to-face conversation also apply to digital and electronic forms of communication with professionals, colleagues, and friends.

Guidance With Respect to Written Records

Written records have a durability and reproducibility distinct from spoken information; there are therefore additional concerns about the protection and handling of paper files or computerized records. These concerns and challenges have become more complex and intense as a result of the digitizing of information. Breaches of confidentiality can occur as a result of the way records are created, stored, or transmitted.

Ordinarily, professionals should not create, update, or store records on their personal electronic devices (e.g., computers and flash drives) or personal online accounts. If a workplace is aware of and allows such off-site handling of records, then privacy safeguards, such as password protection and anonymized client identifications, should be meticulously observed. Records on portable devices should not be opened and read in public places such as coffee shops or on public transportation.

All therapists who practice independently and all businesses should have clear written policies concerning client records. Workplace policies concerning records management should typically address:

- record accuracy and content;
- record storage, both electronic and paper;
- ownership of records;
- record access—both with respect to personnel who may read and manipulate the record and with respect to rights of access by clients;
- record review and retention and related statutes of limitation;
- transfer of information, including transfer by electronic means;
- procedures for handling requests for information by someone other than the client or the client's representative;

- use of client records for research;
- destruction of material removed from records.

These policies should be observed without variance. Failure to comply with the requirements designed to protect client records not only puts client welfare at risk but also makes the practitioner vulnerable to ethics complaints and legal action.

It is particularly important for professionals serving clients in institutions and facilities to be aware of who owns the record. Usually, in a medical setting, the medical facility owns the record. In a private practice, the individual who is legally responsible for the practice owns the record. In a school setting, the school district owns the record. A report prepared by a speech-language pathologist or audiologist in the course of employment in a particular setting is not owned by that speech-language pathologist or audiologist, and he or she may not remove or copy such confidential records while employed, upon termination of employment, or if the practice closes.

It is important for the professional to be aware of what information is necessary and appropriate for inclusion in the client's legal record and to exercise professional judgment in making notations in the client's record.

Appropriate steps must be taken to ensure the confidentiality and protection of electronic and computerized client records and information. All information should be password protected, and only authorized persons should have access to the records and information. Computerized records should be backed up routinely, and there should be plans for protecting computer systems in case of emergencies.

STUDENT PRIVACY ISSUES

Discussion

There are many academic programs that prepare audiologists and speech-language pathologists for entry into the field of communication sciences and disorders. At all levels of professional education, students and student clinicians have privacy rights that educators must respect. Many of these rights are specifically protected by federal law (FERPA, for example), and there may also be relevant state statutes. But, once again, safeguarding the privacy of information entrusted to a teacher, program administrator, or institution is an ethical and not just a legal obligation. According to Principle of Ethics IV of the Code of Ethics, "Individuals shall honor their responsibilities to the professions and their relationships with colleagues and students." Professional regard for students and student clinicians involves respecting each student as the arbiter of what personal information may be divulged and to whom it may be divulged.

Guidance With Respect to Students in Classes

Most academic institutions have very specific policies regarding access to, storage of, and release of confidential student academic and disciplinary records. Academic institutions are less likely to have written policies concerning appropriate conversations and communications among educators with respect to their students. Students do, however, have a right to assume that the knowledge that the faculty have of their academic achievements and personal situations will not be widely or carelessly shared. Verbal and electronically mediated discussion of a student's performance should be carefully restricted to those directly responsible for the student's education. Student performance and personal disclosures should not be discussed in public places, such as elevators, hallways, cafeterias, coffee shops, or campus transportation vehicles. Graded student work and records of student achievement must be carefully safeguarded; access to grades in electronic files stored on mobile devices should be password protected if the device is carried outside of the faculty member's campus office. Sensitive personal information that a faculty member may possess should not be shared at all in the absence of a clear and compelling need to know on the part of the person making inquiries.

Guidance With Respect to Student Clinicians

Maintaining the confidentiality of information is a complex challenge in the case of student clinicians. Those who supervise student clinicians must ensure the privacy of client and student clinical records and should model high regard for client privacy and best practices in recording, securing, and storing client records. Supervisors and mentors must treat the performance, records, and evaluations of student clinicians as confidential.

Supervisors of student clinicians must be familiar with the rules for viewing and sharing client information in a teaching setting. For example, a student supervisor's discussion of a patient record for the purposes of education in a university clinic is not a violation of confidentiality, but a student's discussion of the same patient with other students or friends would constitute a violation of confidentiality.

When student clinicians work with clients, persons unrelated to the client may request information about the client's communication problem. Requests might come from an off-site clinic supervisor, Clinical Fellowship mentor, or a professional who supervises student teachers. Patient or client information cannot be disclosed without a signed release.

CONFIDENTIALITY IN RELATION TO PEERS AND COLLEAGUES

Discussion

Issues of confidentiality also arise for ASHA members and certificate holders in their relationships with colleagues as a result of information they obtain as they serve in roles such as site visitor, consultant, supervisor, administrator, or reviewer of documents such as manuscripts, grant proposals, and fellowship applications. All of these roles allow access to peer information of a personal and confidential nature. These activities are covered broadly under Principle of Ethics IV, which calls upon ASHA members and certificate holders to honor their obligations to "colleagues" and "members of other professions and disciplines."

Guidance

Information about colleagues and professional peers that is gathered or revealed in the course of evaluations, assessments, or reviews should be treated with the same care and respect that are appropriate to information about clients and research subjects.

When a colleague shares sensitive information or when one participates in committees or other groups that discuss sensitive or controversial matters, participants should clarify in a candid conversation what level of confidentiality is expected and scrupulously maintain the desired level. Records of such conversations should be appropriately secured with agreement as to their storage and disposal.

Matters that may result in disciplinary action by some body, board, or institution deserve special comment. Individuals reporting or responding to alleged violations of codes of ethics or professional codes of conduct are also dealing with confidential matters and acting in a confidential relationship with the adjudicating body. It would be prudent to consider all aspects of a matter confidential until a final decision is rendered. Once a final determination has been reached, it is important for the adjudicating body to clarify what information can now be shared and what information must remain confidential.

Adjudicating bodies themselves typically follow rules of confidentiality (some dictated by law and regulation, some dictated by the organization's internal governance policies and procedures) while the case is under consideration.

With respect to disclosure of decisions by adjudicating bodies, individuals need to inform themselves of pertinent laws and organizational policies. It would not be prudent simply to assume that the outcome can in all cases be made public. Even when the outcome can be made public, it is often the case that earlier filings, testimony, and deliberations must be maintained in confidence.

ASHA members who either place a complaint before the ASHA Board of Ethics or find themselves responding to such a complaint have specific responsibilities to preserve the confidentiality of all materials relevant to the adjudication of complaints. Principle of Ethics IV, Rule N, is specific about this ethical obligation and refers the reader to the policies and procedures of the Board of Ethics for further information.

Source: American Speech-Language-Hearing Association. (2013). *Confidentiality.* Available from http://www.asha.org/policy.© Copyright 2013 American Speech-Language-Hearing Association. All rights reserved. Reprinted with permission.

APPENDIX 3–E

SLPA Ethical Dilemma Scenarios

Scenario 1: You are a newly hired speech-language pathology assistant (SLPA) in a public school setting. This is your first SLPA position and your first job in a public school. Your supervisor trained you for approximately 1 week, consisting of showing you paperwork and having you observe her providing services to students. She then became seriously ill and has taken an extended medical leave. The district supervisor has asked you to work until they can find a replacement supervisor for you, including providing treatment services to the students on the supervisor's caseload.

Scenario 2: You are an SLPA in a public school setting and attending graduate school for your master's degree in SLP. You have been employed as an SLPA for approximately 6 months under the supervision of an SLP. There is an opening for an SLP position at another school site, and the district supervisor tells you they would like to hire you for this position. She says that they will request a "waiver" for you to work in this position as an SLP, but in the meantime, she indicates that they need you to begin working in this position immediately, so until the paperwork is official, you will need to perform evaluation and treatment at the new school setting.

Scenario 3: You are an SLPA working in a medical setting that bills Medicare for services provided to patients. Your supervisor has trained you to work with individuals in this setting and you feel relatively competent in doing so, under her supervision. One day she mentions to you that SLPA services are not "billable" under Medicare, but she states that this setting allows you to provide services, as long as the paperwork indicates that the SLP provided the services. As such, your supervisor tells you not to document your services in official records but to let her know the status of the treatment sessions and she will enter that information into the system for you.

Scenario 4: You are an SLPA working in a private practice. Your supervisor has trained you to work with individuals in this setting and you feel competent doing so under her supervision. You are assigned a new client to work on treatment goals addressing memory and attention. When you read the client's chart, you see that she is HIV positive. You are pregnant and concerned that you will contract HIV/AIDS, so you tell your supervisor that you do not feel comfortable working with this client.

Scenario 5: You are an SLPA working in a public school setting. You have been working in this setting for 3 months. Thus far, you have received excellent training. You have a close relationship with one particular student and her family. The student's mother does not get along with your supervising SLP. As a result, the student's mom approaches you one afternoon and asks to speak with you about her child's goals, progress, and future recommendations for the student. She tells you that you "know her child best," and as such, she wants to know your opinion, not your supervisor's opinion, on the topic.

CHAPTER 4
Professional Conduct

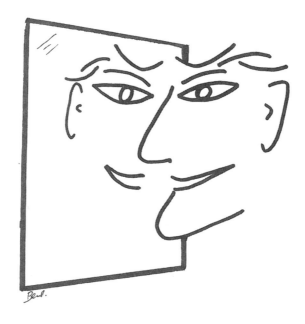

*Learn from yesterday, live for today, hope for tomorrow.
The important thing is not to stop questioning.*
Albert Einstein (renowned physicist)

Being employed as a speech-language pathology assistant (SLPA) means that you enter into a professional community, one in which you are expected to conform to community-accepted standards for professional conduct. Although your training will provide you with the technical skills and competencies needed to perform the duties of an SLPA, there are still "soft skills" required to interface successfully within this professional community and to establish your credibility as an SLPA (American Speech-Language-Hearing Association [ASHA], n.d., paragraph 2). ASHA (n.d.) recommends five tips to establishing your credibility as an SLPA, including the following:

1. Maintain a positive and pleasant attitude.
2. Project a professional image.
3. Convey a willingness to learn new things.
4. Demonstrate initiative.
5. Exhibit a sense of organization.

Broken down further, many of these skills have behaviors that fall under the categories of appearance, communication (verbal and written), self-assessment, and conflict resolution. You, of course, remain an individual with unique characteristics and contributions, but in any setting, there will be expectations of you in each of these areas. Actively seeking to improve your skills in these areas will enhance your effectiveness, project professionalism, and increase your credibility as an SLPA. The sections that follow provide additional detail in each of these areas.

APPEARANCE

Your appearance is one aspect of your ability to establish credibility (ASHA, n.d.; Piasecki, 2003). This does not mean that all SLPAs, in all environments, dress and look alike, but it does mean you should have a professional appearance. This includes wearing clean, neat, and suitable clothing (ASHA, n.d.; Piasecki, 2003). Wearing clothing that is clean and neat are minimal requirements in any setting, but SLPAs often ask, "What is 'suitable' clothing?" For example, must you wear a suit and tie, are jeans acceptable, can you wear jewelry, is perfume appropriate, and so on? In every setting, what is suitable clothing will vary, but generally, if you adhere to the following principles, you will be able to project a professional image and meet the appearance standards of your particular setting:

1. *Check the written policies in your setting on professional attire.* Many settings have specific rules and regulations that require you to dress a certain way. Make sure you familiarize yourself with these rules and follow them in selecting suitable attire. In some settings, such as medical settings, you may be asked to wear a uniform, such as a lab coat, scrubs, or other setting-specific attire (Piasecki, 2003).

2. *Fit your clothing to your duties.* Think about what you will be expected to do and what physical positions you will be in throughout your day. SLPAs may be in a variety of different positions throughout their day, from being seated behind a desk or table, to sitting and playing on the floor with young children, to working in playgroups or other community environments (e.g., grocery stores, parks, libraries), to walking on medical floors, and many other possible positions. Match your clothing to the physical tasks you will be asked to perform. Consider safety and comfort in this decision. Generally, closed-toe and low-heeled shoes allow for the greatest safety in a variety of settings. Clothing that allows you to move freely in a variety of positions also optimizes safety.

3. *Blend into your environment and do not be a distraction.* Use those in your environment who are respected professionals as a general guideline. Look to your superiors for examples of what is expected. Importantly, do not wear clothing or accessories that will be distracting or draw attention to you. Remember that as an SLPA, you interface with a variety of individuals. Your attire should not be a distraction to your clients or others in your work environment. The emphasis should be on what you do and not what you are wearing.

4. *Be conservative.* This aligns with not being a distraction (above), but also pertains to revealing and tight-fitting

clothing. Cultural norms vary in what is acceptable in this area (Piasecki, 2003). In all settings, you should err on the side of being more conservative, which usually translates to wearing clothing that reveals less skin and not wearing clothing that is excessively tight or form fitting.

In addition to attire, you should also consider personal hygiene practices. It goes without saying that good personal hygiene is a minimum requirement (Piasecki, 2003). However, consider as well personal hygiene products. Because SLPAs work with a variety of individuals, you should limit the use of heavily scented personal products, such as perfumes, scented sprays, and body lotions. Some clients may be sensitive to these products or may have adverse medical reactions to them (Piasecki, 2003). Similarly, some clients may be sensitive to the scent of smoke (Piasecki, 2003). If you smoke, you should take steps to ensure this odor is not present when you perform your duties as an SLPA.

You should also consider carefully body jewelry (nose, brow, or lip rings) and exposed tattoos. In some settings they are acceptable, while in others they may be a source of distraction and detract from the performance of your duties. Generally, it is best to minimize or conceal tattoos and body jewelry (Piasecki, 2003).

Last, some employers may require you to wear a nametag, denoting your position and any other relevant employment information (e.g., department) (Piasecki, 2003). ASHA recommends that SLPAs identify themselves verbally, in writing and/or with titles on name badges (ASHA, 2013). Some state licensure standards for SLPAs also have specific regulations about nametags and identification

as an SLPA. You should check with your supervisor on how to obtain an identification badge that meets these standards and make sure that it is visible on your clothing when you are performing your duties as an SLPA.

As with any aspect of your conduct, if you are unsure about what is acceptable appearance in your setting, contact your supervisor for suggestions and guidance.

COMMUNICATION

Verbal Communication

As professionals who specialize in speech and language, SLPAs are expected to have a high level of proficiency in the area of communication. Verbal communication will be the cornerstone of much of your daily interactions with clients and coworkers in most settings (McNamara, 2007). Defining "professional" communication is not an easy task, as the form and content of communication vary, given the topic, the communication partner(s), and the setting (van Servellen, 1997). Generally, however, there are a few principles that guide communication in professional settings. First and foremost, remember that communication in employment settings is typically more formal, both in form and content, than you would use in daily interactions, for example, with family and friends outside of work settings. A few tips to remember in enhancing the effectiveness of your verbal communication and in maintaining the formality of this communication are as follows:

1. Address individuals in your environment accordingly. When working with adult clients, it is generally acceptable

to address them as Mr., Mrs., Miss, Dr., and so on depending on their life role (Piasecki, 2003). With any age individual, client, or coworker, avoid pejorative terms such as sweetie, honey, and so forth (Piasecki, 2003). If you are unclear how someone prefers to be addressed, it is appropriate and courteous to ask him or her.

2. Speak clearly and at a rate appropriate for your communication partner(s). Use vocal loudness that is matched to the tone of the conversation (e.g., softer for personal, sensitive, or private matters) (van Servellen, 1997).

3. Avoid the use of slang and profanity in work settings.

4. Be a good listener. Use active listening strategies, such as not interrupting someone when he or she is speaking (van Servellen, 1997). Commenting (as appropriate) on what the speaker is saying will also let the speaker know that you understand and are paying attention to what he or she has to say.

5. Be mindful of your non-verbal communication and body language. Use a welcoming body language, which includes smiling (as appropriate), maintaining good eye contact, not fidgeting when you are speaking or being spoken to, holding your arms and legs in an uncrossed position, and maintaining an appropriate distance in terms of personal space (Piasecki, 2003; van Servellen, 1997).

6. Be culturally sensitivity to differences in communication styles (van Servellen, 1997). Chapter 5 provides additional information in this area.

In the context of service provision, effective verbal communication is critical (van Servellen, 1997). Jargon refers to the technical terms used by a group of professionals. When working with clients and their families, you will want to be especially careful to reduce jargon in your verbal communication and avoid the use of highly technical terms and descriptions. This will increase comprehension in communication with the individuals you serve and will ensure that you do not intimidate or offend the individuals you interact with by using words they do not share in common with you.

As an SLPA, service provision will require that you are able to comprehend specific aspects of spoken language and, in some cases, produce an accurate model of these structures. In terms of accents and nonstandard dialects held by professionals in the field of speech-language pathology, ASHA (1998) states that "there is no research to support the belief that audiologists and speech-language pathologists who speak a nonstandard dialect or who speak with an accent are unable to make appropriate diagnostic decisions or achieve appropriate treatment outcomes" (para. 8). Rather, ASHA recommends that if a professional speaks a nonstandard dialect or speaks with an accent, this will *not* affect treatment if:

- The individual has the required level of knowledge about normal and disordered communication.
- The individual has the expected level of clinical case management skills.
- If modeling is necessary, the individual is able to model the target phoneme, grammatical feature, or other aspect of speech and language that characterizes the client's particular problem.

If any of these factors affect your clinical services, speak with your supervisor about remediating these skills so that you can provide effective treatment.

Written Communication

Written communication is also an integral part of your daily interactions in the field of speech-language pathology (Goldfarb & Serpanos, 2009). Similar to high expectations in the area of verbal communication, as a professional specializing in speech and language, SLPAs are expected to be proficient in their written communication skills. These skills develop with time and training, but as an SLPA, you should be vigilant in developing and enhancing your skills in the area of written communication. Note writing, as discussed in Chapter 9, is one of the primary modes of written communication required of an SLPA. Chapter 9 contains helpful tips for ensuring accuracy of your written clinical notes. SLPAs may be required to write other documents as well. An important practice in ensuring excellent written communication is to *proof your work, proof your work, and proof your work again*. This is the advantage of written communication in that it is tangible and can be carefully reviewed and rewritten to achieve a high level of performance. This, of course, means that you must plan in advance and allow time for careful proofing. Below are a few additional suggestions to help you have effective and professional written communication.

1. *Proof your written language carefully to ensure it is free of errors in grammar and spelling.* Using spell check and grammar check is a minimum step in proofing your written work, but realize that there is no substitute for careful review and close proofreading of any written documents you generate, for any purpose. If you are working in an electronic format, printing a hard copy version to proof may help you catch errors. Reading your written work aloud may also increase the accuracy of your proofing skills.

2. *Use formality in your written communication.* Generally, brief but complete sentences are required in most forms of written communication. You should avoid the use of slang, colloquialism (e.g., he is *gonna* need, the clinician tried to *get across* the idea), and clichés (e.g., using *tried-and-true* methods, not the client's *cup of tea*) (Hegde, 1998). Similarly, in formal documents, you should spell out contractions (e.g., *haven't* should be written as *have not*, *can't* as *cannot*) (Hegde, 1998).

3. *Ensure your written content is comprehensible to an unfamiliar reader.* Do not assume the reader of your written document knows what you know or shares a similar background on a given topic. When you proof your written work, view it from the perspective of a *new* person reading *new* information. Will what you have written make sense and have sufficient detail for a new person reading new information to understand? If the answer is no, rewrite your document to ensure the content is understandable to an unfamiliar reader.

4. *Use standard forms of medical abbreviations and phonetic notation.* If you do not know the standard abbreviation for a word, spell out the entire word. Appendix 4–A contains a list of common medical abbreviations. Many

online sources are also available to search for standard medical abbreviation. Appendix 4–B contains a list of common International Phonetic Alphabet (IPA) symbols. More information about IPA symbols and their use is also available in Chapter 13. Many word-processing programs contain font libraries with IPA symbols. You can also access IPA symbols for electronic use through online keyboards, such as http://ipa.typeit.org/

5. *Learn from your mistakes.* You will receive feedback from your supervisor about the content and form of your written communication. You should save all comments and suggestions and incorporate these recommendations into all future documents. An excellent way to improve your written form is to make a list of the errors you have made and refer to that list when you proof new documents. Similarly, you can use lists of commonly misused (Appendix 4–C) and misspelled words (Appendix 4–D) and textbooks and online sources for common grammatical errors to help refine your writing skills over time.

One area that requires additional attention is electronic forms of written communication, including e-mails and social networking tools, such as Facebook, Twitter, and so on. As Chapter 3 discussed, all professional communication about the clients you serve is to be held in complete confidence. ASHA's position on confidentiality is contained in Appendix 3–D in Chapter 3. It is critical that you only communicate electronically to or about a client as specifically instructed by your supervisor. Many settings have specific rules and regulations about what type of written information can be sent electronically and how this information is to be transmitted. You should not use personal e-mail accounts for this purpose, nor should you ever post anything about your clients on social networking sites. Remember, too, social networking tools, such as Facebook and Twitter, often serve as a source of information about you to those you interact with professionally, including your clients and their families, your coworkers, and current and prospective employers. Box 4–1 contains helpful tips regarding social media etiquette.

Disability-Sensitive Communication

Last, communication in all forms, whether verbal or written, must be sensitive to the needs and rights of people with disabilities. You should use *person-first language* when communicating with or referring to individuals with disabilities (Centers for Disease Control and Prevention, n.d.). This means referring to the person first and their disability second, such as the "person with aphasia" or "individuals with seizure disorders," not "the aphasic person" or "the epileptic." Similarly, you should not indicate that the person with a disability has suffered or is a victim in some way from their disability (Centers for Disease Control and Prevention, n.d.). This means not using phrases such as "the client suffers from a hearing loss," "the patient suffered a stroke," or "the client is afflicted with multiple sclerosis." Instead, you could say, "the client experienced a stroke," or "the patient has a diagnosis of multiple sclerosis." In addition, if you are referring to a person *without* a disability, do not refer to that person(s) as "normal" (Centers for Disease Control and Prevention, n.d.). That implies that the individual with a disability is not normal. Instead,

Box 4–1. Social Media Etiquette

■ *Pick a professional screen name.*
■ *Create a professional profile and maintain a separate personal profile.* Keep your professional contacts separate from your personal contacts, and "do not send winks, pokes, virtual martinis, or invitations for your business contacts" (Ritch & McGary, n.d., para. 3).
■ *Be careful with what you post online in any form.* Only post information that will portray you in a positive light to all who view, including your supervisor(s), employers, and your clients and their families. Be sure to use privacy settings to limit who can view your personal information, but remember this is not an absolute fail-safe for keeping unflattering information private. The best course of action is to use restraint in posting anything online.
■ *Be respectful in all online communication.* In other words, "acknowledge people when they ask a question, apologize if you offend someone, and never ever spam, flame, or trash someone else online" (Ritch & McGary, n.d., para. 3).

state that the individual(s) is without a specific disability, such as "individuals without aphasia," "individuals without visual impairments," and so on.

Using the correct terminology to refer to a disability is also important. According to the World Health Organization (WHO, 2012), *disability* "is an umbrella term, covering impairments, activity limitations, and participation restrictions" (para. 2). Impairment is a problem in body function or structure, whereas an activity limitation is the difficulty an individual encounters in executing a task or action because of a specific impairment(s). Participation restriction refers to a problem experienced in life situations due to an impairment and activity limitation. Using these classifications, the WHO accounts for the role that personal and environmental factors (not just a person's impairment) play

in participation restriction. Importantly, the WHO emphasizes that disability is a universal human experience, in that all human beings can experience a decrement in health and thereby some degree of disability.

In addition, as an SLPA, you will need to be able to effectively communicate with individuals with a variety of disabilities. In doing so, it is critical that you view all individuals as unique in their needs, desires, and preferred methods of communication. Box 4–2 describes core principles in communicating with individuals with disabilities that can be used as a starting point for developing your skills in this area (North Dakota Center for Persons With Disabilities, n.d., p. 7). Remember that each time you meet someone with a disability, as with any person you meet, view it as an opportunity to

Box 4–2. Communicating With Individuals With Disabilities

I. *Speak directly to the person, rather than through a companion or sign language interpreter who may be present.*

II. *Offer to shake hands when introduced.* People with limited hand use or an artificial limb can usually shake hands, and offering the left hand is an acceptable greeting.

III. *Always identify yourself, and others who may be with you, when meeting someone with a visual disability.* When conversing in a group, remember to identify the person to whom you are speaking. When dining with a friend who has a visual disability, ask if you can describe what is on his or her plate.

IV. *If you offer assistance, wait until the offer is accepted.* Then listen or ask for instructions.

V. *Treat adults as adults.* Address people with disabilities by their first names only when extending that same familiarity to all others. Never patronize people in wheelchairs by patting them on the head or shoulder.

VI. *Do not lean against or hang on someone's wheelchair or pet a service animal.* Bear in mind that people with disabilities treat their chairs as extensions of their bodies. And so do people with guide dogs and help dogs. Never distract a service animal from its job without the owner's permission.

VII. *Listen attentively when talking with people who have difficulty speaking and wait for them to finish.* If necessary, ask short questions that require short answers, or a nod of the head. Never pretend to understand; instead, repeat what you have understood and allow the person to respond.

VIII. *Place yourself at eye level when speaking with someone in a wheelchair or on crutches.*

IX. *Tap a person who has a hearing disability on the shoulder or wave your hand to get his or her attention.* Look directly at the person and speak clearly, slowly, and expressively to establish if the person can read your lips. If so, try to face the light source and keep hands, drinks, and food away from your mouth when speaking. If a person is wearing a hearing aid, don't assume that they have the ability to discriminate your speaking voice. Never shout at a person. Just speak in a normal tone of voice.

X. *Relax.* Don't be embarrassed if you happen to use common expressions, such as "See you later" or "Did you hear about this?" that seem to relate to a person's disability.

Source: North Dakota Center for Persons With Disabilities (n.d.). *Communicating effectively with people who have a disability.* Retrieved from http://www.labor.state.ny.us/workforcenypartners/forms/communication.pdf. Used with permission from the North Dakota Center for Persons With Disabilities, a university-affiliated program at Minot State University, Minot, North Dakota.

get to know that person and to find out firsthand his or her preferred methods of communication.

SELF–ASSESSMENT AND SELF–IMPROVEMENT

Self-assessment, or self-evaluation as it is sometimes called, is the process of evaluating your own skills and abilities and then, importantly, seeking avenues for improvement (Moon-Meyer, 2004). This is critical to becoming a highly skilled SLPA and is also part of professional conduct. SLPAs who seek self-improvement, through self-assessment, act in the best interest of the clients they serve by ensuring the highest quality of care. As discussed in Chapter 3, this is the cornerstone of ASHA's Ethical Principle 1 (Responsibility to Clients Served and Research Participants). SLPAs who engage in self-assessment and self-improvement will continue to grow in their skills over time and thereby reach high levels of proficiency. The evaluations of others, especially your supervisor, will be important in shaping this proficiency, but SLPAs who rely solely on others in their environment to improve their performance will ultimately be limited in their professional growth. Self-assessment and self-improvement can include *any* aspect of your performance as an SLPA, including your clinical skills and those skills outside the clinical realm, such as your interpersonal, written and verbal communication, conflict resolution skills, and so on.

The first step in self-improvement is self-assessment. This requires that you carefully observe and reflect on *your* behaviors. If you are open to the fact that no one is perfect, observation and reflection about your own behaviors will usually reveal potential areas of improvement. Using audio or video recordings can be helpful in evaluating your own behaviors during clinical sessions (Moon-Meyer, 2004). Reflection and taking notes on a task immediately after completion can also be used. Remember, though, that if you are writing notes about what you do as an SLPA, as discussed in Chapter 3, you must do so in a way that protects the confidentiality of your clients. This generally means not recording any identifying information about clients in these written notes and using pseudonyms if you directly reference a client in your written notes. Largely, your notes in the area of self-assessment should be about you, but in some cases, a confidential reference to a clinical interaction may be used to set the context for your narrative. Similarly, if you are recording a clinical session (audio or video), be sure to follow the policies in your setting for doing so, requesting permission, using required formats and protecting these recordings as confidential information.

Individuals new to the process of self-assessment often struggle with what exactly to observe about their own performance or where to begin in the self-assessment process. ASHA forms are available that can be used as a starting point in the self-evaluation of intervention sessions (see Appendix 4–E and 4–F). Remember, though, that self-assessment can be in any area of performance, not just service delivery.

In addition to rating yourself using pre-determined categories and self-rating scales, another good way to further focus your self-assessment is to observe and write down an aspect of a task you performed that was: (a) successful and (b) not successful (Crago, 1987). Once you do this, the next step is to identify what about your own behaviors and actions may have contributed to an area of success and/or an area of difficulty. This is particularly applicable to clinical sessions but can be applied to any aspect of your professional duties as an SLPA. The topics discussed in Chapter 10 are an excellent starting point for areas to assess in the clinical realm.

A reflection journal can be used to record information about your performance in the areas of successful and unsuccessful performance, as well as your own contributions to these outcomes. It can then also be extended to reflecting on how to improve or change your own behaviors for a more successful outcome, as well as a place to record goals and progress in accomplishing self-improvement. Box 4–3 contains an example of an entry in a reflection journal. The CD of this text contains a blank version.

In many ways, an entry in a reflection journal is similar to a note an SLPA may write about a client's performance as they both describe subjective and objective details about a given task or interaction, but an important distinction is that reflection journals focus on your own performance. There is often crossover, however, between discussion of the client's performance and discussion of our own performance. For example, the notes that SLPAs write about a client often include a section devoted to future plans from the SLPA's perspective. As such, observing and recording your own behaviors may help you generate ideas of things to modify in future sessions with a client. This concept is discussed in greater detail in Chapter 9.

Once you have reflected on areas to improve, do not stop there. Set a goal for improvement and continue to monitor your performance in this area, making adjustments until you achieve the desired outcome. Dating your reflection journal entries will allow you to track overall patterns and change over time. You might also consider developing your own "data collection" methods for tracking specific behaviors over time. Chapter 9 discusses data collection methods for tracking client behaviors. Employing similar methods on your own performance is an excellent way to document progress and to improve over time. In addition, if there are more overarching goals that emerge from your self-reflection, such as additional education and/or training in a specific area, write down these goals and work with your supervising speech-language pathologist (SLP) and/or your mentor in developing a plan for improvement in these areas. Last, some additional ideas in the areas of self-assessment and self-improvement include the following:

- Review setting specific methods used to evaluate you (Dowling, 2001). Generally, there will be a set of standards by which you are evaluated for employment purposes, including in many cases a list of clinically related skills you are expected to perform. Chapter 1 contains several examples of SLPA performance measures (Chapter 1, Appendices 1–H to 1–L). Look to these evaluation tools for ideas of specific areas to target in self-assessment/self-improvement.
- Observe experienced clinicians (Dowling, 2001). For SLPAs, this usually means your supervising SLP. It may also mean observing other professionals, such as teachers, occupational therapists,

Box 4–3. Sample Reflection Journal Entry

Date: *2/14/2013*
Task(s): *10:00 a.m. Small Group Session (JL, AS, TM)*

Successes:
JL and AS participated fully and had high levels of accuracy for target sounds. The session ended on time. The students appeared to enjoy the session and were eager to begin. I felt relaxed and was able to stay focused on each student's targets during the session.

Difficulties:
TM was distracted during the session. He left the table several times to look out the window. I wasn't sure how to shape this behavior, other than reminding him that he needed to participate. I had difficulty keeping track of errors and the number and type of cues I gave for sound production. When I listened to the audio recording of the session, I provided many more models than I had noted on my data sheet. I also said "okay" twice when JL's target sound was not correct. The time spent explaining the session's activities took too long (10 minutes). The students argued about which activity to do first and who would start in each activity.

Areas (Ways) to Improve:
1. *Increase structure of the session at the onset. Make sure to briefly instruct the students in the rules of the activity. Don't allow them to choose the order of the activities. Rotate who goes first per session or have them draw from a deck of cards and whoever gets the highest card goes first.*
2. *Improve data collection methods. Get additional examples of data collection sheets used for group sessions. Check with supervisor about her methods for effectively and quickly noting both errors and cues in group settings. Possibly, rearrange the data collection sheet in advance with a column to place an X under each type of cue. Place a sticky note reminder on my data collection sheet for next time reminding me not to say "okay." Listen to the audio recording from next week's session to record the number of "okays."*
3. *Close the blinds in the room or move the table so the students aren't distracted by the things happening outside the window.*

and psychologists, who engage in activities with clients in your setting that are applicable to what you do. It could also mean observing more experienced SLPAs. This can be done once you have identified an area to improve, as a source of additional techniques in this area, or as a source of ideas for areas of self-assessment.

- ■ Immerse yourself in the professional community of SLPs and related professionals. This means attending regional or national conferences and workshops in your clinical service area and participating in applicable training and workshops offered in your setting. This will provide you with state-of-the art information applicable to the field of speech-language pathology and related topics that may stimulate ideas for self-assessment or serve as a resource for self-improvement. In fact, as discussed in Chapter 1, one of ASHA's expectations is that SLPAs will "actively pursue continuing education and professional development activities" (ASHA, 2013, Expectations of an SLPA, para. 1). Some state regulating bodies may also require formal or informal documentation regarding continuing education (CE) to maintain certification, licensure, or credentials as an SLPA.

As with any long-term goal, it is best to start small with a few attainable goals and work up from there. Similarly, do not attempt to reflect on every task you perform as an SLPA all at once. Start with tasks that are more structured or more in need of improvement and work up from there. Do not expect to achieve perfection overnight, if ever. The entire point of this process is to view self-improvement as a career-long goal, no matter your proficiency.

CONFLICT RESOLUTION

As an SLPA, no matter the setting, you will be required to work collaboratively with a variety of individuals, including your supervising SLP, as well as other SLPAs and SLPs in your specific setting. You will also collaborate with individuals from other disciplines. Table 4–1 contains a listing of some types of professions that SLPAs may work with across a variety of settings (Cascella, Purdy, & Dempsey, 2007).

Conflict occurs when individuals or groups disagree. Conflict is inevitable in any workplace setting (Victors, 2009). How conflicts are addressed will have a dramatic impact on their outcome (Culbertson, 2008). There are four possible outcomes to conflict, as listed in Figure 4–1. The most desirable outcome, when possible, is a win/win outcome for all involved. The best way to accomplish this outcome is to first set aside personal feelings and view the conflict objectively from the perspective of everyone involved.

Good interpersonal skills are also at the heart of positive conflict resolution (Gerrard, Boniface, & Love, 1980). Interpersonal skills are "those skills that promote good relationships between individuals" (p. 2). Several guiding principles to resolving conflict effectively include the following:

1. *Employ active listening and good communication skills.* Communicate openly, clearly, and directly about the conflict, expressing your feelings, but do so in a way that respects the feelings of others. Using the communication tips discussed previously will help as well in situations of conflict.
2. *Seek resolutions to conflict, when possible, that result in a positive outcome*

Table 4–1. Professional Colleagues Across Settings

	Birth to 3 Years Settings	Educational Settings	Medical Settings
Audiologist	X	X	X
Chaplain			X
Childcare worker	X		
Dietician			X
Neuropsychologist			X
Nurse	X	X	X
Nurse's aide			X
Occupational therapist	X	X	X
Pediatric development specialist	X	X	
Physical therapist	X	X	X
Physician	X	X	X
Recreational therapist			X
Rehabilitation therapist			X
School counselor		X	
Social worker	X	X	X
Special education teacher	X	X	
Teacher (general education)	X	X	X

Source: Cascella, Purdy, & Dempsey, 2007, p. 263.

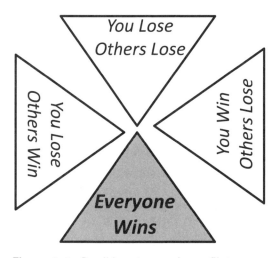

Figure 4–1. Possible outcomes in conflict.

for all involved. Let go of the need to be right or an attachment to a specific outcome (McCready, 2007). Place the conflict in perspective. Do not trivialize or avoid conflict, but also do not make conflict out of trivial matters (Culbertson, 2008).

3. *Be sensitive to the feelings of others and be ready to move on and work collaboratively once a conflict has been resolved.* Do not make the conflict personal. From the outset, separate facts from feelings and opinions (McCready, 2007). Avoid placing blame for conflict (McCready, 2007). At all stages,

consider the feelings of everyone involved and do not hold a grudge (Hull, 2003). This means being willing to admit if you are wrong and apologizing and forgiving others who err or have done something wrong.

In addition, Chapter 3 addresses ethical dilemmas and offers suggestions for addressing ethical conflict. These strategies are helpful in problem solving and helping to make decisions during any conflict, not just those that pose an ethical dilemma.

REFERENCES

American Speech-Language-Hearing Association (ASHA). (n.d.). *Five tips to become a more credible assistant*. Retrieved from http://www.asha.org/associates/Five-Tips-to-Become-a-More-Credible-Assistant/

American Speech-Language-Hearing Association (ASHA). (1998). *Students and professionals who speak English with accents and nonstandard dialects: Issues and recommendations* [Technical report]. Retrieved from http://www.asha.org/policy

American Speech-Language-Hearing Association (ASHA). (2013). *Speech-language pathology assistant scope of practice*. Retrieved from http://www.asha.org/policy

Cascella, R., Purdy, M. H., & Dempsey, J. J. (2007). Clinical service delivery and work settings. In R. Paul & P. Cascella (Eds.), *Introduction to clinical methods in communication disorders* (pp. 259–302). Baltimore, MD: Paul H. Brookes.

Centers for Disease Control and Prevention. (n.d.). *Communicating with and about people with disabilities*. Retrieved from http://www.cdc.gov/ncbddd/disabilityandhealth/pdf/DisabilityPoster_Photos.pdf

Crago, M. (1987). Supervision and self-exploration. In M. Crago & M. Pickering (Eds.), *Supervision in human communication disorders: Perspective on a process* (pp. 137–167). San Diego, CA: Singular.

Culbertson, R. (2008). Conflict: Your role in how it ends. *Perspectives on Administration and Supervision, 18*(3), 99–104.

Dowling, S. (2001). *Supervision: Strategies for successful outcomes and productivity*. Needham Heights, MA: Allyn & Bacon.

Gerrard, B. A., Boniface, W. J., & Love, B. H. (1980). *Interpersonal skills for health professionals*. Reston, VA: Reston Publishing.

Goldfarb, R., & Serpanos, Y. C. (2009). *Professional writing in speech-language pathology and audiology*. San Diego, CA: Plural.

Hegde, M. N. (1998). *A coursebook on scientific and professional writing for speech-language pathologists*. San Diego, CA: Singular.

Hull, R. H. (2003). The art of interpersonal persuasion. *ASHA Leader*. Retrieved from http://www.asha.org/Publications/leader/2003/031007/031007f.htm

McCready, V. (2007). Supervision of speech-language pathology assistants: A reciprocal relationship. *ASHA Leader*. Retrieved from http://www.asha.org/Publications/leader/2007/070508/f070508b/

McNamara, K. (2007). Interviewing, counseling, and clinical communication. In R. Paul & P. Cascella (Eds.), *Introduction to clinical methods in communication disorders* (203–236). Baltimore, MD: Paul H. Brookes.

Moon-Meyer, S. (2004). *Survival guide for the beginning speech-language clinician*. Austin, TX: Pro-Ed.

North Dakota Center for Persons With Disabilities. (n.d.). *Communicating effectively with people who have a disability*. Retrieved from http://www.labor.state.ny.us/workforceny partners/forms/communication.pdf

Piasecki, M. (20 03). *Clinical communication handbook*. Malden, MA: Blackwell.

Ritch, S., & McGary, M. (n.d.). *Social media etiquette for professionals*. Retrieved from http://www.asha.org/associates/Social-Media-Etiquette-for-Professionals/

van Servellen, G. (1997). *Communication skills for health care professionals*. Gaithersburg, MD: Aspen.

Victor, S. (2009, November). *Supervision and conflict resolution*. Paper presented at ASHA 2009 Annual Convention, New Orleans, LA.

World Health Organization. (2012, November). *Disability and health: Fact sheet N°352*. Retrieved from http://www.who.int/mediacentre/factsheets/fs352/en/

APPENDIX 4–A

Common Medical Abbreviations (ASHA, n.d.)

Aa
ADL activities of daily living
A&O alert and oriented
A/P anterior-posterior
AROM active range of motion
ASAP as soon as possible

Bb
b.i.d. twice a day
BP blood pressure
BR bed rest
BS breath sounds
B/S bedside
bx biopsy

Cc
with (c with bar above it)
CA cardiac arrest
CA, ca carcinoma
CAD coronary artery disease
CBC complete blood count
CC chief complaint
CHI closed head injury
c/o complains of
CPR cardiopulmonary resuscitation
CT computerized tomography
CV cardiovascular
CVA cerebral vascular accident
CXR chest x-ray

Dd
d/c discontinue

DC discharge
DNK do not know
DNT did not test
DOB date of birth
d/t due to
Dx diagnosis

Ee
EENT eye, ear, nose, throat
ENT ear, nose, throat
ETOH ethanol (alcohol)
exam examination

Ff
FH family history
f/u follow-up

Gg
GCS Glasgow Coma Scale
GERD gastroesophageal reflux disease
GSW gunshot wound

Hh
H/A headache
HBP high blood pressure
HEENT head, eyes, ear, nose, throat
H_2O water
h/o history of
H&P history and physical
HR heart rate
HTN hypertension
Hx history

Ii

ICCU intensive coronary care unit

ICU intensive care unit

imp. impression

Ll

LBW low birth rate

LE lower extremities

LOC loss of consciousness, level of consciousness

LOS length of stay

LUE left upper extremity

Mm

MBSS modified barium swallow study

MCA middle cerebral artery

MRI magnetic resonance imaging

MVA motor vehicle accident

Nn

NG nasogastric

NICU neonatal intensive care unit

NKA no known allergies

NPO nothing by mouth

Oo

O_2 oxygen

OM otitis media

OME otitis media with effusion

ot. ear

Pp

PE physical examination

Ped. Pediatrics

PEG percutaneous endoscopic gastrostomy

PET positron emission tomography

PH past history

PMH past medical history

p.o. by mouth

PRN as often as necessary, as needed

Qq

Q every

q.h. every hour

q.i.d. four times a day

Rr

rehab. rehabilitation

RLA Rancho Los Amigo Scale

R/O rule out

ROM range of motion

RUE right upper extremity

Ss

SCI spinal cord injury

SH social history

SOAP subjective, objective, assessment, and plan

SOB shortness of breath

s/s signs and symptoms

Tt

TB tuberculosis

TBI traumatic brain injury

TIA transient ischemic attack

TKR total knee replacement

Tx treatment, traction

Uu

UCD usual childhood diseases

UCHD usual childhood diseases

Source: American Speech-Language-Hearing Association (ASHA). (n.d.). *Common medical abbreviations.* Retrieved from http://www.asha.org/uploadedFiles/slp/healthcare/Medicalabbreviations .pdf#search=%22common%22

APPENDIX 4–B

Common International Phonetic Alphabet (IPA) Symbols

CONSONANTS:

IPA SYMBOL	EXAMPLE
/p/	Happy
/m/	Mother
/h/	Hello
/n/	Never
/w/	Wednesday
/b/	Baseball
/k/	Kite
/g/	Golf
/d/	Deliver
/t/	Tuesday
/ŋ/	Pink
/f/	Fall
/j/	Yellow
/r/	Carrot
/l/	Balloon
/s/	Saturday
/tʃ/	Church
/ʃ/	Shoe
/z/	Zoo
/dʒ/	Jewel
/v/	Volcano
/θ/	Thumb
/ð/	That
/ʒ/	Vision

VOWELS:

IPA SYMBOL	EXAMPLE
/i/	See
/ɪ/	Insect
/ʊ/	Foot
/u/	Boot
/e/	Bed
/ə/ Unstressed	Around
/ɜ/	Turn
/ɔ/	Lawn
/æ/	Apple
/ʌ/ Stressed	hut
/ɑ/	Father

R-COLORED VOWELS:

IPA SYMBOL	EXAMPLE
/ɝ/ Stressed	Her
/ɚ/ Unstressed	Color

DIPHTHONGS:

IPA SYMBOL	EXAMPLE
/eɪ/	Play
/eə/	Their
/əʊ/	Boat
/ɪə/	Here
/ɔɪ/	Coin
/ʊə/	Tour
/aɪ/	Sky
/aʊ/	House

APPENDIX 4–C

Commonly Misused Words and Phrases

Effect	Alternate	Incidence
■ *a distinctive impression <the color gives the* effect *of being warm>* ■ *the creation of a desired impression <her tears were purely for* effect> ■ *the conscious subjective aspect of an emotion considered apart from bodily change* Affect ■ *something that inevitably follows an antecedent (as a cause or agent)* ■ *an outward sign* ■ *a set of observable manifestations of a subjectively experienced emotion <patients . . . showed perfectly normal reactions and* affects>	■ *occurring or succeeding by turns <a day of* alternate *sunshine and rain>* ■ *arranged one above or alongside the other* ■ *every other : every second <he works on* alternate *days>* Alternative ■ *offering or expressing a choice <several* alternative *plans>* ■ *different from the usual or conventional <*alternative *lifestyle>*	■ *rate of occurrence or influence <a high* incidence *of crime>* Prevalence ■ *the degree to which something is prevalent; especially: the percentage of a population that is affected with a particular disease at a given time*
Were ■ *past 2d singular, past plural, or past subjunctive of* BE We're ■ *we are* Where ■ *at, in, or to what place <*where *is the house> <*where *are we going>*	Farther ■ *at or to a greater distance or more advanced point <got no* farther *than the first page> <nothing could be* farther *from the truth>* ■ *to a greater degree or extent <see to it that I do not have to act any* farther *in the matter>* Further ■ *in addition :* MOREOVER ■ *to a greater degree or extent <*further *annoyed by a second intrusion> <my ponies are tired, and I have* further *to go>*	Their ■ *of or relating to them or themselves especially as possessors, agents, or objects of an action <*their *furniture> <*their *verses> <*their *being seen>* They're ■ *they are* There ■ *in or at that place <stand over* there> ■ *to or into that place <went* there *after church>* ■ *at that point or stage <stop right* there *before you say something you'll regret>*

145

Abduct	Elicit	Its
■ *to draw or spread away (as a limb or the fingers) from a position near or parallel to the median axis of the body or from the axis of a limb*	■ *to draw forth or bring out <hypnotism elicited his hidden fears>*	■ *of or relating to it or itself especially as possessor, agent, or object of an action <going to its kennel> <a child proud of its first drawings> <its final enactment into law>*
Adduct	■ *to call forth or draw out (as information or a response) <her remarks elicited cheers>*	**It's**
■ *to draw (as a limb) toward or past the median axis of the body*	**Evoke**	■ *it is*
■ *to bring together (similar parts) <adduct the fingers>*	■ *to call forth or up: <evoke evil spirits>*	
	■ *to bring to mind or recollection <this place evokes memories>*	
	■ *to re-create imaginatively*	

Except	You're	Principal
■ *with the exclusion or exception of <daily except Sundays>*	■ *you are*	■ *most important, consequential, or influential:* CHIEF *<the principal ingredient> <the region's principal city>*
Accept	**Your**	NOTE: This can also be a title, such as *<Mr. Thomas is* Principal *of Thomas Jefferson Elementary School.>*
■ *to receive willingly <accept a gift>*	■ *of or relating to you or yourself or yourselves especially as possessor or possessors <your bodies>, agent or agents <your contributions>, or object or objects of an action <your discharge>*	**Principle**
■ *to be able or designed to take or hold (something applied or added) <a surface that will not accept ink>*	■ *of or relating to one or oneself <when you face the north, east is at your right>*	■ *a comprehensive and fundamental law, doctrine, or assumption*
■ *to give admittance or approval to <accept her as one of the group>*		■ *a rule or code of conduct*
■ *to endure without protest or reaction <accept poor living conditions>*		■ *habitual devotion to right principles <a man of principle>*
■ *to recognize as true :* BELIEVE *<refused to accept the explanation>*		
■ *to make a favorable response to <accept an offer>*		
■ *to agree to undertake (a responsibility) <accept a job>*		
■ *to assume an obligation to pay; also : to take in payment <we don't accept personal checks>*		

Personnel

- a body of persons usually employed (as in a factory or organization)
- a division of an organization concerned with personnel

Personal

- of, relating to, or affecting a particular person : PRIVATE, INDIVIDUAL <personal ambition> <personal financial gain>
- done in person without the intervention of another; also : proceeding from a single person
- carried on between individuals directly <a personal interview>
- relating to the person or body
- relating to an individual or an individual's character, conduct, motives, or private affairs often in an offensive manner <a personal insult>
- intended for private use or use by one person <a personal stereo>

Then

- at that time
- soon after that : next in order of time <walked to the door, then turned>
- following next after in order of position, narration, or enumeration
- being next in a series <first came the clowns, and then came the elephants>
- in addition : BESIDES <then there is the interest to be paid>

Than

- used as a function word to indicate the second member or the member taken as the point of departure in a comparison expressive of inequality; used with comparative adjectives and comparative adverbs <older than I am> <easier said than done>
- used as a function word to indicate difference of kind, manner, or identity ; used especially with some adjectives and adverbs that express diversity <anywhere else than at home>
- rather than —usually used only after prefer, preferable, and preferably
- other than

Too

- BESIDES, ALSO <sell the house and furniture too>
- to an excessive degree : EXCESSIVELY <too large a house for us>
- to such a degree as to be regrettable <this time he has gone too far> : VERY <didn't seem too interested>

Two

- being one more than one in number
- being the second —used postpositively <section two of the instructions>

To

- used as a function word to indicate movement or an action or condition suggestive of movement toward a place, person, or thing reached <drove to the city> <went to lunch>
- used as a function word to indicate direction <a mile to the south>
- used as a function word to indicate contact or proximity <applied polish to the table> <put her hand to her heart>
- used as a function word to indicate the place or point that is the far limit <100 miles to the nearest town>
- used as a function word to indicate relative position <perpendicular to the floor>
- used as a function word to indicate purpose, intention, tendency, result, or end <came to our aid> <drink to his health>

To (*continued*)

- *used as a function word to indicate the result of an action or a process <broken all to pieces> <go to seed> <to their surprise, the train left on time>*
- *used as a function word to indicate position or relation in time: as*
- *a : BEFORE <five minutes to five>: TILL <from eight to five>*
- *used as a function word: (1) to indicate a relation to one that serves as a standard <inferior to her earlier works> (2) to indicate similarity, correspondence, dissimilarity, or proportion <compared him to a god>*
- *used as a function word to indicate agreement or conformity <add salt to taste> <to my knowledge>*
- *used as a function word to indicate a proportion in terms of numbers or quantities <400 to the box> <odds of ten to one>*
- *used as a function word to indicate that the following verb is an infinitive <wants to go> and often used by itself at the end of a clause in place of an infinitive suggested by the preceding context <knows more than she seems to>*

Medical Prefix	**Medical Prefix**	**Medical Prefix**
Inter-	A-/An-	Hypo-
■ *Among* <inter*dental*>	■ *Not, without, or less* <*alexia*> <*aphonia*> <an*emia*> <an*oxia*>	■ *under*
■ *In the midst of; within* <inter*oceptor*>		■ *beneath*
		■ *down* <hypo*blast*> <hypo*dermic*>
Intra-	Dys-	■ *less than normal or normally* <hyp*esthesia*> <hypo*tension*>
■ *within* <intra*galactic*>	■ *abnormal, difficult, or impaired* <dys*chromia*> <dys*pnea*><dys*function*>	
■ *during* <intra*day*>		Hyper-
■ *between layers of* <intra*dermal*>		■ excessively <hyper*sensitive*>
		■ excessive <hyper*emia*> <hyper*tension*>

Definitions provided from Merriam-Webster. (2003). *Merriam-Webster's collegiate dictionary* (11th ed.). Springfield, MA: Author.

APPENDIX 4–D

Commonly Misspelled Words in English

A
acceptable
accidentally
accommodate
acquire
acquit
amateur
apparent
argument

B
believe

C
calendar
category
changeable
column
committed
conscience
conscientious
conscious
consensus

D
definite (ly)
discipline

E
embarrass (ment)
equipment
exceed

existence
experience

F
foreign

G
gauge
guarantee

H
harass
height
hierarchy
humorous

I
ignorance
immediate
independent
indispensable
inoculate
intelligence

J
judgment

L
leisure
liaison
library
license

M
maintenance
maneuver
millennium
minuscule
mischievous
misspell

N
neighbor
noticeable

O
occasionally
occurrence

P
pastime
perseverance
personnel
possession
precede
privilege
pronunciation
publicly

Q
questionnaire

R
receive/receipt
recommend

referred
reference
relevant
restaurant
rhyme
rhythm

S
schedule
separate
supersede

T
threshold
twelfth

U
until

Excerpts from http://grammar.yourdictionary.com/spelling-and-word-lists/misspelled.html

APPENDIX 4–E

Self-Evaluation of Intervention Sessions—Educational Setting

Note: This form may be used in conjunction with the Direct Observation Skills Brief Checklist.

Date/Time of Session:

_____

Rate the following on a scale of 1 (disagree) to 5 (agree).

1. I maintained an appropriate relationship with the student throughout the session. ○1 ○2 ○3 ○4 ○5

2. I was self-confident in this session. ○1 ○2 ○3 ○4 ○5

3. I considered the student's needs in selecting my materials and interacting with this student. ○1 ○2 ○3 ○4 ○5

4. I considered the student's cultural/linguistic needs in selecting my materials and interacting with this student. ○1 ○2 ○3 ○4 ○5

5. I used language appropriate for the student's age and education. ○1 ○2 ○3 ○4 ○5

6. I was courteous and respectful with this student. ○1 ○2 ○3 ○4 ○5

7. I was punctual for the session. ○1 ○2 ○3 ○4 ○5

8. I was prepared for the session. ○1 ○2 ○3 ○4 ○5

9. I was dressed appropriately for this session. ○1 ○2 ○3 ○4 ○5

10. I used time efficiently during this session. ○1 ○2 ○3 ○4 ○5

11. I completed the assigned tasks during this session. ○1 ○2 ○3 ○4 ○5

12. I accurately determined correct vs. incorrect responses. ○1 ○2 ○3 ○4 ○5

13. I provided appropriate feedback to the student. ○1 ○2 ○3 ○4 ○5

14. The work area was appropriate for this student. ○1 ○2 ○3 ○4 ○5

15. I was aware of my professional boundaries during this session. ○1 ○2 ○3 ○4 ○5

16. I documented the results of the session appropriately. ○1 ○2 ○3 ○4 ○5

17. I shared the results with my supervision. ○1 ○2 ○3 ○4 ○5

Comments:

SLPA Signature: _____

Source: Reprinted with permission from *Practical Tools and Forms for Supervising Speech-Language Pathology Assistants.* © 2013. American Speech-Language-Hearing Association. All rights reserved.

APPENDIX 4–F

Self-Evaluation of Intervention Sessions—Medical Setting

Note: This form may be used in conjunction with the Direct Observation Skills Brief Checklist.

Date/Time of Session:

_____

Rate the following on a scale of 1 (disagree) to 5 (agree).

1. I maintained an appropriate relationship with the patient throughout the session ○ 1 ○ 2 ○ 3 ○ 4 ○ 5

2. I was self-confident in this session. ○ 1 ○ 2 ○ 3 ○ 4 ○ 5

3. I considered the patient's needs in selecting my materials and interacting with this patient. ○ 1 ○ 2 ○ 3 ○ 4 ○ 5

4. I considered the patient's cultural/linguistic needs in selecting my materials and interacting with this patient. ○ 1 ○ 2 ○ 3 ○ 4 ○ 5

5. I used language appropriate for the patient's age and education. ○ 1 ○ 2 ○ 3 ○ 4 ○ 5

6. I was courteous and respectful with this patient. ○ 1 ○ 2 ○ 3 ○ 4 ○ 5

7. I was punctual for the session. ○ 1 ○ 2 ○ 3 ○ 4 ○ 5

8. I was prepared for the session. ○ 1 ○ 2 ○ 3 ○ 4 ○ 5

9. I was dressed appropriately for this session. ○ 1 ○ 2 ○ 3 ○ 4 ○ 5

10. I used time efficiently during this session. ○ 1 ○ 2 ○ 3 ○ 4 ○ 5

11. I completed the assigned tasks during this session. ○ 1 ○ 2 ○ 3 ○ 4 ○ 5

12. I accurately determined correct vs. incorrect responses. ○ 1 ○ 2 ○ 3 ○ 4 ○ 5

13. I provided appropriate feedback to the patient. ○ 1 ○ 2 ○ 3 ○ 4 ○ 5

14. The treatment environment was appropriate for this patient. ○ 1 ○ 2 ○ 3 ○ 4 ○ 5

15. I was aware of my professional boundaries during this session. ○ 1 ○ 2 ○ 3 ○ 4 ○ 5

16. I documented the results of the session appropriately. ○ 1 ○ 2 ○ 3 ○ 4 ○ 5

17. I shared the results with my supervision. ○ 1 ○ 2 ○ 3 ○ 4 ○ 5

Comments:

SLPA Signature: _____

Source: Reprinted with permission from *Practical Tools and Forms for Supervising Speech-Language Pathology Assistants.* © 2013. American Speech-Language-Hearing Association. All rights reserved.

CHAPTER 5

Cultural and Linguistic Diversity

Carolyn Conway Madding

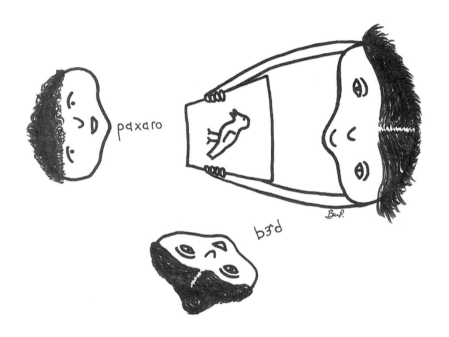

*I know there is strength in the differences between us.
I know there is comfort where we overlap.*

Ani DiFranco (American singer, songwriter, poet, and women's rights advocate)

DIVERSITY OVERVIEW: IMPORTANT STATISTICS

The United States has been a land of immigrants from its inception, resulting in a demographic collage that demonstrates great diversity. In fact, this country is often referred to as the most diverse nation on earth. The U.S. Bureau of the Census (2012) projects that the percentage of racial/ethnic minorities will increase to more than 30% of the population by 2015. With diversity comes the challenge of integrating a multitude of cultures and languages into the fabric of American life.

Perhaps the most formidable task is faced in the field of education, in the effort to provide schooling and special services to children speaking myriad languages and coming from a diversity of cultures.

According to the U.S. Bureau of the Census (2012), more than 57 million persons in the United States older than 5 years speak a language other than English in the home. Seventeen of these home languages encompass 500,000 or more speakers (Table 5–1). The majority representation, however, lies within the Spanish-speaking community, numbering approximately 36 million individuals.

The impact of language variations on municipalities, school districts, hospitals, and other community resources will continue to require adaptation in the foreseeable future. Many cities in the United States, as well as small towns, must accommodate to provide best services. Consider these cities with percentages of the population older than 5 years who speak a language other than English in the home (Box 5–1).

Regardless of the professional service area covered by speech-language pathologists (SLPs) and speech-language pathology assistants (SLPAs), encountering language and cultural diversity will be a certainty. The American Speech-Language-Hearing Association (ASHA) has therefore provided guidelines for assessment, intervention, and family interactions (ASHA, 2004). All speech-language professionals should follow ASHA's mandate for appropriate service provision to linguistically and culturally diverse (CLD) clients and students and avail themselves of continuing education (CEU) opportunities related to CLD populations. The sections of this chapter to follow, as well as the definitions at the end of this chapter, provide an overview of several important terms and concepts needed to

Table 5–1. Speakers of Languages Other Than English in the United States

Ranking	Language
1	Spanish (36 million)
2	Chinese—*all dialects*
3	Tagalog
4	French
5	Vietnamese
6	German
7	Korean
8	Arabic
9	Russian
10	Other Asian languages
11	African languages
12	Italian
13	Portuguese
14	Indic languages
15	French Creole
16	Polish
17	Hindi (560,000)

Source: U.S. Bureau of the Census, 2012.

Box 5–1. Major U.S. Cities and Percentages of Individuals (Older Than 5 Years) Who Speak a Language Other Than English
(U.S. Bureau of the Census, 2012)

El Paso, Texas	73%
Los Angeles, California	61%
San Jose, California	55%
New York, New York	48%
San Francisco, California	45%
Houston, Texas	45%

serve CLD populations. After you finish reading this chapter, test your knowledge of this content with the questions in Appendix 5–A (answers provided).

DEFINITIONS, DISCUSSION, AND THE IMPORTANCE IN SERVICE PROVISION

According to Battle (2002), culture refers to "the behaviors, beliefs, and values of a group of people who are brought together by their commonality" (p. 3). Within the confines of the United States, myriad cultures exist, following their own ways of life. Cultural groups may not only be different from each other in their lifestyles and beliefs but may also speak languages other than English, specific to their groups. Due to the characteristics of life and language, they differ both culturally and linguistically from other groups and from so-called mainstream culture. In contrast, some cultural enclaves may speak English but may maintain a *heritage language* for in-group communication and may live within a blend of cultures, consisting of the mainstream and the specific group from which they arise.

On the contrary, however, are those diverse cultural groups that speak English, or a *dialect* of English, as their native/heritage language but differ only in their cultural attributes from so-called mainstream Euro-Americans. They would be designated as culturally diverse but *not* linguistically diverse.

Dialects

In addition to numerous non-English languages spoken in the United States, dialectal variations of English abound, as well. Dialects are rule-governed variations of a language. They may be spoken by a regional, ethnic, or socioeconomic group. Although dialects of a language are often intelligible to those outside the dialectal group, they may nevertheless vary in form, content, and use. Consider the regional dialects associated with Boston, New Orleans, and New York, as examples. On the other hand, there is Cajun, a dialect of an ethnic, Southern regional group, and African American English, shared by some in widespread African American communities.

Standard American English is the prevalent term for the mainstream dialect of the United States. This is the dialect used in most educational settings and in the media. On the other hand, there are many who speak using a nonmainstream dialect. As dialects are rule governed, just as is Standard American English, they do not represent a language deficit, nor should they be described as inferior or substandard. According to ASHA, all dialects represent a functional and effective tool of expression in English.

It is ASHA's position, therefore, that no dialect of American English should be considered as a speech or language disorder (ASHA, 2003). Speakers of American English dialects do not present with language disorders but rather with language differences/dialectal differences. As such, they are not to be treated by SLPs or SLPAs. If an individual is referred for a screening or assessment and a culturally/linguistically appropriate assessment shows a dialectal difference from Standard American English, no further intervention is warranted.

Similarly, if a referred client/student is *bilingual* or is an English language learner, influences of the individual's non-English language should not be construed as a deficit in English but as a *language difference*. As such, the client/student is not within the scope of treatment for the SLP or the SLPA. If the family or client wishes to produce English that is more consistent with Standard American English, a specialist in accent modification should be privately engaged. English language learners in the schools should be enrolled in special courses to assist them in the development of English but should not be placed on the caseload of the SLP unless they present with a speech or language disorder in their native language, as well as in the emergence of English.

To differentiate between a language difference and a *language disorder*, the SLP must assess the client/student in all languages spoken. A true language disorder will exist across languages as it is a language-learning disability. Box 5–2 contains helpful information for use in addressing speech/language disorders in linguistically and culturally diverse populations. If, however, assessment results show problems in only one language, they are indicative of a language difference, not a language-learning disability.

Cultural Competence/Cultural Literacy

For those professionals who work with students/clients in any setting, a knowledge and understanding of linguistic and cultural diversity is mandatory for successful intervention. As stated by Lipson and Dibble (2005), "Health care profes-

---

Box 5–2. Speech/Language Disorders in Linguistically and Culturally Diverse Populations

- Most children, even those presenting with language disorders, have the capacity and facility to learn more than one language (ASHA, 2012a).
- Learning two languages will not confuse the child, although dual-language development may be prolonged. Learning more than one language does not represent a cognitive overload, so long as both languages are supported (Genesee, 2003).
- Bilingualism represents a positive effect and supports the acquisition of a second language (Uchikoshi & Maniates, 2010).
- Bilingual children with language-learning disorders will experience problems learning and using *both languages* (Roseberry & Connell, 1991). Thus, a bilingual child must be assessed in each of his or her languages to differentiate between a language difference and a language disorder.
- Parents should be encouraged to maintain and model the home language, as this is their best language model (Mumy, 2012).
- Parents should never be told to stop using the home language or to switch to English in the home. This is both culturally and linguistically inappropriate and violates ASHA's mandate (ASHA, 2004).

sionals cannot provide good care without assessing both cultural group patterns and individual variation with a cultural group" (p. xi). This can be accomplished through *ethnographic methods*, adept listening, and careful, considerate interviewing techniques. According to Westby, Burda, and Mehta (2003), speech-language professionals "need to see the world through the eyes of the individuals they serve. Ethnographic interviewing provides a means of asking the right questions in the right ways to accomplish this" (p. 1). Ethnographic interviewing, through the clinician's open-ended questions, allows the client, student, or family to offer glimpses of their life and culture (Westby et al., 2003). To provide effective services to students/clients, professionals must be attuned to all possible aspects of diversity, taking into consideration any issues related to racial/ethnic groups, language, dialect, religion, sexual orientation, age, and country of origin.

Professionals are not required to speak the language of those referred for screening, assessment, or treatment, but understanding the basics of the culture is indeed important, even though the interactions may be through the use of an *interpreter*. The ability to understand and relate effectively with individuals from different cultures and language groups is frequently referred to as *cultural competence* (Hoodin, 2011) or cultural literacy (Haynes, Moran, & Pindzola, 2012).

Cultural competence within a group other than one's own does not ensue spontaneously with the ability to speak, listen/comprehend, and read and write a nonnative language. A person must have experience within the community, often but not necessarily in tandem with language proficiency, to develop cultural competence. According to Westby, professionals do not

have to speak or understand the language of their clients/students but need the ability to empathize with them. Furthermore, she states, "Learning how to 'read' cultures adds to your skill set . . . and also allows you to learn more about yourself" (as cited in Rowden-Racette, 2013, p. 53).

When the SLPA decides to learn a second language, however, to work more empathically and appropriately with individuals over time, certain restrictions apply. One of those is that the nonnative speaker varies from the native/heritage language speaker in that language and culture may be learned linearly, that is, over time. Conversely, the native speaker learns the culture and language cohesively as a developmental process. Thus, she or he is often unaware of the enmeshing of language and culture. The professional who is learning the language and culture of another group must invest time to be both linguistically and culturally competent (Madding, 2002). Cultural and linguistic competence will often be appreciated by individuals and families being served but should not be construed as in-group acceptance.

In summary, language is the principal means through which the socialization process takes place (Madding, 1999). Culture and language are therefore inextricably intertwined during a child's development (Madding, 2000). To become culturally competent as a person outside the group requires time, attention to cues, and an intense interest in the culture and language. SLPAs, as part of the professional team addressing the needs of each client/student, should avail themselves of opportunities to learn as much as possible about the cultural and language background of every client. Awareness is the first principle, followed by interest, investigation, and learning. SLPAs will be pleasantly surprised when clients react favorably to an interest in their culture, as well as when respect is shown for cultural values. Learning the language of the client, or having the ability to greet the client in her or his heritage language, represents a significant step in the continuum of cultural competence acquisition.

To learn more about a culture, we must first recognize the characteristics, values, and beliefs of our own culture. Then we can begin to ascertain the ways in which the behaviors and beliefs of others differ from each other and from the one with which we are most familiar. Appendix 5–B contains cultural consciousness activities to help you explore your own cultural mores or rules. Acknowledging your own culture but respecting what is honored and cherished by others is of utmost importance in the practice of speech-language pathology.

We can learn about other cultures and languages through the Internet, from books and journal articles, and from *cultural informants*. The latter are those from the cultural community who can answer questions and provide information that will help the SLPA to approach and interact with clients, students, and families in a culturally appropriate manner. The cultural informant must be knowledgeable about the specific client's/student's culture and language community (ASHA, 2004).

LANGUAGES OTHER THAN ENGLISH

According to the U.S. Bureau of the Census (2012), there are more than 57,097,847 individuals in the country, age 5 years and older, whose native language is other than English. Due to the free movement of populations within the United States,

professionals in every state may encounter clients/students from any of these languages. It is therefore an educational priority to know which languages are at the top of this list and to become acquainted with their basic characteristics and related cultural distinctions when a student/client is referred to the SLP and the SLPA. See Table 5–1 for languages spoken by the largest number of people in the United States, excluding English (from the largest group, at approximately 36 million, to the last on the list, at 560,000 speakers). Some countries from which these languages derive are also listed in Table 5–2.

Languages and Countries— A Guide for the Professional

SLPs and SLPAs can access phonemic inventories for many different languages and dialects at the following ASHA website: http://www.asha.org/practice/multicultural/Phono. Cultural profiles and resources for service providers for a variety of groups are also included, as well as videos of assessment and treatment of bilingual individuals. Phonemic inventories are available for the following languages listed in Table 5–1: Arabic, Mandarin, Cantonese, Haitian (French) Creole, Hindi, Korean, Russian, Spanish, Tagalog, and Vietnamese. Phonemic information for African American English and dialects of several other languages also reside at this website (ASHA, n.d.-a).

BILINGUAL SLPS AND SLPAS (DEMOGRAPHICS AND STATISTICS)

In a data snapshot of ASHA *bilingual service providers* in the United States, year-end 2011, ASHA (2012b) reported there were

Table 5–2. Languages and Countries of Origin

Language	Countries of Origin
Spanish	Mexico, El Salvador, Nicaragua, Cuba, Puerto Rico (U.S. Commonwealth), Dominican Republic, other countries in Central and South America, and Spain
Chinese (Mandarin, Cantonese, and other dialects)	China, Hong Kong, Taiwan, Singapore, Malaysia, Vietnam, and other Asian countries
Tagalog	Philippines
French (including Patios and Cajun)	Canada, Haiti, France, French Islands in the Pacific and Caribbean, Vietnam, and some African countries
Vietnamese	Vietnam
German	Germany, Austria, and Switzerland
Korean	North and South Korea
Arabic	Egypt, Saudi Arabia, Palestine, Jordan, Kuwait, Lebanon, Libya, Oman, Qatar, Morocco, United Arab Emirates, Yemen, Tunisia, Syria, Djibouti, and others
Russian	Russia, Mongolia, and countries of the Soviet Union
Other Asian Languages:	
Pashtu	Afghanistan
Armenian	Armenia
Bengali	Bangladesh and India
Khmer	Cambodia
Urdu	India and others
Bahasa Indonesia	Indonesia
Farsi	Iran
Japanese	Japan
Burmese	Myanmar (Burma)
Nepali	Nepal
Thai	Thailand
Turkish	Turkey
African languages	Amharic (Ethiopia), Tigrinya (Eritrea), Kiswahili (Kenya, Tanzania), Afrikaans (South Africa), Hausa, Yoruba, and Igbo (Nigeria). The official language in many African countries is English, French, or Portuguese.
Italian	Italy
Portuguese	Portugal, Brazil, Angola, Cape Verde, and others
Indic languages	Bengali, Marathi, Gujarati, Urdu, Pashtu, Nepali, Punjabi, and others
French Creole	Haiti
Polish	Poland
Hindi	India

a total of 6,282 bilingual, ASHA-certified SLPs, of whom 3,790 were Spanish bilingual ASHA-certified SLPs. The largest contingent of bilingual ASHA-certified SLPs who lived in the United States were in Texas (1,077), New York (1,006), California (857), and Florida (608). Of these, the Spanish-language service providers numbered as follows: Texas (946), New York (457), California (488), and Florida (472). Some bilingual clinicians may not be registered with ASHA. Nevertheless, statistics show the overall dearth of bilingual SLPs, with the subsequent conclusion that many bilingual and non-English-speaking clients/students cannot possibly be served directly, without interpretation, in their home or native language.

ASHA reported the primary work settings of bilingual service providers to be almost equally represented by educational and health care settings (ASHA, 2012b). There was no delineation of the non-Spanish-language speakers, nor were data available with regard to bilingual SLPAs.

THE SLPA AS AN INTERPRETER/TRANSLATOR

As a solution to the relatively small corps of bilingual SLPs to serve CLD populations, ASHA (2004) encourages the development of collaborative relationships with *interpreters* and *translators*. A bilingual SLPA may provide a valuable service to her or his supervising SLP and to the clients served, either as a direct service provider under supervision or as an interpreter/translator. See definitions at the end of the chapter for differentiation between an interpreter and translator. In fact, ASHA's 2013 SLPA scope-of-practice document acknowledges this role, stating that provided adequate training, planning, and supervision, SLPAs may perform the following tasks (ASHA, 2013, Service Delivery, para. 1):

1. Assist the SLP with bilingual translation during screening and assessment activities exclusive of interpretation.
2. Serve as interpreter for patients/clients/students and families who do not speak English.
3. Provide services under SLP supervision in another language for individuals who do not speak English and English-language learners.

Your Role as an Interpreter/Translator

To serve as a qualified interpreter or translator, as an SLPA, you must carefully follow guidelines provided by ASHA (2004) and others who have written extensively in this area. Box 5–3 provides an overview of these requirements. Subsequent to gaining thorough background knowledge of your role as interpreter/translator, you may begin to work in this capacity, under the guidance of your supervising SLP.

How to Prepare for Your Role as an Interpreter/Translator

Box 5–4 outlines helpful tips in preparing to work as an interpreter/translator.

WORKING WITH AN INTERPRETER/TRANSLATOR

When you are assigned to work with a client/student who is bilingual or whose

Cultural and Linguistic Diversity **163**

Box 5–3. Basic Requirements to Serve as Interpreter/Translator (ASHA, 2004; Langdon, 2002)

1. Native or near-native proficiency in the student's or client's native language or dialect
2. Ability to provide accurate and complete oral interpretation or written translation
3. Familiarity with and respect for the student's/client's culture and language community
4. Knowledge of professional terminology
5. Maintenance of client/student/family confidentiality of information
6. High-level oral and written proficiency both in English and the non-English language
7. Maintenance of neutrality between yourself and the client/student/family
8. Ability to provide interpretation without addition, subtraction, or commentary
9. Knowledge of assessment and therapeutic techniques, with special emphasis on those to be used with bilingual or non-English-speaking clients/students

---

Box 5–4. Helpful Tips in Preparing to Work as an Interpreter/Translator

1. Although you may be bilingual, do not volunteer or allow yourself to be solicited as an interpreter or translator unless you meet all the minimum requirements listed in Box 5–3. SLPs and other team members may urge you to take on the role when they learn of your bilingual skills. Be honest about your abilities and maintain adherence to basic requirements, as listed in Box 5–3.
2. Do not serve as an interpreter/translator if you are not from the same language community or cultural background as the client/student. Examples of mismatches: You are Mexican American and the client is from Spain or Argentina; you are Egyptian American and your client is from Yemen; you are Mexican American and your client is from a rural, indigenous community in Guatemala. Mismatches such as these may result in inaccurate interpretations, translations, and/or cultural misunderstandings.

language is not one you speak, your first step is to consult with your supervising SLP. As your supervisor, the SLP is legally and ethically responsible for all clients/students on the caseload and delegates tasks to you, as the SLPA (ASHA, 2013). You must have the compliance and permission of the SLP before you can seek the interpreter/translator you need for appropriate intervention (ASHA, 2013). ASHA mandates for service provision express the importance of contacting a qualified interpreter/translator to assist in your interactions with the client/student.

Choosing an Interpreter/Translator

Many school districts, hospitals, and other service sites maintain a bank of interpreters and translators. Inquire if such a list exists and whether the interpreters/translators meet the basic requirements listed in Box 5–4. In cases where no resources are available, it is incumbent upon the supervising SLP to locate and train an interpreter. A cultural informant may assist in locating an appropriate interpreter/translator or one who is willing to be trained. Employment facilities may provide stipends for interpreters and translators. If no remuneration is available, however, you may need to locate someone who is willing to volunteer his or her services. Family members, and most especially children, should not be solicited for this task, for many reasons. Among those may be a vested interest in the case of the client, difficulty in being impartial, and the tendency to cue the client. Children may be embarrassed, cannot be counted on to maintain confidentiality, and do not possess the maturity to follow the basic requirements to be an interpreter/transla-

tor. Whenever possible, choose a trained professional.

Using an Interpreter/Translator

Box 5–5 provides helpful tips when working with an interpreter/translator, including guidelines for before, during, and after treatment sessions.

CHAPTER DEFINITIONS AND OTHER RELEVANT DEFINITIONS

Bilingual: A bilingual individual is one who possesses the ability to use more than one language effectively (Bhatia & Ritchie, 2006). A bilingual person may be fully competent in oral language without the ability to, read, or write in more than one language. Furthermore, a person who comprehends and follows-through with instructions in a language other than her or his native language, even though she or he does not speak in the second language, is at least marginally bilingual.

Bilingual Service Provider: The American Speech-Language-Hearing Association, Office of Multicultural Affairs, provides the following definition:

> Speech-language pathologists and audiologists who present themselves as bilingual for the purposes of providing clinical services must be able to speak their primary language and to speak (or sign) at least one other language with native or near-native proficiency in lexicon (vocabulary), semantics (meaning), phonology (pronunciation), morphology/syntax (grammar), and pragmatics (uses) during clinical management (ASHA, 1989).

Box 5–5. Helpful Tips in Working With an Interpreter/Translator (ASHA, n.d.-b)

Before the Session

1. Meet with the interpreter/translator. Plan sufficient time to review the procedures, goals, professional terminology, and to develop rapport.
2. Remind the interpreter/translator to avoid nonverbal cues such as intonational changes or hand gestures.
3. Ensure that the interpreter/translator will maintain confidentiality.
4. Ask the interpreter/translator to take notes.
5. Inquire about specific cultural or linguistic information that may assist you in working with the client, such as greetings in the client's language.

During the Session

1. Define your role as the SLPA and introduce the interpreter to the client.
2. Talk directly to the client and not to the interpreter.
3. The interpreter should also look at the person to whom she or he is speaking (i.e., the client and then responsively to you).
4. Use short, concise sentences to allow for careful, thorough interpretation.
5. Allow sufficient time for the interpreter to respond in the other language to the client and to relay the message back to you in English.
6. Check to see that the interpreter is taking notes to provide you with nonverbal information during the wrap-up session.

Wrap-Up Session

1. Plan sufficient time at the end of your session to review with the interpreter.
2. If the client or family has brought in written material, ask the interpreter to make a translation for you. This could be done after the session.
3. Review the session and answer any questions the interpreter/translator may have.
4. Thank the interpreter/translator and congratulate them on a job well done.

Biliterate: A biliterate person is one who speaks, reads, and writes effectively in more than one language.

Cultural Informant: A cultural informant is a person with whom a professional may consult to learn more about a cultural and/or linguistic community. The cultural informant should be a member of that community. To avoid bias, more than one cultural informant may be used. The goal in using information about the community is to optimize services for the client (ASHA, 2004). The informant may provide information relative to child-rearing, language and dialect usage, and attitudes toward disabilities (Anderson, 2002).

Dialect: A dialect is defined as "a rule-governed variation of a language spoken by a definable group of people characterized by their culture, ethnicity, or geographical region" (Haynes, Moran, & Pindzola, 2012, p. 426).

Ethnicity: Ethnicity is variously defined as the affiliation with a population group, having a common cultural heritage or nationality, and distinguished by customs, characteristics, languages, and common history.

Ethnographic Methods/Ethnography: An ethnographic method allows an individual to observe and conscientiously collect information about the life and culture of a specific group. Observations and data collection occur over time and can reveal the mores, beliefs, and interactional styles of a group. Ethnographical or qualitative study is descriptive and thus can be especially useful in understanding linguistically and culturally diverse communities (Brice, 2002). "Ethnography is the social research style that emphasizes encountering unfamiliar worlds and making sense of them" (Agar, 1986, p.12).

Heritage Language: A heritage language is one spoken by a family and/or cultural group, sometimes referred to as the native or home language, and usually the first language to which a child is exposed.

Interpreter: An interpreter is a bilingual person specially trained to translate *oral* communication or manual communication systems (sign language) from one language to another (ASHA, 2004).

Language Difference: As opposed to a language disorder, a language difference is characterized by variations from Standard American English in phonology, morphology, syntax, semantics, and pragmatics, as the result of the influence of another language or dialect.

Language Disorder: A language disorder is defined as "impaired comprehension and/or use of spoken, written and/or other symbol systems. The disorder may involve: (1) the form of language (phonology, morphology, syntax), (2) the content of language (semantics), and/or (3) the function of language in communication (pragmatics) in any combination" (ASHA, 1993).

Translator: A translator is a bilingual person specially trained to translate *written* text from one language to another (ASHA, 2004).

REFERENCES

Agar, M. (1986). *Speaking of ethnography.* Newbury Park, CA: Sage.

American Speech-Language-Hearing Association (ASHA). (n.d.-a). *Phonemic inventories across languages.* Retrieved from http://www.asha.org/practice/multicultural/Phono/

American Speech-Language-Hearing Association (ASHA). (n.d.-b). *Tips for working with an interpreter.* Retrieved from http://www.asha.org/practice/multicultural/issues/interpret/

American Speech-Language-Hearing Association (ASHA). (1989). *Bilingual service provider database registration form.* Retrieved from http://www.asha.org/Forms/Bilingua-Service-Provider-Form/

American Speech-Language-Hearing Association (ASHA). (1993). *Definitions of communication disorders and variations.* Retrieved from http://www.asha.org/policy/RP1993-00208

American Speech-Language-Hearing Association (ASHA). (2003). *American English dialects* [Technical report]. Retrieved from http://www.asha.org/policy

American Speech-Language-Hearing Association (ASHA). (2004). *Knowledge and skills needed by speech-language pathologists and audiologists to provide culturally and linguistically appropriate services.* Retrieved from http://www.asha.org/policy

American Speech-Language-Hearing Association (ASHA). (2012a). *The advantages of being bilingual.* Retrieved from http://www.asha.org/about/news/tipsheets/bilingual/

American Speech-Language-Hearing Association (ASHA). (2012b). *Demographic profile of ASHA members providing bilingual services August 2012.* Retrieved from http://www.asha.org/uploadedFiles/Demographic-Profile-Bilingual-Spanish-Service-Members.pdf

American Speech-Language-Hearing Association (ASHA). (2013). *Speech-language pathology assistant scope of practice.* Retrieved from http://www.asha.org/policy/SP2013-00337/

Anderson, R. (2002). Practical assessment strategies with Hispanic students. In A. Brice (Ed.), *The Hispanic child: Speech, language, culture and education* (pp. 143–184). Boston, MA: Allyn & Bacon.

Battle, D. (2002). Communication disorders in a multicultural society. In D. Battle (Ed.), *Communication disorders in multicultural populations* (3rd ed., pp. 33–70). Stoneham, MA: Butterworth-Heinemann.

Bhatia, T., & Ritchie, W. (Eds.). (2006). *The handbook of bilingualism.* Cambridge, UK: Blackwell.

Brice, A. (2002). Clinician as a qualitative researcher. In A. Brice (Ed.), *The Hispanic child: Speech, language, culture, and education* (pp.85–99). Boston, MA: Allyn & Bacon.

Genesee, F. (2003). Rethinking bilingual acquisition. In J. Dewaele, A. Housen, & L. Wei (Eds.), *Bilingualism: Beyond basic principles* (pp. 204–229). Clevedon, UK: Multilingual Matters.

Haynes, W., Moran, M., & Pindzola, R. (2012). *Communication disorders in educational and medical settings: An introduction for speech-language pathologists, educators, and health professionals.* Sudbury, MA: Jones & Bartlett Learning.

Hoodin, R. (2011). *Intervention in child language disorders: A comprehensive handbook.* Sudbury, MA: Jones & Bartlett Learning.

Langdon, H. (2002). Language interpreters and translators: Bridging communication with clients and families. *ASHA Leader, 14–15.*

Lipson, J., & Dibble, S. (2005). *Culture and clinical care.* San Francisco: University of California San Francisco Nursing Press.

Madding, C. (1999). Mama é hijo: The Latino mother-infant dyad. *Multicultural Electronic Journal of Communication Disorders, 1*(2). Retrieved from http://www.asha.ucf.edu/madding3.html

Madding, C. (2000). Maintaining focus on cultural competence in early intervention services to linguistically and culturally diverse families. *Infant-Toddler Intervention: Transdisciplinary Journal, 10*(1), 9–18.

Madding, C. (2002). Socialization practices of Latinos. In A. Brice (Ed.), *The Hispanic child: Speech, language, culture, and education* (pp. 66–84). Boston, MA: Allyn & Bacon.

Mumy, A. P. (2012). *Tips for parents raising bilingual children: When the home language differs from the community language.* Retrieved from http://blog.asha.org/2012/08/16/tips-for-parents-raising-bilingual-children-when-the-home-language-differs-from-the-community-language/

Roseberry, C., & Connell, P. J. (1991). The use of invented language rule in the differentiation of normal and language-impaired Spanish speaking children. *Journal of Speech and Hearing Research, 34,* 596–603.

Rowden-Racette, K. (2013) Knowing others, knowing yourself. *ASHA Leader,* 53.

Uchikoshi, Y., & Maniates, H. (2010). How does bilingual instruction enhance English achievement? A mixed-methods study of Cantonese-speaking and Spanish-speaking bilingual classrooms. *Bilingual Research Journal, 33*(3), 364–385.

U.S. Bureau of the Census. (2012). *Statistical abstract of the United States.* Washington, DC: U.S. Department of Commerce.

Westby, C., Burda, A., & Mehta, Z. (2003, April 29). Asking the right questions in the right ways. *ASHA Leader,* pp. 1–8.

APPENDIX 5–A

Chapter Review Self–Test

		T/F
1.	*Interpreter* and *translator* are synonymous terms.	
2.	Interpreters should tell non-English-speaking families to speak to their children in English.	
3.	Being bilingual means that an individual will be an appropriate interpreter or translator.	
4.	Acquiring cultural competence is an ongoing process.	
5.	Only a bilingual speech-language pathology assistant may work with a non-English-speaking client/student.	
6.	The interpreter/translator should be acquainted with the procedures of the upcoming session before it begins.	
7.	It is the speech-language pathology assistant's role to train and prepare the interpreter.	
8.	The interpreter/translator must be neutral, ethical, and maintain confidentiality.	
9.	A bilingual child may have a language disorder in just one of his or her languages.	
10.	A student with a dialectal difference from the mainstream should receive speech-language services in order to develop Standard American English.	

Answers: 1. F; 2. F; 3. F; 4. T; 5. F; 6. T; 7. T; 8. T; 9. F; 10. F.

APPENDIX 5–B

Cultural Consciousness Activities

1. Think about your own culture (specific to the geographic and familial environment in which you were raised) and list five rules or mores of your culture. (Examples: father is head of the house; church on Sunday is a must, etc.)

2. Thinking of your responses to Question 1, can you think of some cultures where the rules/mores are different?

3. Describe an ideal family in the culture of your childhood.

4. Describe the attitude of your culture toward disabilities.

5. Check the culturally linked attitudes and behaviors that are associated with your culture:

   ____ Punctuality

   ____ Elders have final authority

   ____ Informal child rearing (few rules)

   ____ Birthright inheritance

   ____ Assertiveness, directness

   ____ High expectations for child

   ____ Formality in family relationships

____ Nuclear family most important

____ Greater family (all relatives) most important—family cohesiveness

____ Independence valued

____ Religious family orientation

____ Respect for elderly

____ All older people considered as parents

____ Matriarchal family structure

____ Patriarchal family structure

____ Competition between siblings valued

____ Equality in family structure

____ Adults defined by occupation

____ Marriage affirmed by children

____ Divorce acceptable

____ Unmarried children should live with parents

____ Privacy valued

____ Freedom of opinion

____ Family democracy

____ Importance of tradition

____ Family above personal gain

CHAPTER 6

Health and Safety

Pei-Fang Hung

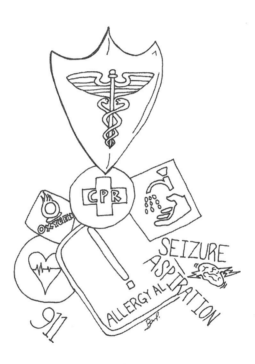

An ounce of prevention is worth a pound of cure.
Benjamin Franklin (scientist/inventor and Founding Father of the United States)

The aim of this chapter is to describe various medical-related matters that a speech-language pathology assistant (SLPA) may encounter when working with clients in various clinical settings, such as child care centers, schools, community clinics, long-term care facilities, private homes, and hospital settings. The purpose is to provide an overview of common medical conditions related to your work as an SLPA and practical information to ensure a safe working environment for both you and the clients you serve. Infection control, standard precautions, first aid, cardiopulmonary resuscitation (CPR), common medical conditions, and precautions are each discussed.

INFECTION CONTROL AND STANDARD PRECAUTIONS

The purpose of infection control is to ensure the protection of individuals who are at risk of acquiring an infection in various settings, such as in the general community or while receiving health care treatment (Centers for Disease Control and Prevention [CDC], 2011). When receiving health care treatment, patients are vulnerable to health care–associated infections (HAIs). According to the U.S. CDC (2011), HAIs affect nearly 2 million individuals every year in the United States and contribute to approximately 80,000 deaths annually.

An infectious disease is caused by pathogens, which are microorganisms that cause diseases to its host (Signore, 2013). The most common pathogens are various bacteria, viruses, fungi, and protozoa (Signore, 2013). These microorganisms are transmitted via several routes. The common routes of transmission include contact, droplet, airborne, vehicleborne, and vector-borne (Box 6–1).

All health care providers, including SLPAs, are responsible for providing safe care to clients. According to the World Health Organization (WHO), infection control refers to the prevention of the spread of infection and ensures the protection of the individuals who might be vulnerable to infection (WHO, 2009). The American Speech-Language-Hearing Association (ASHA) also includes infection control within program operation in its policy documents: *Quality Indicators for Professional Service Programs in Audiology and Speech-Language Pathology: Section III. D. Physical Facilities, Equipment, and Program Environment* (ASHA, 2005).

SLPAs may be exposed to a variety of infectious diseases during the performance of their duties. As such, it is critical that you protect yourself and your clients from the spread of disease in all forms. If you do not take effective precautions against infection, you are at high risk of becoming infected. Similarly, without effective protection, there is a high possibility that the infectious disease can further spread to your clients, colleagues, family members, and the community at large. Therefore, infection control is *essential* to all health care providers, including SLPAs.

Standard precautions (previously known as universal precautions) are "the minimum infection prevention practices that apply to all patient care, regardless of suspected or confirmed infection status of the patient, in any setting where healthcare is delivered" (CDC, 2011, Adhere to Standard Precautions, para. 1). Standard precautions are designed to protect health care providers and to prevent infections from being spread. Key standard precautions important to an SLPA include hand hygiene, use of personal protective equipment, safe handling of potentially contaminated equipment or surfaces, and respiratory hygiene/cough etiquette.

Hand Hygiene

Hand hygiene is the most important way to prevent infection and to reduce the risk of spreading infections (WHO, 2009). For a comprehensive review of hand hygiene, please refer to the *WHO Guidelines on Hand Hygiene in Health Care* (WHO, 2009).

Box 6–1. Common Routes of Microrganism Transmission (CDC, 2011)

Contact Transmission

Contact transmission is divided into direct and indirect contact. Two examples of contact transmissible infectious agents include methicillin-resistant *Staphylococcus aureus* (MRSA) and vancomycin-resistant enterococcus (VRE).

- *Direct contact transmission* refers to the transfer of infectious agents through direct physical contact with an infected individual. An example of direct body-to-body physical contact includes touching an infectious person.
- *Indirect contact transmission* involves the transfer of infectious agents through making physical contact with contaminated items and surfaces. Examples of indirect contact include touching contaminated doorknobs, computer keyboards, or handles.

Droplet Transmission

Droplets are produced after talking, coughing, or sneezing. Infectious droplets may travel through air but cannot remain suspended in the air because they are larger particles (>10 micrometers). When these pathogens drop, they can contaminate the environment and cause indirect contact transmission.

Airborne Transmission

Airborne transmission occurs when very small particles (<10 micrometers) that contain infectious agents spread in the air and these microorganisms enter the respiratory tract and cause infection, such as tuberculosis (TB). Airborne transmission does not require face-to-face contact with an infected individual.

Vehicle–Borne Transmission

Vehicle-borne transmission is a type of indirect transmission of an infectious agent that occurs when microorganisms are transmitted by consuming or contacting contaminated items, such as food or water sources.

Vector–Borne Transmission

Vector-borne transmission occurs when pathogens are transmitted through vectors, such as mosquitoes, flies, or rats.

Good hand hygiene includes hand washing with water and soap and the use of alcohol-based hand rubs.

For SLPAs, hand hygiene should be performed during the following conditions (WHO, 2009) but not limited to:

- Before and after treating a client
- After touching blood, body fluids, or any contaminated items even when gloves are worn
- Immediately after removing personal protective equipment, such as gloves
- Immediately if skin is contaminated and/or injury occurs
- After activities involving personal body functions, such as blowing one's nose.

Also, SLPAs should encourage clients to perform hand hygiene at the beginning of the therapy session, prior to handling task materials, or after activities involving personal body functions.

Table 6–1 summarizes the proper steps in hand washing and hand rubbing, as recommended by WHO and the CDC. Figures 6–1 and 6–2 illustrate these procedures.

Personal Protective Equipment

When there is a risk of coming in contact with nonintact skin, mucous membranes, or body fluids, personal protective equipment is required. According to the Occupational Safety and Health Administration (OSHA, 2003), personal protective equipment refers to equipment that is designed to protect the wearer from injury (CDC, 2011). Examples of personal protective equipment include gloves, goggles, helmets, and protective clothing. The most commonly worn personal protective equipment is gloves. Gloves should be worn when there is a risk of getting in contact with nonintact skin, mucous membranes, or body fluids. Gloves act as a barrier between the skin and potentially hazardous agents, so wearing gloves should not replace good hand hygiene. For SLPAs, the following are several com-

Table 6–1. Steps for Proper Hand Washing and Hand Rubbing

Hand Washing	Hand Rubbing
1. Remove hand and arm jewelry.	1. Remove hand and arm jewelry.
2. Wet hands with warm water and apply soap.	2. Apply between 1 and 2 full pumps of alcohol-based hand sanitizer onto one palm.
3. Rub all aspects of hands for a minimum of 15 seconds, concentrating on the fingertips, between fingers, the back of hand, and the base of thumbs.	3. Spread product over all surfaces of hands, concentrating on the fingertips, between fingers, the back of hand, and the base of thumbs.
4. Rinse and dry hands thoroughly with an air dryer or with a paper towel.	4. Rub hands until product is dry.
5. Turn off taps with paper towel.	

Source: CDC, 2011; Interorganizational Group for Speech Language Pathology and Audiology, 2010.

How to Handrub?

RUB HANDS FOR HAND HYGIENE! WASH HANDS WHEN VISIBLY SOILED

Duration of the entire procedure: 20-30 seconds

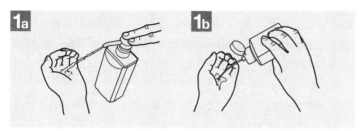
Apply a palmful of the product in a cupped hand, covering all surfaces;

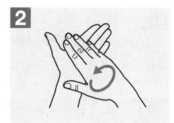
Rub hands palm to palm;

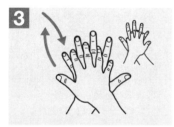
Right palm over left dorsum with interlaced fingers and vice versa;

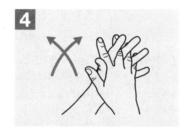
Palm to palm with fingers interlaced;

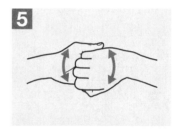
Backs of fingers to opposing palms with fingers interlocked;

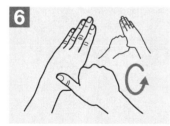
Rotational rubbing of left thumb clasped in right palm and vice versa;

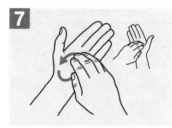
Rotational rubbing, backwards and forwards with clasped fingers of right hand in left palm and vice versa;

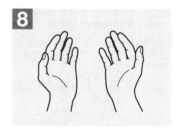
Once dry, your hands are safe.

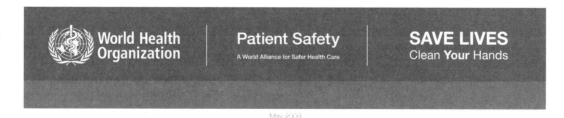

Figure 6–1. Illustration of appropriate hand-rubbing procedures. Copyright World Health Organization (WHO). Used with permission.

How to Handwash?

WASH HANDS WHEN VISIBLY SOILED! OTHERWISE, USE HANDRUB

Duration of the entire procedure: 40-60 seconds

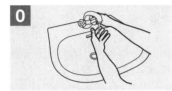

0. Wet hands with water;

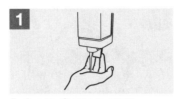

1. Apply enough soap to cover all hand surfaces;

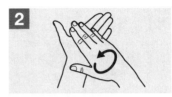

2. Rub hands palm to palm;

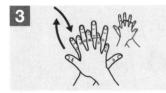

3. Right palm over left dorsum with interlaced fingers and vice versa;

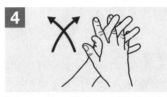

4. Palm to palm with fingers interlaced;

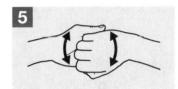

5. Backs of fingers to opposing palms with fingers interlocked;

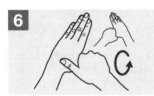

6. Rotational rubbing of left thumb clasped in right palm and vice versa;

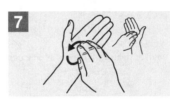

7. Rotational rubbing, backwards and forwards with clasped fingers of right hand in left palm and vice versa;

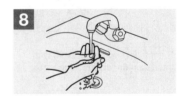

8. Rinse hands with water;

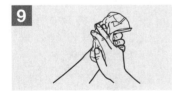

9. Dry hands thoroughly with a single use towel;

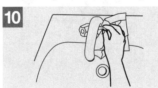

10. Use towel to turn off faucet;

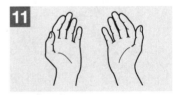

11. Your hands are now safe.

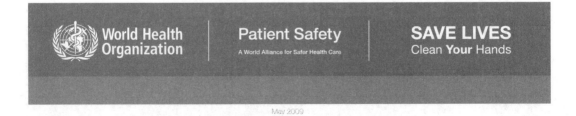

World Health Organization | Patient Safety — A World Alliance for Safer Health Care | SAVE LIVES Clean Your Hands

May 2009

Figure 6–2. Steps of appropriate hand washing. Copyright World Health Organization (WHO). Used with permission.

mon situations that may require you to wear gloves:

- Assisting with an oral peripheral examination or oral hygiene
- Handling dirty materials
- Working with clients who are immune compromised or when additional precaution is needed (e.g., clients with *Clostridium difficile* infection)
- Assisting with feeding and swallowing treatment activities.

In addition, using gloves correctly is essential (CDC, 2013b). First, it is important to select the proper glove material. For example, vinyl gloves are designed for personal care, and latex gloves are for sterile invasive procedures. Avoiding latex gloves should be considered to prevent latex allergies. Second, be sure to use the correct size of gloves and do not reuse single-use disposable gloves. Last, before touching a clean environment, or when the activity or procedure is completed, gloves should be removed immediately.

To protect your eyes, nose, and mouth from the splash of a potentially infectious material or body fluids, you can use eye protectors (e.g., goggles), masks, and face shields (Siegel, Rhinehart, Jackson, Chiarello, & the Healthcare Infection Control Practices Advisory Committee, 2007). Preferred masks include the National Institute for Occupational Safety and Health (NIOSH)–certified N95 filtering facepiece respirators (Figure 6–3) or the P100 filtering facepiece respirators with the elastomeric facepiece seal (CDC, 2013a).

Safe Handling of Potentially Contaminated Equipment or Surfaces

As an SLPA, you may be asked to participate in cleaning and disinfection of treatment materials and the clinical environment. Sterilization is often not required. Cleaning refers to the physical removal of foreign material, such as dust, soil, or secretion by using water and detergents (CDC, 2008). Disinfection refers to the elimination of harmful microorganisms living on

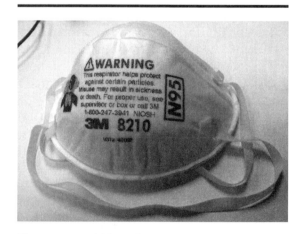

Figure 6–3. 3M N95 Filtering facepiece respirators. Image courtesy of Wikimedia Commons.

the surface of objects, but disinfection does not destroy all microorganisms, especially some bacterial spores (CDC, 2008).

Cleaning usually involves soap and water to remove soil, dust, or foreign material. High-traffic areas, such as furniture in the therapy room, should be cleaned frequently. Treatment materials should be placed on shelves and in bins after use. Shelves and bins should be kept clean and dust free.

For low-level disinfection, SLPAs can apply Environmental Protection Agency (EPA)-registered disinfectant on equipment or surfaces and let solution sit for at least 1 minute before wiping (CDC, 2008). While using the disinfectant, wear rubber gloves to protect hands from irritation and wash hands immediately afterward. When EPA-registered disinfectant is not available, SLPAs may use a fresh chlorine bleach solution. The formula of diluted bleach solution is 1 tablespoon of bleach to 1 quart (4 cups) of water. The CDC and the Healthcare Infection Control Practices Advisory Committee (HICPAC) provide guidelines on environmental infection control measures. A copy of the cleaning and disinfection guidelines for schools is available in Appendix 6–A. Additional information on this topic can also be found on the CDC's website (http://www.cdc.gov/hai/).

Respiratory Hygiene/Cough Etiquette

According to the CDC and HICPAC (CDC, 2012), respiratory etiquette should be implemented for all individuals with signs and symptoms of a respiratory infection. The following measures are used to contain respiratory secretions:

- Cover nose and mouth when coughing or sneezing.

- Use tissues to contain respiratory secretions and dispose of them immediately in the nearest waste receptacle after use.
- Perform hand hygiene after having contact with respiratory secretions and contaminated objects/materials.

Additional information on this topic can also be found on the CDC's website (http://www.cdc.gov/flu/professionals/infectioncontrol/resphygiene.htm).

FIRST AID AND CARDIOPULMONARY RESUSCITATION

In case of an emergency, an SLPA should be trained in first aid and cardiopulmonary resuscitation (CPR) to respond appropriately. This section discusses the general rules about first aid and CPR and how to get certified.

General Rules About First Aid

First aid refers to providing the initial care or management for an injury or illness (American Red Cross, 2013). In most treatment settings, a first aid kit is available, which contains items to handle an emergency. In the United States, OSHA requires all job sites and workplaces to have first aid kits available for use. This kit is typically stored in a place where it is easily accessible for adults but out of reach of children. As an SLPA, you should know where this kit is and what items are available.

Key items should be included in a first aid kit (Cronan, 2010): first aid manual, sterile gauze pads, adhesive tapes, adhesive bandages, antiseptic wipes, alcohol wipes, antibiotic ointment, antiseptic solution, pain killers, tweezers, scissors, safety pins, disposable instant cold packs, thermometers, plastic nonlatex gloves, and a flashlight with extra batteries. The kit should be checked on a regular basis to replace low-stock items and medicines that may have expired and to check if the flashlight works properly and there are backup batteries available.

CPR Certification

According to American Heart Association (AHA, 2010), CPR is an emergency procedure that manually ensures blood can continue circulating in the body after an individual has a cardiac arrest. All the cells in our body require oxygen and nutrients to survive, and these are carried in the blood. When a cardiac arrest happens, the heart stops beating. Blood then stops circulating, and breathing ceases after a few minutes. A cardiac arrest can be caused by a heart attack, other heart diseases, drugs, blood loss, head injury, or heart rhythm disturbance. CPR is an emergency procedure to keep the blood flowing in the body, but it cannot restart the heart. Further measures, such as defibrillator, are needed to restart the heart.

In general, CPR involves chest compression and rescue breaths (AHA, 2010). Chest compression manually pumps the heart to continue blood flowing throughout the body. Rescue breaths supply air to the lungs and can be performed either by mouth-to-mouth resuscitation or by using a device. CPR training is easy, and it is extremely important for SLPAs to get CPR certification to react to emergency situations. The American Red Cross and American Heart Association offer many training courses for CPR and first aid certification. For more information on CPR, visit the American Red Cross website (http://www.redcorss.org) and the AHA (http://www.heart.org). Local fire departments also offer CPR training courses that are certified by the AHA.

COMMON MEDICAL CONDITIONS

When an SLPA is working with a client/patient, medical emergency situations can occur. This section covers several medical conditions that an SLPA might encounter when providing care or treatment. By understanding the symptoms and causes of these medical conditions, SLPAs can react to the medical emergency accurately and seek medical attention immediately.

Stroke

According to the National Stroke Association (2013), stroke is the fourth leading cause of death in the United States. A stroke, also known as cerebrovascular accident (CVA), occurs when the blood supply to part of the brain is suddenly interrupted or when a blood vessel in the brain bursts, spilling blood into the brain or the spaces surrounding the brain. There are two kinds of stroke: ischemic stroke and hemorrhagic stroke. An ischemic stroke is caused by an obstruction of a blood vessel that supplies blood to the brain. The obstruction can result from cerebral thrombosis or embolism. Cerebral thrombosis refers to the formation of a blood clot inside a blood vessel that blocks the vascular circulation in the brain. A cerebral embolism happens when a clot breaks off from another part of body and travels to the brain, resulting in the obstruction of a blood vessel in the brain. A hemorrhagic stroke happens when a weakened blood vessel ruptures. The weakened blood vessel can result from a blood vessel malformation, such as arteriovenous malformation, or a cerebral aneurysm.

When the vascular circulation in the brain is blocked or interrupted, neurons (brain cells) can no longer receive the oxygen and nutrients they need from the blood supply. This results in the death of neurons and the loss of abilities controlled by that brain area. How an individual with a stroke is affected depends on where the stroke occurs in the brain and how much of the brain is damaged. For example, a small stroke may cause only minor weakness of an arm or leg, whereas a larger stroke can result in paralysis (total loss of function) on one side of the body. A stroke can damage many important brain functions, such as speech, language, movement, vision, or memory. Stroke is one of the main causes of many acquired speech-language related disorders, such as aphasia, dysarthria, apraxia of speech, and other cognitive-linguistic disorders (ASHA, 2013). Stroke is a medical emergency, and prompt treatment is crucial. Box 6–2 summarizes possible signs and symptoms of a stroke. If a person is experiencing these symptoms, an SLPA should call 911 and get immediate medical attention. Early intervention can minimize brain damage and potential complications.

Heart Attack

Similar to a stroke, a heart attack, also known as a myocardial infarction, happens when the blood vessels, that supply blood to the heart, are blocked (National Institutes of Health [NIH], 2013b). When the flow of oxygen-rich blood is blocked or interrupted, that section of the heart cannot get oxygen and nutrients and the muscles of that section of the heart begin to die. Coronary heart disease (CHD) is the most common cause of a heart attack. CHD is a result of the buildup of plaque inside the coronary arteries, the major oxygen-rich blood supply to the heart.

As an SLPA, if someone is experiencing symptoms of a heart attack, you should get medical attention immediately by dialing 911 or a local emergency number. Box 6–3 lists the common symptoms of a heart attack. The chest pain may move from the chest to other parts of the body, such as shoulder, arms, back,

---

Box 6–2. Common Symptoms and Signs of a Stroke
(National Stroke Association, 2013)

- Sudden numbness or weakness of the face, arm, or leg, especially on one side of the body
- Sudden confusion, trouble speaking or understanding
- Sudden trouble seeing in one or both eyes
- Sudden trouble walking, dizziness, loss of balance or coordination
- Sudden severe headache with no known cause

> ### Box 6–3. Common Symptoms of a Heart Attack (NIH, 2013b)
>
> - Chest pain or discomfort (because the heart is not getting enough blood)
> - Shortness of breath
> - Fatigue with activity
> - Sweating
> - Nausea

or neck. Acting fast for a heart attack can limit damage to the heart. According to the NIH (2013b), treatment for a heart attack works best when given right after the symptoms occur.

Airway Obstruction

Airway obstruction means a blockage in the airway, either upper airway or lower airway (NIH, 2013a). The upper airway includes the nasal cavity, pharynx, and larynx, and the lower airway refers to the trachea, bronchial tree, and lungs. Airway obstruction can prevent air from getting into the lungs (partially or totally). This can be fatal and requires immediate medical attention. Airway obstruction is classified as chronic airway obstruction or acute airway obstruction.

Chronic airway obstruction takes a long time to develop. Examples of chronic airway obstruction are chronic obstructive pulmonary disorders (COPD), emphysema, and abscesses in the airway. Acute airway obstruction occurs quickly. The common cases that SLPAs might encounter include inhaling, swallowing, or choking on a foreign object, allergic reactions, or a small object lodged in the nose. Children are at higher risk of foreign object obstruction than are adults (American Society for Gastrointestinal Endoscopy, 2011). Therefore, make sure to keep small items away from children when working with them and constantly monitor them for any unsafe behaviors, such as trying to put small toys into the nose or mouth or swallowing a big piece of food without chewing.

The symptoms of airway obstruction depend on the location of obstruction. Box 6–4 lists common symptoms of airway obstruction. When any of these symptoms is noticed, get medical help immediately.

> ### Box 6–4. Common Symptoms of an Airway Obstruction (NIH, 2013a)
>
> - Difficulty with breathing
> - Wheezing breathing noise
> - Change of skin color (bluish color)
> - Panic
> - Gasping for air

If trained personnel are available onsite, the Heimlich maneuver can be performed for someone choking on a foreign object and CPR can be used for someone who is not breathing.

Seizures

A seizure is caused by sudden disorganized and abnormal electrical activity in the brain, so the person's muscles contract and relax repeatedly (U.S. National Library of Medicine, 2012). There are many different types of seizures. Seizures can result from many medical conditions, such as brain injury, stroke, brain tumor, liver or kidney failure, high fever, low blood sugar, or drug abuse. Specific symptoms of seizures depend on what part of the brain is involved. They occur suddenly. Box 6–5 lists common symptoms of a seizure. Symptoms may stop after a few seconds or minutes, usually lasting no longer than 10 to 15 minutes. Table 6–2 lists a few things that should be considered during and after a seizure.

Box 6–5. Common Symptoms of a Seizure
(U.S. National Library of Medicine, 2012)

- Brief blackout with confusion, drooling, eye movement, grunting, or snoring
- Sudden falling
- Uncontrollable muscle spasms with jerking limbs or shaking of the entire body
- For mild cases, there might be no body shaking and the person may seem to be staring into space

---

Table 6–2. What to Do During and After a Seizure

During a Seizure	After a Seizure
• Stay calm and try to time the seizure.	• Make sure to check for any injuries or difficulty of breathing.
• If the seizure lasts longer than 3 minutes or if the person is pregnant, call 911.	• Provide a safe area for the person to rest and do not give him or her anything to eat or drink until he or she is fully conscious and oriented.
• Remove objects that might hurt the person and provide postural support to prevent further injury.	
• If the person is on the ground, position him or her on his or her side to avoid saliva or vomit going into the airway.	
• Do not attempt to open the mouth and put anything in the mouth, since this could pose a choking hazard (O'Hara, 2007).	
• Do not attempt to give anything to drink or eat while the person is having a seizure (O'Hara, 2007).	

Source: Chillemi & Devinsky, 2011.

Severe Allergic Reactions

Most of the time, people experience minor allergic symptoms when having allergic reactions. However, when a severe allergic reaction happens, it can be rapid and potentially life threatening (NIH, 2013a). Allergic symptoms occur when a person's own immune system reacts to normally harmless substances. According to the NIH (2013a), the most common allergy triggers include certain food, medication, pollen, dust mites, mold, insect stings, and latex. Mild allergic symptoms are mild eye irritation, localized skin rash, and congestion. Severe allergic reactions include generalized swelling, wheezing, nausea, vomiting, fast heartbeat, and difficulty breathing.

Before working with a client, an SLPA should review the client's medical history thoroughly to find out if she or he has a known allergy. Make sure to avoid the exposure of common allergic triggers. Severe allergic reactions require immediate medical treatment. If someone starts to have a significant allergic reaction, such as difficulty breathing or increased heart rate, call 911 or immediately go to the nearest emergency room.

> ### ADDITIONAL THINGS TO CONSIDER: WORKING WITH CLIENTS WITH SPECIAL MEDICAL NEEDS

SLPAs might have to work with clients who have special medical needs. It is important to understand these specific needs and provide reasonable accommodation. This section discusses the precaution that SLPAs should be aware of when working with clients who have special medical needs.

Oxygen Use

SLPAs might work with clients who need to use oxygen. Oxygen is used for individuals who cannot keep appropriate oxygen levels in their blood. Oxygen is a prescribed drug, and it can improve respiration and decrease the work of heart (National Heart, Lung, and Blood Institute, 2011). Oxygen is delivered through the use of an oxygen mask or a nasal cannula (Figure 6–4B). The common types of oxygen systems are oxygen concentrators, gas cylinders, liquid oxygen systems, and portable oxygen concentrators (American Lung Association, 2013). Oxygen concentrators are used in the home (Figure 6–4A). While a concentrator is running, it can make oxygen and give the user an indefinite supply of oxygen. Oxygen cylinders are painted green, which is the universal color for medical oxygen cylinders. They come in many different sizes depending on the needs of the patient/client. In general, they range from 2 to 6 feet in height. Once the cylinder is empty, it needs to be refilled by trained personnel. The liquid oxygen system is self-contained and has a large reservoir. Liquid oxygen is stored in the system and needs to be refilled, usually weekly. Portable oxygen concentrators are similar to the home oxygen concentrators, but they are smaller in size, more portable, and better for travel than home oxygen concentrators (American Lung Association, 2013).

Although oxygen is nonflammable, it makes things burn much faster than usual. Thus, smoking is prohibited in the room where oxygen is in use. "NO SMOKING" signs are commonly placed in treatment rooms where oxygen is being used. Make sure to keep oxygen 6 feet away from any heat sources, such as heat ducts, radiators, space heaters, fireplaces, matches, and

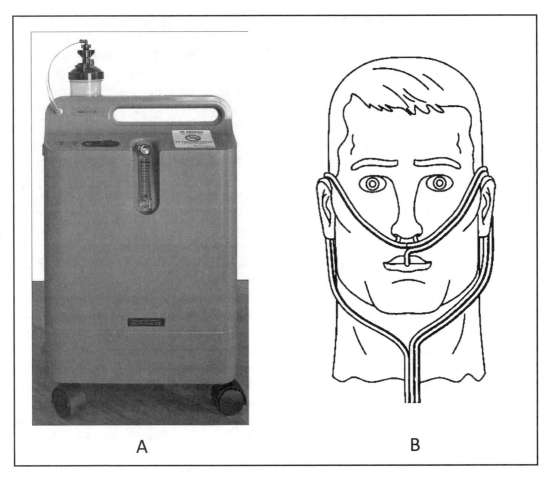

Figure 6–4. A. EverFlo oxygen concentrator (Respironics) and **B.** Nasal cannula. Images courtesy of Wikimedia Commons.

lighters. If the client uses a gas cylinder, keep the tank in its stand to avoid rolling or falling. It may cause injury or damage to the client or persons nearby. Also, SLPAs should pay attention to the oxygen tubing because the client may get tangled in the tubing or trip over the tubes. This might interfere with oxygen circulation.

Dysphagia and Aspiration Precautions

Dysphagia is the medical term for swallowing difficulty. Individuals with dysphagia experience difficulty in transmitting food or liquid from mouth to stomach due to the tongue, throat (pharynx and larynx), or esophagus not working probably (Groher & Crary, 2010). Dysphagia can result from numerous medical conditions, such as stroke, head injury, progressive neurodegenerative diseases (e.g., Parkinson disease), oral/pharyngeal/esophageal cancers, or other esophageal diseases. These neurologic diseases can impair the nerves and muscles used for swallowing, resulting in difficulties in moving food or liquid from the mouth to the stomach.

Cancers can cause reduced movement of the tongue, pharynx, or larynx. Esophageal disorders can cause the esophagus to become narrower than usual so food or liquid cannot travel along the esophagus smoothly. Common symptoms and signs of dysphagia are summarized in Box 6–6.

Individuals with dysphagia are at high risk of aspiration. Aspiration refers to the entry of food or liquid into the larynx or lungs. Due to the difficulties in transmitting food or liquid from the mouth to the stomach, the chances of food or liquid entering the airway increase. Things that can be inhaled into larynx or lungs include food, liquid, saliva, vomited stomach contents, and stomach acid. These things can cause substantial damage to lungs and result in pneumonia, lung abscess (a collection of pus in the lungs), airway obstruction, and even death.

ASHA addresses dysphagia in its SLPA scope of practice document (2013, Responsibility Outside the Scope for SLPAs, para. 1), stating that SLPAs, may *not*:

a. perform procedures that require a high level of clinical acumen and technical skill (e.g., vocal tract prosthesis shaping or fitting, vocal tract imaging and oral pharyngeal swallow therapy with bolus material);

b. tabulate or interpret results and observations of feeding and swallowing evaluations performed by SLPs;

c. develop or determine the swallowing strategies or precautions for patients, family, or staff.

As a care provider though, it is important you maintain a safe environment for the individuals you serve. This means when working with individuals with dysphagia, you are aware of the risk of aspiration and follow any aspiration precautions recommended by the supervising speech-language pathologist (SLP). Aspiration precautions typically involve one or more of the following:

- Sit in an upright position when eating food or drinking liquid.
- Only consume the recommended food and liquid consistency, such as finely chopped food and thickened liquid.

Box 6–6. Common Symptoms and Signs of Dysphagia
(Groher & Crary, 2010)

- Increasing time for chewing
- Need to swallow multiple times
- Drooling or liquids leaking through the nose
- Difficulty or discomfort when swallowing
- Coughing or choking when swallowing
- Difficulty with breathing during feeding
- Feeling of food stuck in the throat
- Frequent clearing of the throat
- Vomiting swallowed food
- Loss of appetite
- Dehydration, malnutrition, or weight loss

- Remind the patient/client to chew well and eat slowly.
- Eliminate distraction, such as turning off the TV or radio.
- Check the person's mouth after eating for any food residue.
- Keep sitting upright for 30 to 45 minutes after eating.

If the client shows significant symptoms or signs of dysphagia, such as coughing or difficulty breathing, ask her or him to stop eating or drinking immediately, seek medical attention, and notify your supervising SLP.

Tube Feeding

When individuals with dysphagia are at a high risk of aspiration, they are no longer able to consume an oral diet safely. Alternative feeding methods are implemented to meet their nutrition and hydration needs while continuing to treat their dysphagia. Feeding tubes are the most common approach of alterative feeding (Hanson et al., 2008). Different types of feeding tubes are available depending on the patient's condition and needs. Nasogastric (NG) tubes and percutaneous endoscopic gastrostomy (PEG) tubes are two frequently used feeding tubes (Groher & Crary, 2010). NG tubes are plastic tubes that are inserted through the nose, pass the throat, and go into the stomach. The placement of PEG tubes requires a small incision in the abdomen to insert the tube into the stomach. NG tubes are for short-term use, whereas PEG tubes can be used for a longer time or even permanently (Gomes et al., 2010).

These feeding tubes do not prevent aspiration from happening, so it is essential for SLPAs to follow aspiration precautions when working with individuals with dysphagia and feeding tubes. Remember to keep clients with aspirations precautions in an upright position, as much as possible, and avoid laying them flat when they are getting continuous feeding. Lying flat increases the risk of food regurgitation and can further result in aspiration. If there is any leakage or blockage of the feeding tubes, contact the individuals' caregiver(s) or trained personnel for further assistance.

Ventilator Use and Tracheotomy

According to the NIH (2013c), a ventilator is a machine that is mainly used in hospitals and can be used in long-term care facilities or the home for long-term use. When an individual cannot breathe independently, a ventilator is used to support breathing. It can get oxygen into the lungs, remove carbon dioxide from the body, and help the patient breathe easier. Many diseases, conditions, and factors can affect lung function. When that happens, the individual might need a ventilator to support her or his breathing. Examples of diseases and conditions that affect breathing include pneumonia, lung diseases, COPD, brain injury, stroke, or laryngeal injuries.

A tracheostomy is a surgical procedure to create a hole that goes through the front of the neck and into the trachea (NIH, 2013c). It can be temporary or permanent. A tube is placed though the hole to provide an airway, and breathing is through the tube rather than through the nose and mouth (Figure 6–5). One common reason for having a tracheostomy is when a ventilator needs to be used for more than a few weeks. The tracheostomy tube can be used to connect to a ventila-

Health and Safety   187

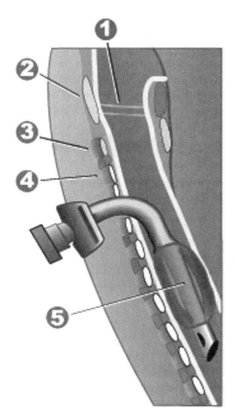

Figure 6–5. Diagram of a tracheostoma and tracheostomy tube. *Note.* 1 = vocal folds; 2 = thyroid cartilage; 3 = cricoid cartilage; 4 = tracheal cartilages; 5 = balloon cuff. Image courtesy of Wikimedia Commons.

tor to support breathing. Another possible reason for using a tracheostomy tube is to help clear mucus or secretion from the lungs.

Because air no longer passes through vocal folds, individuals who have a tracheostomy cannot produce a voice easily. There are many ways to assist individuals in producing sound for speech. Certain tracheostomy tubes can redirect airflow to produce speech. Many different types of valves also can be used to redirect the airflow for voicing. Trained SLPs can recommend options for communication and provide training to clients in the use of different devices to meet their communication needs.

REFERENCES

American Heart Association (AHA). (2010). 2010 AHA guidelines for CPR & ECC. *Journal of Circulation, 122*(18). Retrieved from http://circ.ahajournals.org/content/122/18_suppl_3.toc

American Lung Association. (2013). *Supplemental oxygen.* Retrieved from http://www.lung.org/lung-disease/copd/living-with-copd/supplemental-oxygen.html

American Red Cross. (2011). *American Red Cross First Aid/CPR/AED participant's manual* (5th ed.). St. Paul, MN: Staywell.

American Society for Gastrointestinal Endoscopy. (2011). *Guideline: Management of ingested foreign bodies and food impactions.* Retrieved from http://www.asge.org/uploadedFiles/Publications_and_Products/Practice_Guidelines/Management%20of%20ingested%20foreign%20bodies%20and%20food%20impactions.pdf

American Speech-Language-Hearing Association (ASHA). (2005). *Quality indicators for professional service programs in audiology and speech-language pathology.* Retrieved from http://www.asha.org/policy

American Speech-Language-Hearing Association (ASHA). (2013). *Stroke.* Retrieved from http://www.asha.org/public/speech/disorders/stroke.htm

Centers for Disease Control and Prevention (CDC). (2008). *Guideline for disinfection and sterilization in healthcare facilities.* Retrieved from http://www.cdc.gov/hicpac/pdf/guidelines/disinfection_nov_2008.pdf

Centers for Disease Control and Prevention (CDC). (2011). *Guide to infection prevention for outpatient settings: Minimum expectations for safe care.* Retrieved from http://www.cdc.gov/HAI/settings/outpatient/outpatient-care-gl-standared-precautions.html

Centers for Disease Control and Prevention (CDC). (2012). *Respiratory hygiene/cough etiquette in healthcare settings.* Retrieved from http://www.cdc.gov/flu/professionals/infectioncontrol/resphygiene.htm

Centers for Disease Control and Prevention (CDC). (2013a). *NIOSH-approved particulate filtering facepiece respirators.* Retrieved from http://www.cdc.gov/niosh/npptl/topics/respirators/disp_part/default.html

Centers for Disease Control and Prevention (CDC). (2013b). *Protocol for hand hygiene and glove use observations.* Retrieved from http://www.cdc.gov/dialysis/prevention-tools/Protocol-hand-hygiene-glove-observations.html

Chillemi, S., & Devinsky, O. (2011). Quick tips: What to do if someone has a seizure. *Neurology Now, 7*(2), 12.

Cronan, K. (2010). *First aid kit.* Retrieved from http://kidshealth.org/parent/firstaid_safe/home/firstaid_kit.html?tracking=83967_G#cat31

Gomes, C., Lustosa, S., Matos, D., Andriolo, R., Waisberg, D., & Waisberg, J. (2010). Percutaneous endoscopic gastrostomy versus nasogastric tube feeding for adults with swallowing disturbances. *Cochrane Database of Systematic Reviews, 10*(11), CD008096. doi:10.1002/14651858

Groher, M., & Crary, M. (2010). *Dysphagia: Clinical management in adults and children.* Maryland Heights, MO: Mosby Elsevier.

Hanson, L., Garrett, J., Lewis, C., Phifer, N., Jackman, A., & Carey, T. (2008). Physicians' expectations of benefit from tube feeding. *Journal of Palliative Medicine, 11*(8), 1130–1134.

Interorganizational Group for Speech Language Pathology and Audiology. (2010). *Infection prevention and control guidelines for speech-language pathology.* Retrieved from http://www.uwo.ca/fhs/csd/files/downloads/pdf/2009_10/Infection%20Prevention%20control%20GuidelinesSLP%20FINAL%20Feb%202010.pdf

National Heart, Lung, and Blood Institute. (2011). *What is respiratory failure?* Retrieved from http://www.nhlbi.nih.gov/health/health-topics/topics/rf/printall-index.html

National Institutes of Health (NIH). (2013a). *What is anaphylaxis?* Retrieved from http://www.niaid.nih.gov/topics/foodAllergy/understanding/Pages/anaphylaxis.aspx

National Institutes of Health (NIH). (2013b). *What is a heart attack?* Retrieved from http://www.nhlbi.nih.gov/health/health-topics/topics/heartattack/

National Institutes of Health (NIH). (2013c). *What is a ventilator?* Retrieved from http://www.nhlbi.nih.gov/health/health-topics/topics/vent/

National Stroke Association. (2013). *Stroke 101 fact sheet.* Retrieved from http://www.stroke.org/site/DocServer/STROKE_101_Fact_Sheet.pdf?docID=4541

Occupational Safety and Health Administration. (2003). *Personal protective equipment.* Retrieved from https://www.osha.gov/Publications/osha3151.html

O'Hara, K. A. (2007). First aid for seizures: The importance of education and appropriate response. *Journal of Child Neurology, 22,* 30S–37S.

Siegel, J., Rhinehart, E., Jackson, M., Chiarello, L., & the Healthcare Infection Control Practices Advisory Committee. (2007). *2007 Guideline for isolation precautions: Preventing transmission of infectious agents in healthcare settings.* Retrieved from http://www.cdc.gov/hicpac/pdf/isolation/Isolation2007.pdf

Signore, A. (2013). About inflammation and infection. *EJNMMI Research, 3*(8). Retrieved from http://www.ejnmmires.com/content/pdf/2191-219X-3-8.pdf

U.S. National Library of Medicine, National Institutes of Health. (2012). *Seizures.* Retrieved from http://www.nlm.nih.gov/medlineplus/ency/article/003200.htm

World Health Organization (WHO). (2009). *WHO guidelines on hand hygiene in health care.* Retrieved from http://www.who.int/gpsc/5may/tools/9789241597906/en/index.html

APPENDIX 6-A
CDC Cleaning and Infection Guidelines (Schools)

School Guide

How to Clean and Disinfect Schools to Help Slow the Spread of Flu

Cleaning and disinfecting are part of a broad approach to preventing infectious diseases in schools. To help slow the spread of influenza (flu), the first line of defense is getting vaccinated. Other measures include covering coughs and sneezes, washing hands, and keeping sick people away from others. Below are tips on how to slow the spread of flu specifically through cleaning and disinfecting.

1. **Know the difference between cleaning, disinfecting, and sanitizing.**

   Cleaning removes germs, dirt, and impurities from surfaces or objects. Cleaning works by using soap (or detergent) and water to physically remove germs from surfaces. This process does not necessarily kill germs, but by removing them, it lowers their numbers and the risk of spreading infection.

   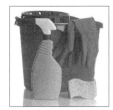

   Disinfecting kills germs on surfaces or objects. Disinfecting works by using chemicals to kill germs on surfaces or objects. This process does not necessarily clean dirty surfaces or remove germs, but by killing germs on a surface after cleaning, it can further lower the risk of spreading infection.

   Sanitizing lowers the number of germs on surfaces or objects to a safe level, as judged by public health standards or requirements. This process **works by either cleaning or disinfecting** surfaces or objects to lower the risk of spreading infection.

2. **Clean and disinfect surfaces and objects that are touched often.**

   Follow your school's standard procedures for routine cleaning and disinfecting. Typically, this means daily sanitizing surfaces and objects that are touched often, such as desks, countertops, doorknobs, computer keyboards, hands-on learning items, faucet handles, phones, and toys. Some schools may also require daily disinfecting these items. Standard procedures often call for disinfecting specific areas of the school, like bathrooms.

   Immediately clean surfaces and objects that are visibly soiled. If surfaces or objects are soiled with body fluids or blood, use gloves and other standard precautions to avoid coming into contact with the fluid. Remove the spill, and then clean and disinfect the surface.

3. **Simply do routine cleaning and disinfecting.**

   It's important to match your cleaning and disinfecting activities to the types of germs you want to remove or kill. Most studies have shown that the flu virus can live and potentially infect a person for only 2 to 8 hours after being deposited on a surface. Therefore, it is not necessary to close schools to clean or disinfect every surface in the building to slow the spread of flu. Also, if students and staff are dismissed because the school cannot function normally (e.g., high absenteeism during a flu outbreak), it is not necessary to do extra cleaning and disinfecting.

   Flu viruses are relatively fragile, so standard cleaning and disinfecting practices are sufficient to remove or kill them. Special cleaning and disinfecting processes, including wiping down walls and ceilings, frequently using room air deodorizers, and fumigating, are not necessary or recommended. These processes can irritate eyes, noses, throats, and skin; aggravate asthma; and cause other serious side effects.

U.S. Department of Health and Human Services
Centers for Disease Control and Prevention
Page 1 of 2
October, 2010

4. Clean and disinfect correctly.

Always follow label directions on cleaning products and disinfectants. Wash surfaces with a general household cleaner to remove germs. Rinse with water, and follow with an EPA-registered disinfectant to kill germs. Read the label to make sure it states that EPA has approved the product for effectiveness against influenza A virus.

If an EPA-registered disinfectant is not available, use a fresh chlorine bleach solution. To make and use the solution:

- Add 1 tablespoon of bleach to 1 quart (4 cups) of water. For a larger supply of disinfectant, add ¼ cup of bleach to 1 gallon (16 cups) of water.
- Apply the solution to the surface with a cloth.
- Let it stand for 3 to 5 minutes.
- Rinse the surface with clean water.

If a surface is not visibly dirty, you can clean it with an EPA-registered product that both cleans (removes germs) and disinfects (kills germs) instead. Be sure to read the label directions carefully, as there may be a separate procedure for using the product as a cleaner or as a disinfectant. Disinfection usually requires the product to remain on the surface for a certain period of time.

Use disinfecting wipes on electronic items that are touched often, such as phones and computers. Pay close attention to the directions for using disinfecting wipes. It may be necessary to use more than one wipe to keep the surface wet for the stated length of contact time. Make sure that the electronics can withstand the use of liquids for cleaning and disinfecting.

Routinely wash eating utensils in a dishwasher or by hand with soap and water. Wash and dry bed sheets, towels, and other linens as you normally do with household laundry soap, according to the fabric labels. Eating utensils, dishes, and linens used by sick persons do not need to be cleaned separately, but they should not be shared unless they've been washed thoroughly. Wash your hands with soap and water after handling soiled dishes and laundry items.

5. Use products safely.

Pay close attention to hazard warnings and directions on product labels. Cleaning products and disinfectants often call for the use of gloves or eye protection. For example, gloves should always be worn to protect your hands when working with bleach solutions.

Do not mix cleaners and disinfectants unless the labels indicate it is safe to do so. Combining certain products (such as chlorine bleach and ammonia cleaners) can result in serious injury or death.

Ensure that custodial staff, teachers, and others who use cleaners and disinfectants read and understand all instruction labels and understand safe and appropriate use. This might require that instructional materials and training be provided in other languages.

6. Handle waste properly.

Follow your school's standard procedures for handling waste, which may include wearing gloves. Place no-touch waste baskets where they are easy to use. Throw disposable items used to clean surfaces and items in the trash immediately after use. Avoid touching used tissues and other waste when emptying waste baskets. Wash your hands with soap and water after emptying waste baskets and touching used tissues and similar waste.

www.cdc.gov/flu/school

1-800-CDC-INFO

PART II

Skills Development

CHAPTER 7
Deciphering Lesson Plans and Goals

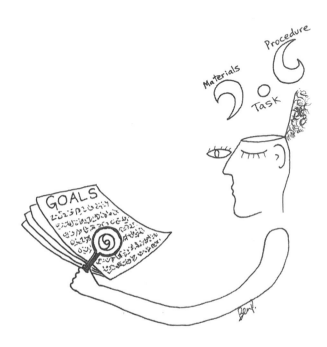

Our goals can only be reached through a vehicle of a plan, in which we must fervently believe, and upon which we must vigorously act. There is no other route to success.

Pablo Picasso (famous artist)

As discussed in Chapter 1, one of the job responsibilities within the scope of duties of a speech-language pathology assistant (SLPA) is to follow treatment plans/protocols developed by the speech-language pathologist (SLP) (American Speech-Language-Hearing Association [ASHA], 2013b). Specifically, ASHA states that SLPAs may execute specific components of a treatment plan if (ASHA, n.d.-a, Key Issues, Scope of SLPAs, para. 1):

- The goals and objectives listed on the treatment plan and implemented by the SLPA are only those within the SLPA's scope of practice and are tasks the SLP has determined the SLPA has the training and skill to perform.
- The SLP provides at least the minimum specified level of supervision to ensure quality

of care to all persons served. The amount of supervision may vary and must depend on the complexity of the case and the experience of the assistant.

Before services can be implemented by an SLPA, it is the responsibility of the supervising SLP to develop an individualized treatment plan for each client. The first step in this process is an assessment (also known as an evaluation). This is conducted solely by an SLP (ASHA, 2013b). If treatment is recommended, a treatment plan is then developed (also by the SLP) in which specific treatment goals are outlined. In some settings, assessment results and a treatment plan are summarized in a single document. In other settings, this information is summarized in separate documents. The appendices of this chapter contain sample reports from an educational setting, including an individualized education plan (IEP) (Appendix 7–A), private practice (Appendix 7–B), and medical settings (Appendix 7–C). In some settings, these documents may be stored in a paper file. In other settings, this information is stored and accessed electronically (Krebs, 2008).

As discussed in Chapter 3, in all settings, these documents and the specifics of a client's treatment are strictly confidential and not to be shared with unauthorized individuals (ASHA, 2013a). You may not bring these documents home to review, nor may you send them or discuss their content with anyone not authorized access to this information. As an SLPA, you should familiarize yourself with the form of documentation used in your setting and how to access this information. If you are asked to provide services to a client, you should review the client's assessment report(s) and treatment plan in detail. Be sure to ask your supervising SLP if you have any questions about this documentation.

LESSON PLANS

After a treatment plan is developed by your supervising SLP, the next step is to explore specific details on how to implement this plan for each individual client. How this information is conveyed to you and the format of this documentation will vary across settings and supervisors. In some settings, a lesson plan is used to outline additional information needed to implement treatment (ASHA, 2009). It may be that you are required to develop a draft of this plan for your supervisor to review, prior to implementing treatment. In other settings, this plan will be developed for you by your supervising SLP. In both instances, collaboration between you and your supervising SLP is required.

The concept of a lesson plan is borrowed from the field of education and was originally designed as a detailed description of the instruction to be provided by a teacher during a given class session (Karges-Bone, 2000). When applied to the field of speech-language pathology, lesson plans highlight important details and procedures for a single treatment session(s) to be provided over a short period (e.g., over 1 or 2 weeks) (Hegde & Davis, 2010; Meyer, 2004). A lesson plan recommended by ASHA (2009) for use by SLPAs contains the core components of the treatment goals (Goals and Objectives), a description of the materials and equipment needed that session (Materials/Equipment), a description of the activity/task to be used (Activity/Task), and columns used to suggest applicable modifications (Make It Easier/Make It More Difficult). Commonly, the column for modifications is also referred to as "Prompts/Modifications." Lesson plans can also include information on the client's performance (Data Collection), either as a description of data to be collected that particular session or, if used during the session, as a summary of the client's actual performance.

An example of a lesson plan containing these components is available in Figure 7–1. Depending on the setting, some or all of these categories may be preferred. The CD of this textbook contains additional blank copies of lesson plans applicable for SLPA use. The sections that follow address each component of this plan in greater detail. It is important that you clearly understand each component of this plan *before* you have any contact with a client. The importance of this cannot be overemphasized. To do this, as the picture and title of this chapter suggests, you must *decipher* this information very carefully.

Goals and Objectives

The Goals and Objectives section of a lesson plan will list the goals and objectives to be targeted during a given treatment session(s). Understanding goals and objectives can be very challenging for a new SLPA as the language used is often unfamiliar and complex. Take heart, though: With time and exposure to this terminology, this process gets easier. Goals and objectives are important because they guide the selection of therapy materials, content, and procedures (Mager, 1997). They also serve as the basis for determining if a behavior has been accomplished and, importantly, provide those involved (including the client and the clinician) a full description of the desired outcome(s) of treatment (Mager, 1997). Furthermore, in some settings, they are also used directly for reimbursement purposes (Cornett, 2010). Although SLPAs do not write or modify goals, it is still valuable to review their format in helping you to *decipher* them.

Defining Goals

Treatment goals are statements of an outcome to be obtained. Traditionally defined, goals describe a behavior to be accomplished over the course of treatment (Roth & Worthington, 2001). Goals may or may not state a terminal behavior to be accomplished but generally are targeted over months or often, as in the case of a school setting, within an academic term. For example, a traditionally defined goal might be, "The client will read at grade level." By their nature, goals are broad statements of behavior; however, increasingly, the term *long-term goal* is used to identify a goal that states the behavior to be accomplished but also includes additional measurable terms (e.g., increase, decrease, maintain) and an expected ending level of performance, such as, "The student will increase the number of conversational topics that he spontaneously initiates (with no verbal or other prompts) in a student-adult conversation from one to four" (Minneapolis Public Schools, 2009). In some settings, the terms *goal* and *long-term goal* are used interchangeably, and in other settings, a general goal is followed by a set of specific long-term goals. The term *annual goal* may also be used to denote a goal that is to be accomplished that year, such as "By (annual IEP date), [the student] will

Client Name: Joseph Jones		Teacher/Room #: Wilson 12			
SLPA: Sarah S. Assistant		Supervising SLP: Samantha A. Supervisor			
Session Date(s): Week of 2/18/2013					
Goal/Objective	Activity/Task	Materials/ Equipment	Make it Easier	Make it More Difficult	Data Collection
Joseph will produce /ʃ/ in the initial positions of words with 90% accuracy, across 10 attempts in 2 separate sessions.	Go Fish: Have Joseph ask for cards with words containing the /ʃ/ in the initial position (e.g., ship, shell, she). If he accurately produces the target, reinforce this by stating yes I have a _____, or, No I don't have a _____ (as applicable), emphasizing the /ʃ/ sound. If he inaccurately produces the target sound, model a correct version and an incorrect version and ask him to clarify by re-attempting (e.g., "did you want a ___ (/ʃ/ accurately produced) or a ___ (/ʃ/ distorted production?")	Go Fish cards containing CVC words with /ʃ/ in the initial position of words (e.g., ship, shell, she) Reminder card with picture of hand over lip to represent /ʃ/ Mirror	Point to the reminder card and/or model lip rounding before each production and after production error. Give him cards with the word written on it and the /ʃ/ underlined	Require him to have accurate production for the target word AND Go Fish When he lays down his pairs, reference it as "shelving" and have him name the pairs he obtained in the sentence, "I'll shelve 2 ___, with correct production of /ʃ/ in shelve and the target word.	+ = Accuracy (no cues/modification) +C= Accurate with cues. Note cues • M = verbal model • V = visual reminder • W = Written word CA = close approximation – = Inaccurate, Despite cues

Figure 7–1. Sample SLPA lesson plan.

listen attentively by using appropriate eye contact, body language, and/or proximity during oral communication in class in [8 out of 10] opportunities" (Porter & Steffin, 2006, p. 13).

Defining Objectives

Objectives accompany goals and are a series of steps needed to accomplish the desired behavior listed in the goal. Objectives are also referred to as short-term objectives or, in some settings, are called *short-term goals* or *benchmarks*. Very precise and measurable language is used in objectives to state not only the behavior to be obtained but at what level, by when, and under what conditions (Meyer, 2004; Roth & Paul, 2007; Roth & Worthington, 2001). Box 7–1 lists three key components of objectives: the performance (or do statement), the condition, and the *criterion* (singular) or *criteria* (plural) (Meyer, 2004; Roth & Paul, 2007; Roth & Worthington, 2001). Appendix 7–D contains examples of goals and objectives from real-world settings.

To decipher goals and objectives, you can ask yourself specific questions about what is written and what additional information is needed, such as the questions listed in Box 7–2. In the area of performance, the performance statement needs to be something that you can actually observe, meaning you can see or hear it (Meyer, 2004; Roth & Paul, 2007). If the performance is not something that you can observe, the objective cannot be implemented. For example, verbs that describe performance, such as *understand, analyze,* and *process,* are not something you can see or hear, and as such, without further clarification, you would have no way of knowing if the client was performing the required task(s). Hence, in

terms of the performance (or do) portion of an objective, you can ask yourself the following:

1. Is the performance stated?
2. What is the performance?
3. Is the performance observable (e.g., can I see it or hear it)?
4. What additional information is needed?

Similarly, a condition statement must be something that you as an SLPA can reproduce.

For example, in an objective targeting pragmatics, the condition of "when speaking with grade-level peers" cannot be replicated in a one-on-one session with the clinician. Similarly, if a fluency goal included a condition of "during episodes of blocking" but you do not know what an episode of blocking is, you would not be able to replicate that condition. As such, it is important to ask yourself the following:

1. Is the condition stated?
2. What is the condition?
3. Can I replicate the condition?
4. What additional information is needed?

Last, the criterion of an objective must be stated in a way that you can measure it. The information you record is often referred to as *data.* As will be discussed, this will be the information that is typically listed under "Data Collection" in the lesson plan. In order for you to measure and record the client's performance on a given task, the criterion portion of an objective must be something that you can effectively measure. For example, if a criterion states, "with fewer than one stuttered word," but you are not familiar with what to count as a stuttered word, you will not be able to record the client's

Box 7–1. Key Components of Behavioral Objectives

Performance: States what a client is expected to do to demonstrate mastery of the objective, including the *quality*[1] and *nature*[1] of performance. This is sometimes referred to as the "do" statement because it states what the client will do (e.g., the client will . . .).[2]

Examples:

Independently say the names of primary colors

Legibly write the numbers 1 to 10

Spontaneously greet members of the social group

Accurately produce the phoneme /t/ in the final positions of words

Condition: States what the client will be provided with (or denied) when performing the behavior, including (as applicable) terms to define the location,[1] with whom,[1] and given what type of assistance.[1]

Examples:

In the community, with a typical peer

During a classroom group-reading activity, given a story starter

In a one-on-one setting, given a verbal model from the clinician

In response to a written command, without verbal cues to initiate

Criterion: States how the objective will be evaluated and in some cases by when the behavior is to be accomplished, including as applicable the frequency, duration, accuracy, latency/speed, and/or intensity of a behavior.[1]

Examples:

With 80% accuracy, given at least 20 attempts

Within 2 minutes of a verbal prompt, in 8 of 10 opportunities

For 2 minutes on two separate occasions

---

performance accurately. Similarly, if the criterion calls for "80% accuracy" in the accurate production of /r/, but you cannot accurately distinguish between correct, partially correct, and incorrect production of /r/, you will not be accurate in recording information about the client's performance. If parts of the criterion are

> **Box 7–2. Deciphering Goals/Objectives: Questions to Ask**
>
> **PERFORMANCE**
>
> Is the performance stated? ☐ YES ☐ NO
>
> What is the performance required? _____
>
> Can I observe the performance? ☐ YES ☐ NO
>
> Additional information needed?
>
> **CONDITION**
>
> Is the condition stated? ☐ YES ☐ NO
>
> What is the condition? _____
>
> Can I replicate the condition? ☐ YES ☐ NO
>
> Additional information needed?
>
> **CRITERION**
>
> Is the criterion stated? ☐ YES ☐ NO
>
> What is the criterion? _____
>
> Can I measure the criterion? ☐ YES ☐ NO
>
> Additional information needed?

missing, it is also impossible to record data accurately. As such, in deciphering the criterion of an objective, ask yourself the following:

1. Is the criterion stated?
2. What is the criterion?
3. Can I measure the criterion (e.g., collect data)?
4. What additional information is needed?

Any time you have a question or need additional clarification, be sure to ask your supervisor *before* you implement any treatment activity. The CD of this textbook contains a sample worksheet with these questions. Appendix 7–D contains sample goals and objectives from real-world settings. The sample reports in Appendices 7–A to 7–C also contain samples of goals and objective. A good way to develop your skills in deciphering goals and objectives is to use these examples to practice your skills in the area of identifying the performance, condition, and criterion and in asking important questions about each.

Activity/Task

The Activity/Task section of a lesson plan will contain information relative to the type of activity or task to be used during treatment in addressing a specific goal or objective. Although objectives are detailed in their format/language, they can often be addressed utilizing a variety of activities or tasks, selected based on the client's interests, age, and specific needs. For example, consider the objective, "The client will request objects by pointing to an icon in his AAC device, in 9 of 10 opportunities." If this is implemented with a 6-year-old boy with autism who likes trains, an activity to target this goal may be to have the client build a train track by requesting different colors and types of trains, track, and other building materials, using a train theme page from his AAC notebook. In contrast, if this same objective is implemented with an adult with aphasia who enjoys cooking, the activity may be to follow a recipe in baking a cake by requesting needed items from the cooking page on her voice output AAC device.

Your supervising SLP will assist you in determining the type of activity/task most appropriate for each client. The chapters that follow on play and literacy (Chapter 12), speech sound remediation (Chapter 13), and group therapy (Chapter 11) each provide some sample tasks and activities in these areas. A review of sample activities across all ages and disorders is beyond the scope of this book; however, here are a few suggestions that will help in familiarizing you with an activity/task prior to implementing treatment:

1. *Self-study.* Before you engage in treatment activities with a new client, you should review treatment information specific to the client's disorder and unique presentation. Many resources, both online and in traditional treatment textbooks in communicative dis-

orders, provide both a general framework of treatment techniques and a list of sample activities/tasks, which may be used given specific treatment objectives or approaches. If you are not familiar with how to access this information, ask your supervising SLP for assistance.

2. *Observe.* Observe your supervising SLP engaging in the activity/task prior to implementing it yourself. This is valuable in helping you understand nuances that are not easily conveyed in a written description. Be sure to take notes during this observation so that you can refer back to them prior to implementing treatment.

3. *Role-play.* Role-play the activity/task with your supervising SLP. This is also an excellent way to become comfortable with implementing an activity/task. Be sure to play the role of the therapist during this role-play, as this is the role you will play when implementing treatment.

4. *Ask questions.* During supervisory conferences, be sure to clarify any questions you may have about a specific activity/task. Ask, too, about the "whys" of the activity/task. This will be of value in understanding the SLP's rationale for selecting that particular activity/task.

Materials/Equipment

The Materials/Equipment section of a lesson plan lists any materials or equipment needed to implement treatment. This could be wide ranging, including items specific to the activity/task itself, such as pictures, worksheets, toys and games, tokens for reinforcement, and so on. This may also include items needed to record a client's performance, such as a specific score sheet, audio recorder, and so forth. When the materials are used specifically in treatment to elicit a target response, this is referred to as *stimuli* (plural) or *stimulus* (singular). As an SLPA, you should ensure you have these items ready and accessible *before* the treatment session begins. Be sure to review your material and equipment well ahead of time to make sure it is in good working order. This ensures that no time is wasted once the session begins in locating missing items or in repairing/troubleshooting malfunctioning equipment. Chapter 10 provides some general principles in selecting appropriate stimuli, as do Chapters 11, 12, and 13. Remember as well, as discussed in Chapter 6, all equipment and materials used must be properly cleaned for use in any treatment session.

Prompts and Modifications (Also Known as Make It Easier/Make It More Difficult)

This section of an SLPA lesson plan includes any suggested modifications to the activity/task that could be employed to reduce or increase task demands, including any recommended prompts or assistance appropriate to the task. Remember, treatment is a dynamic process. It may be that a given activity or task needs to be adjusted slightly to increase the client's participation and thereby address the desired objective. These modifications are not intended to alter the treatment goals or objectives but rather meant to enhance participation in the designated activity/task. As with all aspects of the client's treatment, these should be discussed with the supervising SLP. Recognize as well that formats of a lesson plan vary across settings, and as such, not all supervising

SLPs will use or require this information on a lesson plan. If not, it will be important for you to discuss this information with your supervising SLP to ensure that you understand how to modify an activity or task appropriately (if needed) so that it remains consistent with the SLP's treatment plan for that particular client. Chapter 10 provides information on prompts and cues, as well as a discussion on the use of reinforcement in shaping behaviors. These are an important part of task/activity modification. Box 7–3 also contains examples of techniques to modify an activity/task, by altering the time constraints, tasks demands, or reinforcement provided. Not all modifications are equally applicable to all objectives, particularly if the modification changes the task sufficient to alter a treatment objective's condition, performance, or criterion. This is not the purpose of these modifications. For example, if the objective was, "The student will use present progressive tense when describing pictures not visible to the clinician in 18 of 20 attempts," but you made the task easier by requiring the client to repeat after you a list of 20 verbs in present progressive tense, the activity would no longer be targeting the desired objective. As an SLPA, you must not modify elements of a treatment activity/task, which alter the treatment plan (ASHA, 2013).

Data Collection

Recording data about the client's performance is critical (Mowrer, 1982). As an SLPA, accurate data collection is particularly important in that you are the eyes and ears for your supervising SLP when you are implementing treatment and she or he is not present to observe the client's

Box 7–3. Potential Modifications in Activity/Task

1. Increase or decrease *time constraints*

   EXAMPLES

   - Give the client more time to respond (make it easier)
   - Require a quicker response (make it more difficult)
   - Give more breaks between responses (make it easier)
   - Require more responses in a shorter period (e.g., fewer breaks) (make it more difficult)

2. Increase or decrease the task *demands*

   EXAMPLES

   - Require a fully correct response (make it more difficult)
   - Accept a partially correct response (make it easier)
   - Require a shorter or less complex response (make it easier)
   - Require a longer or more complex response (make it more difficult)

3. Increase or decrease the *reinforcement* provided

   EXAMPLES

   - Provide reinforcement after every response (make it easier)
   - Provide intermittent reinforcement (make it more difficult)
   - Provide tangible reinforcement (make it easier)
   - Provide token reinforcement (make it more difficult)

performance. The Data Collection section of a lesson plan could include a description of any specific or important aspects of the information to be recorded that session. In some cases, lesson plans may also include spaces for you to record the data from a specific session on the lesson plan itself. In that case, the lesson plan doubles as a data collection sheet as well. Data collection is discussed in detail in Chapter 8. Chapter 9 addresses how to summarize this information effectively in a note about treatment.

REFERENCES

American Speech-Language-Hearing Association (ASHA). (n.d.-a). *Speech-language pathology assistants*. Retrieved from http://www.asha.org/Practice-Portal/Professional-Issues/Speech-Language-Pathology-Assistants/

American Speech-Language-Hearing Association (ASHA). (n.d.-b). *Writing measurable goals and objectives*. Retrieved February 9, 2013, from http://www.asha.org/uploadedFiles/Writing-Measurable-Goals-and-Objectives.pdf

American Speech-Language-Hearing Association (ASHA). (2009). *Practical tools and forms* for supervising speech-language pathology assistants. Rockville, MD: Author.

American Speech-Language-Hearing Association (ASHA). (2013a). *Confidentiality.* Retrieved from http://www.asha.org/policy

American Speech-Language-Hearing Association (ASHA). (2013b). *Speech-language pathology assistant scope of practice.* Retrieved from http://www.asha.org/policy

Cornett, B. S. (2010, August). Health care reform and speech-language pathology practice. *ASHA Leader.* Retrieved from http://www.asha.org/Publications/leader/2010/100803/Health-Care-Reform-SLP.htm.

Hegde, M. N., & Davis, D. (2010). *Clinical methods and practicum in speech-language pathology* (5th ed.). Clifton Park, NY: Delmar.

Karges-Bone, L. (2000). *Lesson planning: Long-range and short-range models for grades K–6.* Boston, MA: Allyn & Bacon.

Krebs, J. M. (2008, September). Paper, paper everywhere? How to go paperless in your private practice. *ASHA Leader.*

Mager, R. F. (1997). *Preparing instructional objectives: A critical tool in the development of effective instruction.* Atlanta, GA: Center for Effective Performance Press.

Meyer, S. M. (2004). *Survival guide for beginning speech-language clinician* (2nd ed.). Austin, TX: Pro-Ed.

Minneapolis Public Schools. (2009). *Consensus points on language goals.* Retrieved from http://www.asha.org/uploadedFiles/Consensus-Points-on-Language-Goals.pdf

Mower, D. E. (1982). *Methods of modifying speech behaviors: Learning theory in speech pathology.* Prospect Heights, IL: Waveland.

Porter, J., & Steffin, B. (2006). *Speech-language pathology goals and objectives written to the California standards.* Retrieved on February 9, 2013, from http://www.csha.org/pdf/SLPGoalsandObjectivesupdate.pdf

Roth, F., & Paul, R. (2007). Communication intervention. In R. Paul & P. Cascella (Eds.), *Introduction to clinical methods in communication disorders* (pp. 157–178). Baltimore, MD: Paul H. Brookes.

Roth, F. P., & Worthington, C. K. (2001). *Treatment resource manual for speech-language pathologists* (2nd ed.). Albany, NY: Delmar.

CHAPTER ENDNOTES

1. ASHA (n.d.-b)
2. Roth and Paul (2007) and Roth and Worthington (2001)

APPENDIX 7-A
Educational Setting—Sample Reports

INITIAL SPEECH-LANGUAGE ASSESSMENT—PRESCHOOL

ABC School District

Initial Speech-Language Assessment Report

Student:	XXXXXXX
DOB:	XXXXXXX
Parents:	XXXXXXX
Address:	XXXXXXX
Assessment conducted by:	XXXXXXXX, CCC-SLP
Assessment dates:	March 16, 2012, March 17, 2012, and March 18, 2012
Report date:	April 2012

Reason for Referral:
This assessment was conducted at the request of the child's parents. Specifically, they reported that XXXXXX is difficult to understand without context, uses short utterances, and is easily frustrated. His parents indicated that XXXXXX's frustration is due at least in part because he is unable to express himself for his wants and needs.

Brief Background Information:
XXXXXX is a 2-year, 11-month-old boy whose primary language is English, although some French is spoken in the home. He resides with his parents and a younger sibling. There is no history of ear infections and no reported serious accidents or illnesses. The family receives private, in-home behavioral therapy to address XXXXXX's disruptive behavior and tantrums.

Behavioral Observations:
XXXXXX presented as a pleasant, inquisitive, and well-behaved child. Good rapport was established with this examiner after a brief "warming up" period. XXXXXX's father remained present during the assessment. XXXXXX participated fully in the assessment process and completed all necessary testing to obtain present levels of speech and language function. Testing took place over three sessions lasting approximately 1 hour each, and XXXXXX received snacks and breaks as needed.

Over the course of assessment, XXXXXX was easily distracted; however, when redirected, he was able to re-engage with this examiner and return to the task. He appeared to put forth his best effort during the course of testing and appeared to understand the directions presented by this examiner.

Assessment Results:

Assessment was conducted at a local elementary school in the speech-language therapy room. Test materials used have been validated for the specific purposes for which they were used. Assessment results are considered a valid estimate of XXXXXX's current level of performance.

Assessments Administered:

Parent Interview

Informal Language Observation

Clinical Assessment of Articulation and Phonology (CAAP)

Receptive One-Word Picture Vocabulary Test (ROWPVT)

Expressive One-Word Picture Vocabulary Test (EOWPVT)

Preschool Language Scales-5 (PLS-5)

Language Sample

Oral-Peripheral Examination

Informal Observation (voice, fluency, and intelligibility)

(See Appendices at the end of the report for test validity statements and test score description)

Articulation:

Speech Production Abilities:

The Clinical Assessment of Articulation and Phonology (CAAP) was administered to assess XXXXXX's speech production. The CAAP is a norm-referenced assessment that measures articulation and phonology in preschool and school-age children ages 2 years, 6 months to 8 years, 11 months. The results of this assessment follow:

Consonant Inventory Score	55
Standard Score	64
Percentile	3

XXXXXX's standard score of 64 is significantly below average.

Performance summary:

Single phonemes: As demonstrated in the following chart, which classifies phonemes by typical age of acquisition, XXXXXX's performance on the CAAP revealed the following specific articulation errors:

Typical Age of Mastery*	Phonemes	Misarticulated Sound/Location	Error Example
4 Years	/p/, /b/, /m/, /n/, /w/, /h/, /k/, /g/, /f/, /d/, /j/	/p/ final position /b/ final position /g/ final position /f/ final positions	[shee] for /sheep/ [we] for /web/ [do] for /dog/ [kni] for /knife/
6 Years	/ŋ/, /t/, /l/, /r/	/ŋ/ final position /t/ initial and final position /l/ final position	[ki] for /king/ [ees] for /teeth/ [da] for /gate/ [heza] for /seal/
7 Years	/sh/, /ch/, /dg/, /th/	/ch/ final position /dg/ final position /th/ (voiceless) initial and final positions	[raw] for /watch/ [ka] for /cadge/ [fum] for /thumb/ [ees] for /teeth/
8 Years	/v/, /s/, /z/, /ð/	/v/ final positions /s/ initial /z/ initial and final /th/ (voiced) initial and final positions	[hi] for /hive/ [heza] for /seal/ [do] for /zoo/ [chee] for /cheese/ [vem] for /them/ [ba] for /bathe/

*Gordon-Brannan and Weiss, 2007.

Stimulability: XXXXXX was stimulable for several erred sounds including /gate/ and /star/, but was unable to produce /thumb/, /them/, or /clown/ given an immediate model.

Phonological processes: Phonological processes are sound production patterns, or simplifications, that are different from typical adult pronunciations and are used by children as they develop their phonological system. A phonological process is considered active if it occurs 40% of the time or more in a given sample. XXXXXX demonstrated the following phonological processes:

Final Consonant Deletion (85%):   [pi] for /pig/

Cluster Reduction (70%):   [fwa] for /flag/

Vocalization (100%):   [koo] for /school/

As indicated above, phonological processes are normal in a child's early speech development, and the above processes, with the exception of vocalization, are found in the speech repertoire in typically developing children. The above noted errors significantly reduce XXXXXX's intelligibility.

<u>Multisyllabic words:</u> In addition to assessment on single-syllable words, XXXXXX was assessed on multisyllabic words, which require additional sequencing, planning, and precision. The error patterns and phonological processes XXXXXX demonstrated on the single-syllable words were mirrored in the multisyllabic words.

Vocabulary Development:

The <u>Receptive One-Word Picture Vocabulary Test</u> (ROWPVT-4) was administered to assess XXXXXX's ability to comprehend age-level vocabulary items. For this assessment, XXXXXX was asked to point to objects, actions, and concepts pictured in a field of four illustrations. XXXXXX demonstrated receptive vocabulary skill within the average range. The results are as follows:

Results of ROWPVT-4

Raw Score	31
Standard Score	98
Percentile	45

The <u>Expressive One-Word Picture Vocabulary Test</u> (EOWPVT) was administered to assess XXXXXX's ability to name specific items (i.e., concepts, objects, and actions) pictured in a field of four illustrations. XXXXXX's ability to use a wide variety of vocabulary items falls in the average range. The results are as follows:

Results of EOWPVT-4

Raw Score	23
Standard Score	92
Percentile	30

Language Functioning:

The <u>Preschool Language Scales-5</u> (PLS-5) was administered to gain insight into XXXXXX's comprehensive developmental language skills. This instrument is interactive and play based and is designed for children from birth through age 7. Items assessed range from preverbal interactional skills to emergent language and early literacy. The results are as follows:

Modality	Standard Score	Percentile
Auditory Comprehension	87	19
Expressive Communication	85	16
Total Language Score	85	16

On the *Auditory Comprehension* portion of the assessment, XXXXXX responded correctly to the following:

- Identification of familiar items (i.e., block, cup, car)
- Understanding of object use (i.e., "show me what you use to drink water")
- Identification of colors (i.e., "show me the blue crayon")

Examples of items XXXXXX was unable to respond to correctly include:

- Recognizing actions in pictures (i.e., "show me the child who is washing")
- Understanding of spatial concepts (i.e., "put box on the table")

XXXXXX's performance on the Auditory Comprehension portion of the PLS-5 falls in the low average range.

On the *Expressive Communication* portion of the assessment, XXXXXX responded correctly to the following:

- Naming objects in photographs
- Using a variety of words (e.g., girl, kids, truck)
- Using words for a variety of functions (e.g., requesting objects, actions, assistance)

Examples of items XXXXXX was unable to respond to correctly include:

- Using different word combinations (i.e., verb + noun/pronoun)
- Using words more often than gestures to communicate

XXXXXX's performance on the Expressive Communication portion of the PLS-5 falls in the low average range.

Performance Summary:
XXXXXX's Total Language score on the PLS-5 falls in the low average range. While XXXXXX performed very comparably across the two modalities, he demonstrated a slight advantage in his ability to comprehend spoken language.

<u>Language Sample</u>
A language sample was obtained on March 16th and March 18th during the parent interview and during the psychological and speech-language assessments. During these sessions, XXXXXX generally played quietly and independently at a table with toys (i.e., cars, trucks, pencils). He interacted verbally with his father to a request (e.g., "cars!") and occasionally to comment (e.g., "the kids"). After some initial reticence, he responded verbally to questions and commands delivered by the school psychologist and this examiner, and demonstrated limited verbal interaction during play sequences with this examiner.

During these observations, XXXXXX did not demonstrate a significant number of spontaneous utterances; as such a formal language sample with a minimum of 50 utterances could not be obtained. However, XXXXXX's limited spontaneous language was analyzed, specifically his observed phrase length and his language form (e.g., inflectional markers, parts of speech, etc.). Overall, XXXXXX used one-word phrases, regular plurals, and negation. Examples of his spontaneous utterances follow:

- "The dogs!"
- "Car!"
- "Truck!"
- "Nana."
- "Boy."
- "No!"

While a formal language sample was not obtained, it can be inferred from his spontaneous language use that XXXXXX uses shorter phrases than would be expected based on criterion-referenced norms of utterance length, which suggest that a child 2 years, 11 months of age typically and consistently uses phrases that contain between 2.5 to 3.5 words (Paul & Norbury, 2012).

During a play sequence scaffolded by this examiner (e.g., playing with cars), XXXXXX consistently produced two-word phrases appropriate to an accompanying action (e.g., "truck go," "truck stop," "truck crash!"). This ability to imitate the modeled language may be suggestive of an emerging expansion of phrase length.

Oral-Peripheral Examination:
The Oral-Peripheral Examination is an exam that views structures organically and functionally for speech production adequacy. External structures and muscles of the face, lips, and jaw were judged to be within normal limits for speech production.

Voice and Fluency:
Voice quality was judged to be age and gender appropriate. No abnormal disfluencies were observed.

Intelligibility:
Per observation by this examiner, XXXXXX was 80% intelligible at the single-syllable, single-word level with context. At the short phrase level, he was 70% intelligible with context and 60% intelligible without context.

Summary and Impressions:
XXXXXX, at 2 years, 11 months of age, presents with a speech and language disorder, as evidenced by significant speech-sound errors and impaired expressive communication abilities. Relative strengths are noted in XXXXXX's receptive language functioning, particularly in the area of receptive vocabulary development. Significant deficits and delays were noted in his speech sound development. These phonological delays are readily apparent and appear to be affecting all areas of expressive language development.

It can be inferred from these findings that XXXXXX's speech and language impairments present no indication of spontaneous recovery and may significantly interfere with his ability to communicate with others, attract adverse attention, and adversely affect his educational performance.

<u>Recommendations:</u>
Members of the Individualized Education Program team need to review the above information along with other pertinent information to determine the Least Restrictive Environment and the most appropriate education setting and interventions to meet the student's education needs.

_____

Speech-Language Pathologist

INDIVIDUALIZED EDUCATION PLAN—ELEMENTARY SCHOOL

EFG School District

☐ Written Translation Requested
Language: English

Individualized Education Program

Last Name XXXXXX
First Name XXXXXX
Student ID XXXXXX
IEP Date 4/14/11
Next IEP 4/14/2012
Last Annual IEP 4/14/2012
Last Eval 4/14/2011
SPED Entry Date 4/15/2011

Purpose of Meeting: ☒ Initial ☐ Annual ☐ Triennial ☐ Transition
☐ Pre-expulsion ☐ Interim ☐ Expanded ☐ Other: _____

DOB: 11/9/2004 ☐ F ☒ M   **Grade**: Kindergarten   **Migrant:** ☐ Yes ☒ No

Home Language: English   **EL:** ☐ Yes ☒ No ☐ Redesignated
Interpreter: ☐ Yes ☒ No

Residency: Parent or Legal Guardian
School Attending: ABC Elementary School

Parent/Guardian: XXXXX

District of Residence: EFG School District
School of Residence: ABC Elementary School

Ethnicity: 1. WHITE____ 2. _____ 3. _____ 4. _____

211

Primary Disability   Eligible for Special Education   ⦿ Yes   O No

O Autism (AUT)	O Hard of Hearing (HH)*	O Other Health Impairment (OHI)
O Deaf-Blindness (DB)*	O Mental Retardation (MR)	⦿ Specific Learning Disability (SLD)
O Deafness (DEAF)*	O Multiple Disability (MD)	O Speech/Language Impairment (SLI)
O Emotional Disturbance (ED)	O None	O Traumatic Brain Injury (TBI)
O Established Medical Disability (EMD)	O Orthopedic Impairment (Ol)*	O Visual Impairment (VI)*

Secondary Disability

O Autism (AUT)	O Hard of Hearing (HH)*	O Other Health Impairment (OHI)
O Deaf-Blindness (DB)*	O Mental Retardation (MR)	⦿ Specific Learning Disability (SLD)
O Deafness (DEAF)*	O Multiple Disability (MD)	O Speech/Language Impairment (SLI)
O Emotional Disturbance (ED)	O None	O Traumatic Brain Injury (TBI)
O Established Medical Disability (EMD)	O Orthopedic Impairment (Ol)*	O Visual Impairment (VI)*

*Low Incidence Disability

Eligibility Statement:

A severe discrepancy exists between intellectual ability and academic achievement in the areas of written expression and listening comprehension. XXX evidences processing disorders in the area(s) of *Attention* (the ability to sustain attention and concentrate on a task or activity) as well as a personal weakness in *Auditory Processing* (the ability to recognize, perceive, and interpret auditory stimuli).

Describe how the student's disability affects involvement and progress in the general curriculum (or, for preschoolers, participation in appropriate activities): He will benefit from small group and individual specialized instruction that is not available in the general class.

For Initial Placement Only

Has the student received prereferral early intervening services in the past 2 years?

☒ Yes   ☐ No

Date of initial referral for special education services: 2/17/2011

Person initiating the referral for special education service: Student study/intervention team

Date district received parental consent: 2/17/2011

Date of initial meeting to determine eligibility: 4/14/2011

PRESENT LEVELS OF ACADEMIC ACHIEVEMENT/ FUNCTIONAL PERFORMANCE

Educational Strengths/Preferences/Interests
He tries to work in small groups. He enjoys working on the computer and uses the DS game at home.

Concerns of parent relevant to educational progress
Mom is concerned about his reading. Mom indicated he had 2 full years of preschool. When he doesn't want to work, he stops working completely.

State Standards

English/Language Arts	□ Adv.	□ Proficient	□ Basic	□ Below Basic	□ Far Below Basic
Mathematics	□ Adv.	□ Proficient	□ Basic	□ Below Basic	□ Far Below Basic
Hist./Soc. Science	□ Adv.	□ Proficient	□ Basic	□ Below Basic	□ Far Below Basic
Science	□ Adv.	□ Proficient	□ Basic	□ Below Basic	□ Far Below Basic

Most Recent Scores

Listening _____ Speaking _____ Reading _____ Writing _____

Fitness/PE Test (Grades 5, 7, & 9 only) _____

Other Assessment Data (e.g., curriculum assessment, other district assessment, etc.)

DRA Level 1, knows 8 of 27 kindergarten sight words, almost all capital and lower case letters

Hearing _____ □ Pass □ Fail □ Other: _____
Vision _____ □ Pass □ Fail □ Other: _____

The **Brief Written Language**- <k.0; Spelling subtest-<k.0; requires the production of single letters and words in response to oral prompts, **Writing Samples** subtest- <k.0; measures the ability to convey ideas in writing; requires the production of meaningful written sentences in response to a variety of task criteria.

213

The **Listening Comprehension** cluster provides a measure of achievement including understanding directions and comprehending oral language. XXX's overall listening comprehension ability is within the low average range. His performances on the Understanding Directions and Oral Comprehension subtests were within the low range.

Cognitive Functioning
The assessments results indicate that XXX meets eligibility criteria for SLD. A severe discrepancy exists between intellectual ability and academic achievement in the areas of written expression and listening comprehension. XXX evidences processing disorders in the area(s) of *Attention* (the ability to sustain attention and concentrate on a task or activity) as well as a personal weakness in *Auditory Processing* (the ability to recognize, perceive, and interpret auditory stimuli).

Communication Development
XXX continues to exhibit decreased speech intelligibility. He exhibits difficulty producing /v/ in all word positions and he produces a frontal distortion for /s/ and /z/ in all word positions. XXX is stimulable for correct production of /v/ in all word positions when given a verbal model. Additionally, XXX exhibits the phonological process of gliding, substituting [w] for /r/ and /l/ in all word positions. Both the SLP and classroom teacher reported that his expressive and receptive language skills appear to be within normal limits. The frontal distortion of /s/ and /z/ and substitution of [w] for /r/ and /I/ is appropriate for his age.

Gross/Fine Motor Development
Gross and fine motor development appears to be within normal limits.

Social Emotional/Behavioral
XXX is social, affectionate, and talkative; however, he is easily distracted. He is respectful of adults and is learning social boundaries from his peers.

Health (including medications information)
XXX has general good health and parents report his hearing and vision are within normal limits.

Vocational
XXX tries to be responsible and is beginning to read the calendar.

Self-Help
XXX can get himself dressed and take care of his personal needs.

Area of need to be addressed in goals and objectives for student to receive educational benefit:

☐ Math Calculations ☐ Math Applications ☐ Reading Fluency ☐ Self-Help Skills

☐ Social Behavior ☐ Attendance ☐ Pre-vocational skills ☒ Writing

☒ Reading Comprehension ☒ Speech and Language ☐ Other: _____

SPECIAL FACTORS TO BE CONSIDERED

Does the student require assistive technology devices and/or services?
☒ No   ☐ Yes

Does the student require low incidence services, equipment, and/or materials to meet educational goals?   ☒ N/A   ☐ No   ☐ Yes

Considerations if the student is blind or visually impaired: ☒ N/A

Considerations if the student is deaf or hard of hearing: ☒ N/A

If the child is an English learner, consider the language needs of the child as those needs relate to the IEP: ☒ N/A

Does student's behavior impede learning of self or others?   ☒ No   ☐ Yes

☐ Behavior Support Plan (BSP) attached
☐ Behavior Intervention Plan (BIP) attached

Statewide Testing

Participation in Math
⊙ Grade Exempt (before Grade 2/after Grade 11)

Participation in English Language Arts
⊙ Grade Exempt (before Grade 2/after Grade 11)

Participation in Writing (4th and 7th grade)
⊙ Grade Exempt

Participation in Science
⊙ Grade Exempt

Participation in History (8th grade)
⊙ Grade Exempt

ANNUAL GOALS

Area of Need: Pre-Academic/ Academic Reading	Measurable Annual Goal #1 By 4/14/12: In the resource room & in the general ed. class, XXX will use the pictures from the story to make predictions about its content with 80% correct each opportunity as measured by work samples & observation record.
Baseline: He has trouble blending words and remembering what he reads.	☒ Enables student to be involved/progress in general curriculum/state standard #C 0.2.2 ☒ Addresses other educational needs resulting from disability ☐ Linguistically appropriate ☒ Person(s) Responsible: *General Education Teacher & RSP*

Area of Need: Pre-Academic/ Academic Reading	Measurable Annual Goal #2
	By 4/14/12: In the resource room & in the general ed. class, XXX will blend vowel-consonant sounds orally to make words or symbol with 80% correct each opportunity as measured by work samples & observation record.
Baseline: He knows sounds of words but he does not consistently blend the words in context or isolated.	☒ Enables student to be involved/progress in general curriculum/state standard #W 0.1.9 ☒ Addresses other educational needs resulting from disability ☐ Linguistically appropriate ☒ Person(s) Responsible: *General Education Teacher & RSP Parents*

Area of Need: Pre-Academic/ Academic Writing	Measurable Annual Goal #3
	By 4/14/12: In the resource room & in the general ed. Class, XXX will determine a reasonable spelling, using pre-phonetic knowledge, letter sounds, and knowledge of letter names with 80% correct each opportunity as measured by work samples & observation record.
Baseline: He tries to write words to form a sentence. He can write a missing word for a sentence given a review of choice of words to write.	☒ Enables student to be involved/progress in general curriculum/state standard #C 0.1.2 ☒ Addresses other educational needs resulting from disability ☐ Linguistically appropriate ☒ Person(s) Responsible: *General Education Teacher & RSP Parents*

Area of Need: Language/ Communication	Measurable Annual Goal #4
	By 4/14/12, XXX will independently produce /v/ in all word positions in sentences with 80% accuracy across 2 consecutive sessions.
Baseline: When on task, produces /v/ in all word positions with 30% accuracy with verbal models.	☐ Enables student to be involved/progress in general curriculum/state standard #_____ ☒ Addresses other educational needs resulting from disability ☒ Linguistically appropriate ☒ Person(s) Responsible: *Speech/Language Specialist General Education Teacher & Parents*

Area of Need:	Measurable Annual Goal #5
Language/ Communication	By 4/14/12, in the speech room, XXX will produce sentences using the correct subjective pronoun to describe pictures and stories with 80% accuracy across two consecutive sessions.
Baseline: XXX exhibits difficulty producing the appropriate subjective pronoun to describe stories and photographs. For example, XXX frequently substitutes him for he and her for she, which distracts the reader from the message.	☒ Enables student to be involved/progress in general curriculum/state standard #S 3.1.4 ☒ Addresses other educational needs resulting from disability ☐ Linguistically appropriate ☒ Person(s) Responsible: *Speech/Language Specialist General Education Teacher & Parents*

SERVICES

Service Options considered: ☒ General Education ☒ DIS ☒ RSP ☐ SDC ☐ NPS
☐ Other _____

Services		Provider	Start/ End Date	Frequency	Duration (Total Minutes)	Location
Specialized academic instruction	I/G	a District of service	4/15/11	(4×) Weekly	30	a Special Education Room
			4/15/12			
Speech & Language	I/G	a District of service	4/15/11	(4×) Weekly	30	a Special Education Room
			4/15/12			

Special Transportation: ☐ Yes ☒ No   **Extended School Year (ESY):** ☐ Yes ☒ No

Programs and services will be provided according to when student is in attendance and consistent with the public school calendar and scheduled services, excluding holidays, vacations, conference schedules, and noninstructional days.

PLACEMENT

Physical Education: ☐ General ☐ Specially Designed (describe) _____
  ☐ APE   ☐ High School PE Requirements (2 years): ☐ Met ☐ In Progress

Service District: <u>EFG School District</u>
School of Attendance: <u>ABC Elementary School</u>
School Type   <u>Public Day School</u>
Federal Setting: <u>Regular Classroom</u>

All special education services provided at student's home school: ☒ Yes ☐ No

Other Agency Services:
  ☐ California Children's Services (CCS)   ☐ Regional Center
  ☐ Probation   ☐ Department of Rehabilitation
  ☐ Dept. of Social Services (DSS)   ☐ Other _____
  ☐ County Mental Health (CMH)

Student Eligible for Mental Health Services under Chapter 26.5   ☐ Yes ☒ No

Mental Health Services Language Included on the IEP   ☐ Yes ☒ No

Transportation: ☐ None   ☒ General   ☐ Special Ed _____

Student Transition:
☒ N/A   ☐ PK to Elementary   ☐ Elementary to Middle School
☐ Middle to High School   ☐ High School to Adult Transition
☐ High School to Post Secondary   ☐ Other _____

GRADUATION PLAN
(Grade 8 and Higher)

Projected graduation date and/or secondary completion date _____
  ☒ Diploma
  ☐ Non-Diploma Certificate

APPENDIX 7-B
Private Practice—Sample Reports

PRIVATE PRACTICE SAMPLE REPORT—CHILD

 ABC Speech Services
Speech & Language Evaluation Report

Name: XXXXXXXXXX   Date of Birth: 4/11/11
Address: XXXXXXXXXX   Chronological Age: 1.9-year-old (21 months)
         XXXXXXXXXX
Date of Report: 2/4/13
Telephone: XXXXXXXX   Assessment Date: 1/22/13
RCOC Service Coordinator: XXXXXXXXX

I. BACKGROUND INFORMATION:
The reason for the referral is to determine XXXXXX's level of functioning in the areas of speech and language. XXXXXX is a 1.9-year-old boy who lives with her mother, father, and baby sister. He was diagnosed with autism by XXXXXX at 16 months of age. At or during birth, XXXXXX may have had a brain injury, which caused left-side weaknesses of his upper and lower extremities and left eye droop (ptosis). Vietnamese is his primary language. Per parent report, there is a family history of autism (two of XXXXXX's cousins). He is currently receiving physical therapy 1 hour per week at XXXXXXX. In the past, he received feeding therapy at XXXXXXX and six sessions of speech therapy at XXXXXX. He has constipation problems and takes Miralax daily. His mom reported some sensory problems such as rubbing objects on his mouth, grabbing her hand repeatedly to rub or lick, and rubbing his face. XXXXXX passed his newborn hearing screening and there are no concerns with his hearing and vision at this time. Please refer to the Regional Center intake summary for further medical and developmental information.

II. ASSESSMENT RESULTS:
XXXXXX's speech, language, pragmatics, and informal cognitive/play skills were assessed using clinical observations, parent report, review of records, <u>Developmental Assessment of Young Children (DAYC)–Cognitive Subtest,</u> and <u>The Rossetti Infant-Toddler Language Scale.</u> The speech and language assessment was conducted in Vietnamese.

219

DAYC–Cognitive Subtest:

Age Equivalent:	23 months
Percentile:	70%ile
Standard Score:	108

The Rossetti Infant-Toddler Language Scale

Pragmatics:	3 months scattering to 9–12 months (86% delay)
Language Comprehension:	15 months with scattering to 33–36 mos. (29%delay)
Language Expression:	12 months with scattering to 33–36 mos. (43% delay)

A. RECEPTIVE LANGUAGE:

In the area of language comprehension, XXXXXX scored solidly at the 15-month level with scattered skills up to the 33- to 36-month level (29% delay). He is able to identify pictures, objects, action words, and body parts upon request. Also, XXXXXX follows one-step commands, recognizes family member names, understands the prepositions "in, on," and responds to simple questions. He does not identify objects by category, understand 50 words, and follow related two-step commands.

B. EXPRESSIVE LANGUAGE:

In the area of language expression, XXXXXX scored solidly at the 12-month level with scattered skills up to the 33- to 36-month level (43% delay). Although he uses up to four-word sentences to communicate wants and needs, his language is mostly scripted. As a result, his language is highly restricted. He does not spontaneously combine novel utterances. He demonstrates both immediate and delayed echolalia. XXXXXX is often off topic and will say random words out of context (e.g., Vietnamese: "girl left home" when he was playing with the farm set). He is good at narrating and stating the obvious (e.g., Vietnamese: "mom go to restroom, open mouth, go upstairs, close door"). When prompted, he is able to request desired toys/food/items (e.g., Vietnamese: "eat cheese, mom open cheese eat, yes eat"). If joint attention is established, then he is able to ask and answer simple questions. He is inconsistent with imitating words. Despite talking a lot, XXXXXX does not engage in a back-and-forth conversation and rarely initiates conversation with others.

C. SPEECH:

Oral structures appear adequate for speech production. XXXXXX used the age-appropriate consonants /p, b, m, w, t, d, n, h/ during the assessment. Speech intelligibility was judged to be 90% to 100%.

D. COGNITIVE/PLAY SKILLS:

According to the Rossetti, XXXXXX's pragmatics skills are at the 3-month level with scattered skills up to the 9- to 12-month level, which is considered significantly below the average range (86% delay). During play, he demonstrates limited interactions, rarely initiates play acts, and has to be prompted to maintain play. He is object oriented and his play is rigid and repetitive. He sees shapes and letters in objects and gets fixed. He is not able to maintain eye contact, vocalize to gain attention, consistently respond to his name, initiate turn-taking routines, and imitate other children. Results of the <u>DAY-C</u> cognitive subtest indicated he is at the 70th percentile, which places him in the average range. He spontaneously names objects, uses pretend objects in play, counts 1 to 20, matches objects by color and shape, and stacks at least six blocks.

III. OBSERVATIONS:

XXXXXX participated in most of the test tasks and activities. His mom sat in during the testing and served as informant. He demonstrates fleeting eye contact, inconsistent joint attention, and flat affect. When excited, XXXXXX exhibits awkward arm and leg movements (e.g., when he got to play with the shape sorter). Per parent report, XXXXXX has compliance issues and tantrums at home (e.g., when there is a change in routine). When around peers, he would look at what the peers are doing but never interact with them.

IV. SUMMARY & RECOMMENDATIONS:

XXXXXX demonstrates an 86% delay in pragmatics (solid at 3 months), a 29% delay in receptive language skills (solid at 15 months), and a 43% delay in expressive language (solid at 12 months). It is recommended that XXXXXX receive 2 hours per week of speech therapy. Per parent report, there are some sensory and behavioral problems at home. It is recommended that XXXXXX receive an OT and ABA evaluation to determine if therapy is warranted.

V. GOALS:

1. XXXXXX will follow related two-step verbal directions with 80% accuracy.
2. XXXXXX will spontaneously produce novel utterances to communicate his wants and needs with 80% accuracy.
3. XXXXXX will consistently imitate words upon request with 80% accuracy.
4. XXXXXX will initiate one-step play acts during pretend play with 80% accuracy.
5. XXXXXX will initiate one to three comments and/or questions during pretend play with 80% accuracy.
6. XXXXXX will appropriately use words to get someone's attention with 80% accuracy.
7. XXXXXX will initiate turn-taking games with 80% accuracy.

XXXXXXXXX
Speech-Language Pathologist

PRIVATE PRACTICE SAMPLE REPORT—CHILD

 ABC Speech Services

Speech & Language Evaluation Report

Name: XXXXXX
Address: XXXXXXXXXX
XXXXXXXXX
Telephone: XXXXXXXX

Date of Birth: 12/13/99
Chronological Age: 12.1-year-old

Date of Report: 2/16/12

I. BACKGROUND INFORMATION:

XXXXXX is a 12.1-year-old girl who is currently home-schooled through XXXXXX Charter School. She is in the sixth grade. She has been receiving speech and language therapy since she was 2¾ years old. She no longer receives occupational therapy. Her hearing and vision are within normal limits. She lives with both of her parents and an older sister. This assessment is for XXXXXX's triennial review.

II. ASSESSMENT RESULTS:

XXXXXX was assessed on 2/6/12 and 2/9/12 for a total of 2.75 hours. Based upon observations, she gave good effort on all of the test items. XXXXXX's speech and language skills were assessed using clinical observations, parent report, records review, <u>Comprehensive Assessment of Spoken Language (CASL),</u> and CELF-4 Pragmatics Profile.

A. LANGUAGE:

<u>Comprehensive Assessment of Spoken Language (CASL):</u>

	Standard Score	Percentile
Nonliteral language	120	91%ile
Meaning from context	117	87%ile
Inference	111	77%ile
Ambiguous sentences	114	82%ile
Pragmatic judgment	107	68%ile

Based upon parent report and observations, XXXXXX tends to perform well on standardized language tests but has difficulty using and generalizing what she knows with different people and across different situations and settings. XXXXXX scored within average range on all subtests. On the nonliteral language subtest, she had to explain the meaning behind the nonliteral language that was given. For example, When Mother heard about the accident, the ground started shifting beneath her feet. What does this mean? XXXXXX responded, "Mother was worried." On the meaning from context subtest, XXXXXX was asked to figure out the meaning of an unusual word from listening to a sentence. For example, Sara got tired of moving her head up and down to follow the *saltations* of the Russian dancers. Explain what *saltations* means. XXXXXX said, "Jumping." On the inference subtest, she had to listen to a story and make an inference and figure out the clues in the story. For example, Darrell and Todd waited patiently in line for a chance to buy two of the remaining tickets for the rock concert. They left the ticket window without tickets. Why? XXXXXX responded, "The tickets were sold out." On the ambiguous sentences subtest, she had to explain two different meanings for an ambiguous sentence. For example, The man followed the tracks for three miles, and then exhaustion overcame him. XXXXXX answered, "Animal tracks and railroad tracks." On the pragmatic judgment subtest, the therapist described some events and XXXXXX had to explain the best thing to say or do in the given situation. For example, It is a hot summer day. MayLee's friend is wearing a heavy jacket. What does MayLee ask her friend? XXXXXX responded, "Why are you wearing a heavy jacket when it's hot outside?"

CELF-4 Pragmatics Profile:
Per parent report, she had a raw score of 99, but her criterion score for her age should be >142 (below average). Some test items that her mom rated as "never" include the following: initiates greetings, introduces others, and apologizes appropriately. Examples of test items that her mom rated as "sometimes" are as follows: asks for clarification during conversations; tells/understands jokes; agrees and disagrees using appropriate language; uses appropriate facial expressions, tone of voice, and body language; and uses nonverbal cues appropriate to the situation.

Clinical observations (social skills group):
During therapy, XXXXXX is able to engage in long reciprocal conversations with adults and peers with preferred topics (e.g., animals, books). She tends to talk about preferred topics and does not realize that other people might not be interested. However, she is only able to maintain non-preferred topics (e.g., shopping, arts & crafts) with peers by making two to eight conversational exchanges. She offers significantly more comments than questions. She needs to work on asking more questions to show the listener that she is interested in what he or she is saying. Also, XXXXXX needs to practice selecting appropriate topics of conversation and play choices based on what she already knows about the other person's likes and dislikes. During conversations with people she knows, she is able to maintain eye contact. However, she avoids eye contact and does not initiate greetings or conversation with new people. XXXXXX reported that she only talks to people she knows and feels that she is too shy and does not know what to say to new people. When we go on fieldtrips (e.g., shopping at the mall, Color Me Mine), XXXXXX demonstrates limited interactions and needs maximum prompting in order for her to talk to her friends.

Also, she tends to avoid talking to other people. For example, she needed to throw away trash at Color Me Mine. She asked me where the trash can was located and I told her to ask the store clerk. Instead of asking the store clerk, XXXXXX just held on to her trash.

In the area of nonverbal communication, XXXXXX is more aware of other people's facial expressions, tone of voice, and hand and body gestures. During structured activities, she is able to read the nonverbal cues and figure out what to do or say when given different social situations with 80% accuracy. However, she continues to have difficulty reading nonverbal cues and responding appropriately to them in real-life situations. In role-playing activities, XXXXXX correctly displays nonverbal cues appropriate to the social situation with 80% accuracy. However, she demonstrates limited range of facial expression (mostly smiling or neutral facial expression) and tone of voice in real-life situations. She rarely uses hand gestures while she is talking. Generalization of learned skills to different people, situations, and settings continues to be difficult for XXXXXX.

Perspective taking (theory of mind concepts) is another area of difficulty. It is difficult for her to take someone else's perspective and infer what the other person might be thinking and/or feeling. As a result, it is difficult for her to alter her verbal and nonverbal language to accommodate to the person or situation. XXXXXX struggles with flexibility in her thinking and assumes that other people think the same way so it is difficult for her to see multiple interpretations. Despite being in multiple group activities (e.g., church, sailing, horseback riding), XXXXXX rarely interacts with her peers. She expresses a desire to have friends but does not know how to go about it. When asked who her friends are, she named her dog and her sister. XXXXXX also named acquaintances at church, in her neighborhood, and after-school activities. She mostly plays with boys who are younger than her (limited talking required). The play choices (e.g., tag, hide & seek) are immature for her age (limited talking required). Her mom reported that XXXXXX has the awareness of what it takes to make friends because she is very bright. She also is willing to integrate with peers but has significant difficulty applying what she knows to real-life situations. Parental concerns include: as social demands increase, XXXXXX will have a harder time making and keeping friends and XXXXXX might be depressed in the future if she does not have true friendships with her peers.

B. SPEECH:
Oral structures and functions are adequate for speech production. XXXXXX is able to correctly produce all of her sounds in all word positions at the conversational level and no longer needs articulation therapy.

III. SUMMARY & RECOMMENDATIONS:
XXXXXX demonstrates delays in the area of social skills/pragmatics. She would benefit from intervention to improve her social language and skills

and interactions with her peers. It is recommended that XXXXXX receive individual speech therapy for .5 hour per week and social skills group for 1 hour per week. It is also recommended that she receives 3 hours total of speech ESY.

IV. NEW GOALS:

1. XXXXXX will appropriately initiate greetings and conversation with new people during structured activities such as school events and after-school activities with 80% accuracy as measured by clinical observations, therapy notes, and parent report across three consecutive sessions.

2. XXXXXX will state appropriate topics of conversation and play choices depending on who she is talking to (e.g., 6 years old vs. 13 years old, boys vs. girls) with 80% accuracy as measured by clinical observations and therapy notes across three consecutive sessions.

3. XXXXXX will maintain the topic of conversation by making at least eight exchanges (emphasis on asking more questions than making comments) with nonpreferred topics with adults and peers with 80% accuracy as measured by clinical observations and therapy notes across three consecutive sessions.

4. XXXXXX will appropriately use a total of five different body gestures, hand gestures, facial expressions, and/or tone of voice per conversation with 80% accuracy as measured by clinical observations and therapy notes across three consecutive sessions.

5. XXXXXX will take someone's perspective and make an inference about what he or she likes or is thinking with 80% accuracy as measured by clinical observations and therapy notes across three consecutive sessions.

6. XXXXXX will problem solve by stating two things that you should do or say and explain the consequences for each solution when given different social situations and/or conflicts with 80% accuracy as measured by clinical observations and therapy notes across three consecutive sessions.

_____

XXXXXXXXXX
Speech-Language Pathologist

APPENDIX 7–C

Medical Setting—Sample Reports

OUTPATIENT SAMPLE REPORT—ADULT

Pt. was seen in the speech clinic for a cognitive evaluation on 01/28/11 sec. to pt. c/o memory problems. Patient is a 25 y/o Army Combat Veteran who was deployed to Afghanistan from 2006–2007 and to Iraq from 2009-2010. Pt. reported that he fell on his head and neck, with LOC for unknown period of time, and was treated in the ER. Pt endorses left-side numbness and neck spasms. Records also indicate subjective complaints of right-side weakness. Pt also reported a syncopal incident after his fingers were cut off in a noncombat accident in the military (see psychosocial hx for details). Pt did not endorse any other hx of head trauma prior to, or during the military.

Pt. endorsed problems with memory and attention. Pt. reported that he has difficulty remembering details of readings, how to complete math problems, new learning in school, dates/events, and tasks. Pt. also reported misplacing important items.

Pt. stated that he is sleeping approximately 3 hours per night without medication and 4–5 hours (broken) with medication. Pt. eats 2 meals per day. Pt. reported that he drinks ETOH 1× per week (usually 4 beers). Pt. drinks ½ cup of coffee every other day. Pt. denied smoking or recreational drugs.

Pt. is currently compensating for memory difficulties by using his Blackberry smartphone; pt. utilizes the calendar application but not the task application. Pt. is currently enrolled in college; however, he is considering withdrawing from school sec. to panic attacks and difficulty learning. Pt. is unsure of goals at this time; pt. reported "living day-to-day." Pt's goals for therapy are to learn tips for memory.

I. Global Positioning System (GPS) Questionnaire:
"Are you having difficulty driving at this time?" and/or "Are you having any difficulty following directions while driving?"

[ ] NO = GPS not indicated. Discontinue assessment.
[x] YES

Comments: Pt. reported zoning out while driving. Pt. owns a GPS but he doesn't use it consistently. SLP encouraged pt. to use the GPS while driving to both familiar and unfamiliar destinations. GPS is not medically indicated.

II. Rivermead Behavioral Memory Test (RBMT-3):
SLP administered the Rivermead Behavioral Memory Test (RBMT-3). The RBMT provides a systematic method of assessing cognitive deficits associated with

XYX Medical Facility
Patient ID: XXXXXX

nonprogressive brain injury and to monitor change over time. This test was standardized on 333 people (172 females, 161 males) ranging in age from 16 to 89. RBMT-3 subtests are converted to subtest scaled scores with a mean of 10 and a standard deviation of 3. In addition to providing scaled scores for the RBMT-3 subtests, a General Memory Index (GMI), representing overall memory performance, is also used. The GMI has a mean of 100 and a standard deviation of 15.

Subtest	Scaled Score
First and Second Names—Delayed Recall	2
Belongings—Delayed Recall	5
Appointments—Delayed Recall	8
Picture Recognition—Delayed Recognition	1
Story—Immediate Recall	4
Story—Delayed Recall	4
Face Recognition—Delayed Recognition	4
Route—Immediate Recall	7
Route—Delayed Recall	7
Messages—Immediate Recall	11
Messages—Delayed Recall	11
Orientation and Date	7
Novel Task—Immediate Recall	7
Novel Task—Delayed Recall	5

Sum of Scaled Scores: 83
General Memory Index: 64 (2.4 SD below mean)
Percentile Rank: 0.8

IMPRESSION: Pt. presented with moderate-to-severe memory deficits. Suspect pt's adjustment issues, lack of sleep, and dx. of PTSD are largely contributing to his cognitive deficits. Neuropsych assessment found similar results. Pt. has begun MH services and was encouraged to continue actively treating PTSD. Pt. would benefit from training to use his Blackberry as a memory aid and organizational tool. Will defer cognitive therapy at this time until mental health issues are better controlled. Pt. might benefit from the College Connection program if he decides to withdraw from school this semester.

RECOMMENDATIONS: 1) SLP scheduled a f/u appt. to review test results and recommendations. 2) If pt. is agreeable, SLP will schedule 1–2 sessions to train pt. to use his Blackberry to improve organization and time management. 3) Pt. was encouraged to use the GPS while driving to both familiar and unfamiliar destinations. 4) SLP encouraged to continue actively treating PTSD.

XYX Medical Facility
Patient ID: XXXXXX

OUTPATIENT SAMPLE REPORT—ADULT

Pt. was seen in the Speech Clinic on 04/23/13 for continued assessment to determine most appropriate treatment plan. Pt. was alert and an active participant in the evaluation. Pt. was fully cooperative with all assessment tasks with no frustration noted. Results are as follows:

SLP administered portions of the Boston Naming Test. Pt. responded accurately to 42% of stimuli presented (14/33 spontaneous responses); 7 of the 14 correct responses were self-corrections. Pt's incorrect responses were typically characterized by phonemic errors (e.g., holipotter for helicopter, mushumber for mushroom). Perseverations of paraphasias were typical; each attempt/repetition was closer to the correct word. Pt. was provided with semantic and phonemic cues; however, pt. was unable to accurately respond following cues. Pt. presented with reduced awareness of phonemic paraphasias; pt. showed potential to improve awareness. SLP verbally provided pt. with the correct response and incorrect response containing a phonemic error. Pt. was able to identify if the word was correct vs. incorrect 75% of the time. Pt. also spontaneously utilized compensatory strategies to improve verbal expression such as gestures, circumlocutions, or substituting the word.

SLP administered the ACLC, which is an assessment of auditory comprehension; normative data are not available for this test. Pt. correctly identified a pictured object/action/adjective from a field of 5 with 78% accuracy (39/50 trials). Pt. identified two-critical elements from a field of four with 50% accuracy (5/10 trials). Pt. identified three-critical elements with 70% accuracy. Suspect improvement with the more complex task is sec. to pt's increased use of strategy of asking for repeats.

IMPRESSIONS: Pt. would benefit from speech therapy to improve auditory comprehension, self-awareness/self-monitoring, and verbal expression. Pt. is motivated to improve communication skills and is stimulable to implement compensatory strategies. Pt. would highly benefit from intensive therapy 5 days per week; unsure if goals can be accomplished as an outpatient. Pt. might also benefit from occupational therapy to address cognitive skills given his high level of functioning prior to injury.

PLAN: SLP will schedule speech and language therapy 5 days per week for a minimum of 4 weeks with goals as follows:

AUDITORY COMPREHENSION

STG 1a: Pt. will correctly identify a pictured object from a field of 4 at 90% accuracy while using compensatory strategies for improved auditory comprehension as needed (e.g., ask for repeat of message, ask for a written cue) across 30 trials and 2 consecutive sessions.

XYX Medical Facility
Patient ID: XXXXXX

STG 1b: Pt. will correctly identify a pictured object from a field of 6 at 90% accuracy while using compensatory strategies for improved auditory comprehension as needed (e.g., ask for repeat of message, ask for a written cue) across 30 trials and 2 consecutive sessions.

STG 1c: Pt. will correctly identify a sequence of 2 pictures from a field of 6 at 90% accuracy while using compensatory strategies for improved auditory comprehension as needed (e.g., ask for repeat of message, ask for a written cue) across 30 trials and 2 consecutive sessions.

STG 1d: Pt. will correctly identify a sequence of 2 pictures from a field of 8 at 90% accuracy while using compensatory strategies for improved auditory comprehension as needed (e.g., ask for repeat of message, ask for a written cue) across 30 trials and 2 consecutive sessions.

SELF–AWARENESS/SELF–MONITORING

STG 2a: Pt. will reduce his perseverative errors to no more than 2 repetitions per word during a picture-naming task with 90% accuracy across 30 trials and 2 sessions.

STG 2b: Pt. will reduce his perseverative errors to no more than 2 repetitions per word during a phrase-level picture-description task with 90% accuracy across 30 trials and 2 sessions.

STG 2c: Pt. will reduce his perseverative errors to no more than 2 repetitions per word during a sentence-level picture-description task with 90% accuracy across 30 trials and 2 sessions.

SELF–AWARENESS/SELF–MONITORING

STG 3a: Pt. will judge the SLP's verbal productions as correct vs. incorrect during a picture-naming task with 90% accuracy across 30 trials and 2 consecutive sessions.

STG 3b: Pt. will judge his verbal productions as correct vs. incorrect during a picture-naming task with 90% accuracy across 30 trials and 2 consecutive sessions.

STG 3c: Pt. will judge his verbal productions as correct vs. incorrect during a phrase-level picture-description task with 90% accuracy across 30 trials and 2 consecutive sessions.

STG 3d: Pt. will judge his verbal productions as correct vs. incorrect during a sentence-level picture-description task with 90% accuracy across 30 trials and 2 consecutive sessions.

XYX Medical Facility
Patient ID: XXXXXX

VERBAL EXPRESSION

STG 4a: Pt. will implement appropriate compensatory strategies to improve verbal expression (e.g., pause to plan, circumlocution, word substitution, use of gestures, writing word) during a picture-naming task in 90% of relevant instances across 2 consecutive sessions.

STG 4b: Pt. will implement appropriate compensatory strategies to improve verbal expression (e.g., pause to plan, circumlocution, word substitution, use of gestures, writing word) during a phrase-level picture-description task in 90% of relevant instances across 2 consecutive sessions.

STG 4c: Pt. will implement appropriate compensatory strategies to improve verbal expression (e.g., pause to plan, circumlocution, word substitution, use of gestures, writing word) during a sentence-level picture-description task in 90% of relevant instances across 2 consecutive sessions.

LONG–TERM GOALS

LTG 1: Pt. will correctly identify a sequence of 3 pictures from a field of 8 at 90% accuracy while using compensatory strategies for improved auditory comprehension as needed (e.g., ask for repeat of message, ask for a written cue) across 30 trials and 2 consecutive sessions.

LTG 2: Pt. will reduce his perseverative errors to no more than 2 repetitions per word during a wh-question response task with 90% accuracy across 30 trials and 2 sessions.

LTG 3: Pt. will judge his verbal productions as correct vs. incorrect during a wh-question response task with 90% accuracy across 30 trials and 2 consecutive sessions.

LTG 4: Pt. will implement appropriate compensatory strategies to improve verbal expression (e.g., pause to plan, circumlocution, word substitution, use of gestures, writing word) during a wh-question response task in 90% of relevant instances across 2 consecutive sessions.

XYX Medical Facility
Patient ID: <u>XXXXXX</u>

OUTPATIENT SAMPLE REPORT—CHILD

XYZ Children's Hospital
Department of Pediatric Rehabilitation
Speech and Language Evaluation Report

RELATED DIAGNOSIS
Ependymoma (*ICD-9-CM:* 191.9)

BACKGROUND INFORMATION
Referral Concerns
XXXXXX was referred for a speech and language evaluation by Dr. Y due to concerns regarding mild cognitive communication deficits. His mother reported no concerns with regards to XXXXXX's speech and language, but she expressed concerns about his attention and memory.

Developmental History
XXXXXX reportedly reached all of his developmental milestones at an age-appropriate time, including gross and fine motor skills, and speech and language.

Social History
XXXXXX lives in an English-speaking home in Utah with his two siblings, parents, and grandparents. He enjoys hanging out with his friends, riding his bike, reading, and playing chess with his older brother.

Educational History
XXXXXX is currently in sixth grade at a local school district. XXXXXX has an active individualized educational program (IEP); he is in a special day class and has recently been placed into a higher reading and language arts class. XXXXXX is reportedly a good student across subjects, and receives good grades. Per parent report, prior to the ependymoma diagnosis, he performed well in school. When not at school, XXXXXX is cared for by his parents and grandparents.

Feeding History
XXXXXX's mother expressed no concerns regarding feeding and feeding history is unremarkable.

MEDICAL HISTORY
Medical history was obtained from a review of his chart. XXXXXX was initially diagnosed with an ependymoma in 2007. At that time, XXXXXX underwent surgical resection followed by radiation. He was not treated with chemotherapy at that time. He was followed continually over the next several years. In January 2010, scans revealed tumor recurrence. At that time he again underwent surgical resection followed by chemotherapy consisting of but not limited to Cisplatin, Vincristine, Cytoxan, and Etopiside. Chemotherapy was completed in June 2010.

In response to his mother reporting frequent episodes of falling, a stat MRI was ordered in July 2010, but no evidence of any abnormal enhancement to suggest tumor recurrence. Per parent report, XXXXXX has a significant visual impairment in his left eye.

EVALUATION

Information for this evaluation was obtained through parent/patient interview, elicitation of behaviors, and clinical observation of skills. The outpatient evaluation took place in a quiet therapy room located at the Pediatric Rehabilitation Department. The following people were present at various points during the evaluation: XXXXXX, his grandmother, his mother, and a speech-language pathologist. The evaluation was completed in English. Due to XXXXXX's visual impairment, when there was a visual stimulus in an assessment, a brightly colored (pink) piece of paper was placed to the left of the page to encourage XXXXXX to make a complete visual scan.

Formal Assessment

Tests Administered

Clinical Evaluation of Language Fundamentals (CELF-4)

The *CELF-4* is a flexible and multiperspective assessment that examines a child's language and communication strengths and weaknesses from ages 5 to 21 years, and 11 months old. Areas assessed include vocabulary, syntax, morphology, pragmatics, memory, comprehension, and expression. XXXXXX's results are detailed below and are gauged to be an accurate reflection of his current skills.

Three subtests from the *Clinical Evaluation of Language Fundamentals, 4th Edition* (*CELF-4*) were administered to assess XXXXXX's language and cognitive skills as they compare to typical peers; Concepts and Following Directions, Word Classes (Expressive), and Word Classes (Receptive).

CELF-4 4/7/13

Subtest	Raw Score	Scaled Score	Percentile	Interpretation
Word Classes, Expressive:	7	7	16th	*Mild*
Word Classes, Receptive:	11	7	16th	*Mild*
Word Classes, Total:	18	9	37th	*Mild*
Concepts and Following Directions	54	13	84th	*High Average*

For these assessments, the mean scaled score for is 10 and the standard deviation is 3. Typical performance ranges between 7 and 13.

Word Classes, Expressive & Receptive:
This subtest examines the child's ability to hold a list of four words in working memory, identify the two words that are most closely related, and then describe their relationship. **For both expressive and receptive language, XXXXXX scored in the mild range compared to his same-age peers.**

Concepts and Following Directions:
This subtest requires the student to identify pictures of geometric shapes in response to orally presented directions. The student must wait for the entire set of directions and then follow the directions in the order that the items were presented. **XXXXXX scored in the high average range compared to his same-age peers.**

Ross Information Processing Assessment–Primary (RIPA-P)

The *Ross Information Processing Assessment–Primary (RIPA-P)* has been designed to assess impairments in information-processing skills in children from 5 to 12 years of age who have experienced neuropathologies that may affect these skills. Due to time constraints, only selected subtests from the *RIPA-P* were administered for this evaluation.

XXXXXX's results are detailed below and are gauged to be an accurate reflection of his current skills. On the individual subtests, XXXXXX's performance ranged between "within normal limits" and "moderate impairment." However, when the subtests were grouped by composite quotient, his performance fell within normal limits. His strongest performance was in his ability to remember the immediate past and his spatial orientation (e.g., the location of United States with respect to the Mexico). He was most challenged when asked to recall general information (e.g., the name of a famous American).

*The RIPA-P has been standardized on individuals with traumatic brain injury. As such, standard measurements of performance, such as standard scores, are not used to represent "average function."

RIPA-P 4/7/13

Subtest	Raw Score	Standard Score	Percentile	Interpretation
Immediate Memory	69	16	98	*Within Normal Limits*
Recent Memory	75	13	84	*Mild*
Recall of General Information	56	10	50	*Moderate*
Spatial Orientation	75	17	99	*Within Normal Limits*
Temporal Orientation	63	12	75	*Mild*
Organization	67	13	84	*Mild*
Problem Solving	69	12	75	*Mild*
Composite Quotients	Sum of Standard Score	Percentile	Quotient	Interpretation
Memory Quotient	39	90	119	*Within Normal Limits*
Orientation Quotient	29	97	127	*Within Normal Limits*

Immediate Memory:
This subtest requires the child to repeat numbers, words, and sentences of increasing length and complexity. Items are presented auditorily. XXXXXX's performance on this subtest can be interpreted to be within normal limits.

Recent Memory:
This subtest requires the child to recall specific new acquired information relative to his or her environment and daily activities. XXXXXX's performance on this subtest reflects a mild impairment.

Recall of General Information:
This subtest requires the child to recall general information in remote memory. The stimuli represent information that is acquired between the ages of 5 and 12. XXXXXX's performance on this subtest reflects a moderate impairment.

Spatial Orientation:
This subtest requires the child to answer questions related to spatial concepts and orientation. XXXXXX's performance on this subtest can be interpreted to be within normal limits.

Temporal Orientation:

This subtest requires the child to answer questions relate to time-based information. XXXXXX's performance on this subtest reflects a mild impairment.

Organization:

This subtest requires the child to recall category members within a 1-minute time limit and recall a category type given three category members. XXXXXX's performance on this subtest reflects a mild impairment.

Problem Solving:

This subtest requires the child to respond to stimulus items containing day-to-day problems. XXXXXX's performance on this subtest reflects a mild impairment.

Test of Narrative Language (TNL)

The Test of Narrative Language (TNL) measures a child's ability to answer literal and inferential comprehension questions. It also is a good measure of how well children use language in narrative discourse. There are three narrative formats: no picture cues, sequence picture cues, and single picture cues. Narrative language abilities require the integration of semantic, syntactic, and pragmatic language for the construction of form—meaning relationships at the sentence and text level. Children who score below 90 on the Narrative Language Ability Index may demonstrate deficits in vocabulary and difficulty with recall, general language comprehension, and syntax. Scores in this range may also be indicative of challenges with social and academic language.

XXXXXX's results are detailed below and are gauged to be an accurate reflection of his current skills. On Narrative Comprehension, XXXXXX answered questions about a story that had been read to him. He performed within the average range on these tasks. On Oral Narration, XXXXXX was expected to retell two stories and create one of his own. He performed within the average range on these tasks. His strongest performance was in his ability to answer familiar, concrete questions about a story (e.g., remembering character names) and in his creativity in the creation of his own fictional story (e.g., the aliens wanted the two kids to take them to see the President of the United States).

TNL 4/7/13

	Raw Score	Standard Score	Interpretation
Narrative Comprehension	31	9	*Average*
Oral Narration	68	13	*Average*
Narrative Language Ability Index	22	65	*Average*

Informal Assessment Administered
Divided Attention Activity Worksheet

This worksheet required XXXXXX to maintain his focus on a task with competing requirements; he had to follow a pattern and trace a line from one target to the next in sequential order (i.e., moving from A–1–B–2–C–3, etc.). XXXXXX was able to complete this worksheet with 95% accuracy. During the task, XXXXXX repeatedly reviewed the written instructions provided on the worksheet to check his accuracy. During one of the reviews, he spotted an error, erased the line in error, and redrew the line correctly. This strategy of review was very effective on this task and may help him with homework assignments that present a greater than average challenge for him.

SKILLS RELATED TO COMMUNICATION

Attention/Behavior

Attention is a key component to developing language. To function appropriately at home and within the classroom, children are expected to focus and attend to their speaker, listen to what is being said, and then utilize and act upon information given (usually instructions or rules).

During the assessment, XXXXXX was able to sustain attention and focus on tasks at hand; he required no repetitions for directions. For example, during one of the narrative tasks, his grandmother entered the room. Although her entry caused a distraction, XXXXXX was able to continue with the task without requiring a review of the information. Further, when asked between assessments if he needed a break, he replied that he did not and continued for another 30 minutes.

Overall, XXXXXX demonstrated appropriate attention and was polite and interacted appropriately with his grandmother, mother, and the speech-language pathologist.

Memory

Memory involves encoding, storing, and retrieving information. These memory skills are important within the classroom and at home because they are required every day when teachers/parents ask their students/children to follow directions related to lessons, assignments, and activities as well as when taking notes and learning vocabulary and related words.

Encoding/Storing/Retrieving for auditory and visual stimuli: On the Concepts and Following Directions subtest, XXXXXX was able to recall directions that increased in length and complexity (e.g., "point to the small orange car" and "point to the small black fish after you point to the big fish and then point to the shoe and ball"). Further, at the end of the session, XXXXXX was able to recall the spelling of the word *bueno* that the speech-language pathologist had talked about early in the session. His performance on this assessment is reflective of his current level of academic performance.

In general, XXXXXX demonstrates appropriate skills with regards to memory.

Executive Functions

Executive functions refer to a child's ability to initiate and stop actions, monitor and change behavior as needed, and plan future behavior when faced with new tasks and situations. Executive functions allow us to anticipate outcomes and adapt to changing situations. The ability to form concepts and think abstractly is often considered a component of executive function.

Per parent report, XXXXXX is very independent and helpful around the house; he is very involved with his siblings and participates in daily chores in addition to his schoolwork. He has demonstrated no problems with his homework. XXXXXX's performance on the Divided Attention Task is reflective of effective executive function.

Within this evaluation and as reported by his family, XXXXXX demonstrates appropriate executive function as evidenced in the results of the individual formal and informal assessments.

Play Skills

Play skills were not evaluated.

COMMUNICATION

Receptive Language

Receptive language refers to XXXXXX's ability to comprehend and process what others are saying. In general, XXXXXX is able to respond appropriately to questions and comments addressed to him. The Word Classes–Receptive subtest of the CELF-4 was administered to assess his receptive language skills in depth. XXXXXX was significantly more challenged by multiple-syllable words (e.g., catastrophe, latitude, and permanent) than by single-syllable words (e.g., joined and sunset).

In general, XXXXXX presents with receptive language skills reflective of a mild impairment.

Expressive Language

Expressive Language refers to XXXXXX's ability to communicate and express his wants, needs, thoughts, and ideas to those around him. In general, XXXXXX is able to express himself appropriately during his daily activities. The Word Classes–Expressive subtest of the CELF-4 and the TNL were administered to obtain an in-depth understanding of XXXXXX's expressive language skills. XXXXXX was able to find relationships between words that were part of his daily life (e.g., pillow/blanket and window/glass) and struggled with words that were more abstract (e.g., connected/joined and achieving/accomplishing).

In general, XXXXXX presents with expressive language skills reflective of a mild impairment.

Oral Motor/Articulation
XXXXXX demonstrated appropriate articulation and motor speech skills.

Voice
Based on informal observations during conversational speech, XXXXXX exhibits appropriate vocal characteristics at this time, including pitch and loudness, which do not impact his overall ability to communicate with others.

Fluency
No abnormal dysfluencies were noted in running speech.

Social Communication/Pragmatics
Pragmatics refers to the way that language is used to communicate with others (the social use of language). Throughout this assessment, and as reported by his family, XXXXXX exhibited appropriate social communication.

In general, XXXXXX presents with appropriate social communication skills. He was polite and respectful in the evaluation. He willingly and actively engaged in conversation with the speech-language pathologist. Per parent report, he is well liked and respected by his peers and teachers.

SUMMARY

XXXXXX is a polite, well-behaved adolescent boy who was referred for a speech and language evaluation due to concerns regarding attention and memory. Results of this assessment indicate that both attention and memory are appropriate for his age and his recovery from an ependymoma.

Per parent report, he is receiving effective support through his IEP and the academic structure of the special day class. Based on these results, it is recommended that XXXXXX continue with his current support system through his school. If he exhibits a change in his academic performance or demonstrates any status changes in speech, language, attention, or memory, it is recommended that he be evaluated again.

Thank you for the opportunity to participate in the assessment of XXXXXX. Please feel free to contact me should you have any questions or concerns regarding the content of this report.

_____

Speech-Language Pathologist

Cc: family, (MD Name) ***, insurance

INPATIENT SAMPLE REPORT—ADULT

XYZ REHABILITATION HOSPITAL
COMMUNICATIVE DISORDERS SERVICE

Medical Diagnosis: Stroke

Date of Onset: April 2002   **Date of Report:** 6/12/02

Speech/Language Pathologist: XXXXXXXXX

Referring Physician: XXXXXX   **Report:** Initial: _X_ Final: _X_

1. **BACKGROUND INFORMATION/PROGRESS REPORT:**
   37 y/o male, well known to speech clinician from previous LBMMC visit rehab center admit. Pt initially presented with altered LDC, nausea, and vomiting, having been out drinking with friends the previous night. Initially nonverbal and unable to sit up. Paramedics were called and reported CGS 1-5-1 and alcohol odor. Pt taken to LB Community Hospital, where a head CT was initially read as a bleed, then re-read as negative. Pt c/o chest pain or palpitations in ER. PMHx: headaches, anxiety, HTN, hyperlipidemia. Follow-up CT revealed occluded **L** internal carotid artery. Pt was d/c'd with residual mod-severe receptive aphasia and severe expressive aphasia, and **R** hemiplegia. SOHx: Pt lives with wife and 4-year-old daughter; with other family members involved.

2. **SPEECH/LANGUAGE/COGNITIVE DIAGNOSIS:** Pt was evaluated in clinic office with his wife present. Portions of the Boston Diagnostic Aphasia Exam (BDAE), the Boston Naming Test, and the Reading Comprehension Battery for Aphasia (RCBA) were given. The following results were obtained:

   Cognition: Difficult to fully assess all areas secondary to expressive language. However, immediate recall of short paragraph was 100% accurate for y/no responses. Problem solving during functional activities is at min assist-to-supervised.

   Speech: Verbal attempts were 100% accurate during nonstructured tasks, such as picture description of "cookie theft" from BDAE. Pt was 20% accurate for verbal attempts in response to automatic phrases in structured task. Imitations of short sentences, verbally presented, were 30% accurate, with apraxic distortions. Pt was 100% accurate for automatics (i.e., counting, days, months).

   Lang.: Pt was 75% to 100% accurate for y/no responses to questions regarding complex ideational material, verbally presented. Pt was 40% accurate reading sentences and pointing to printed/ picture from field of 3.

3. **PROGNOSIS:** ____ Excellent _X_ Good _X_ Fair ____ Guarded ____ Poor
   Secondary to: above results and pt's progress over time

4. **RECOMMENDATIONS:**
Speech/Language/Cognitive therapy <u>3×</u> times weekly for <u>4</u> weeks.

5. **GOALS:**
<u>**Patient/Family**</u>: To talk.   **Discharge Goals Met:** _____ Yes _____ No

<u>**Treatment:**</u>
↑ reading comprehension of survival words/signs to min assist (75%–80% acc.).

↑ automatic speech thru melodic intonation therapy to mod assist.

↑ naming of family members & common household items to mod assist.

Thank you for referring this patient.

NAME: XXXXX

M.D.: XXXXX

MMC NO.: XXXXX   **AGE:** <u>37</u>

_____

Speech-Language Pathologist

APPENDIX 7–D

Sample Goals and Objectives

ADULT LANGUAGE DISORDERS

Target Area: Spoken Language Expression

Objective 1: Given a visual prompt (e.g., picture) and not more than three cues (e.g., written, semantic, phonemic), the patient will say the names of familiar <u>people</u>, in 7 of 10 opportunities.

Objective 2: Given a visual prompt (e.g., picture) and not more than three cues (e.g., semantic, phonemic) in a clinic setting, the patient will say the name of 10 familiar <u>places</u> in 7 of 10 opportunities.

Objective 3: Given a visual prompt (e.g., picture) and not more than three cues (e.g., semantic, phonemic) in a clinic setting, the patient will say the name of 10 familiar <u>objects</u> in 7 of 10 opportunities.

Objective 4: Given a visual prompt (e.g., picture) and not more than three cues (e.g., semantic, phonemic) in a clinic setting, the patient will say the name of 10 familiar <u>activities</u> in 7 of 10 opportunities.

Target Area: Multimodality Communication

Goal: To improve communicative effectiveness, XXX will switch communication modalities to writing, drawing, or description when word retrieval difficulties occur in conversation.

Objective 1: In response to word retrieval difficulties, XXX will switch communication modalities to writing, drawing, or description during picture description in 8 of 10 opportunities.

Objective 2: In response to word retrieval difficulties, XXX will switch communication modalities to writing, drawing, or description during conversation in 8 of 10 opportunities.

Target Area: Auditory Comprehension

STG 1a: Pt. will correctly identify a pictured object from a field of four at 90% accuracy while using compensatory strategies for improved auditory comprehension as needed (e.g., ask for repeat of message, ask for a written cue) across 30 trials and two consecutive sessions.

STG 1b: Pt. will correctly identify a pictured object from a field of six at 90% accuracy while using compensatory strategies for improved auditory comprehension as needed (e.g., ask for repeat of message, ask for a written cue) across 30 trials and two consecutive sessions.

STG 1c: Pt. will correctly identify a sequence of two pictures from a field of six at 90% accuracy while using compensatory strategies for improved auditory comprehension as needed (e.g., ask for repeat of message, ask for a written cue) across 30 trials and two consecutive sessions.

STG 1d: Pt. will correctly identify a sequence of two pictures from a field of eight at 90% accuracy while using compensatory strategies for improved auditory comprehension as needed (e.g., ask for repeat of message, ask for a written cue) across 30 trials and two consecutive sessions.

AUGMENTATIVE AND ALTERNATIVE COMMUNICATION

Target Area: AAC Use

Goal: The student will access his *Proloquo2go* app on his iPad to make requests during speech therapy sessions.

> *Objective 1:* When verbally prompted once (e.g., "Turn on your iPad."), the student will follow visual instructions to turn on his iPad and open the *Proloquo2go* app, in four of five opportunities, during speech therapy sessions.

> *Objective 2:* When verbally prompted once (e.g., "What should we do next?"), the student will access his *Proloquo2go* app on his iPad to make requests, in four of five opportunities, during speech therapy sessions.

Target Area: Functional/Expressive Communication

By May 2014, during daily activities and routines, XXX will use her AAC device for functional communication (e.g., protesting, requesting, stating opinions), given

visual supports in four of five opportunities across 3 trial days, as measured by observation and data collection.

Target Area: Receptive Language

By May 2014, during daily activities and routines, XXX will use her AAC device to answer familiar yes/no questions, given visual supports in four of five trials across 3 trial days as measured by observation and data collection.

By May 2014, during daily activities and routines, XXX will use her AAC device to answer familiar "who" and "what" questions given visual supports in four of five trials across 3 trial days as measured by observation and data collection.

By May 2014, during structured speech-language activities, XXX will use her AAC device to answer basic "wh" comprehension questions (i.e., who, what doing, where, when) related to a short passage/story, given visual supports as needed in four of five trials over three consecutive sessions as measured by observation and data collection.

AUTISM SPECTRUM DISORDERS

Target Area: Play

Goal: The client will perform sequences of common play scripts (e.g., restaurant, store, library), in response to a video self-model in the clinic setting.

> *Objective 1:* The client will imitate a minimum of four actions and four verbalizations of imaginative play sequences of common play scripts (e.g., restaurant, store, library), following a video self-model, in at

least two play scripts, in the clinic setting.

Target Area: Social Skills

Goal: To improve social skills, the client will demonstrate appropriate use of social rules in conversations with familiar and unfamiliar communication partners.

Objective 1: When presented with a visual stimulus (i.e., video modeling), the client will demonstrate appropriate use of social rules (e.g., greetings, introductions, and asking questions) given moderate (3–5) verbal cues and gestures, in three of five opportunities with the clinician in the clinic setting.

Objective 2: When presented with a visual stimulus (i.e., video modeling), the client will demonstrate appropriate use of social rules (e.g., greetings, introductions, and asking questions) given minimal (1–2) verbal cues and gestures, in four of five opportunities with the clinician in the clinic setting.

Target Area: Language

By December 2012, during naturalistic activities (e.g., play, snack, library), given no more than two prompts (e.g., visual, phonemic, questioning), XXX will produce semantic relations within the modifier + object category, using at least two-word utterances, with 70% accuracy,

By December 2012, during two of three naturalistic activities (e.g., play, snack, library), with more than two prompts (e.g., visual, phonemic, questioning), XXX will produce semantic relations within the negation + object category, using at least two-word utterances, with 70% accuracy.

CHILD LANGUAGE DISORDERS

Target Area: Auditory Comprehension

Goal: The student will follow one- to two-step instructions with verbal prompts.

Objective 1: The student will follow one- to two-step instructions in 40% of opportunities with verbal and visual prompts.

Objective 2: The student will follow one- to two-step instructions in 50% of opportunities with verbal and visual prompts.

Objective 3: The student will follow one- to two-step instructions in 50% of opportunities with verbal prompts.

Target Area: Preliteracy / Phonology

Goal: To improve preliteracy skills, the client will demonstrate increased phonological awareness by segmenting monosyllabic words.

Objective 1: To improve preliteracy skills, the client will demonstrate increased phonological awareness by categorizing (e.g., Which one begins with a different sound: *feet, five, soup, fat?*) in response to print and verbal cues in 7 of 10 opportunities.

Objective 2: To improve preliteracy skills, the client will demonstrate increased phonological awareness by deletion (e.g., Say *trip* without the /t/) in response to print and verbal cues in 7 of 10 opportunities.

Objective 3: To improve preliteracy skills, the client will demonstrate increased phonological awareness by substitution (e.g., Replace the /m/ in *man* with /f/) in response to print and verbal cues in 7 of 10 opportunities.

Objective 4: To improve preliteracy skills, the client will demonstrate increased phonological awareness by manipulation (e.g., Say the word *stop*. Now move the /s/ to the end of the word and say it again) in response to print and verbal cues in 7 of 10 opportunities.

Target Area: Morphology

By May 2009, during pretend play activities, following therapist recasts, XXX will produce *-ing* verbs (e.g., children are singing) in at least 10 utterances across three sessions.

By May 2009, during pretend play activities, XXX will complete cloze procedures to produce *-ing* verbs (e.g., we are . . .) in at least 10 utterances across three sessions.

By May 2009, during pretend play activities, the client will spontaneously produce *-ing* verbs (e.g., puppy jumping) in at least 10 utterances across three sessions.

Target Area: Pragmatics

Goal: The client will produce appropriate sentences for a variety of social functions (e.g., requesting, turn-taking, repairing conversational breakdowns).

Objective 1: The client will produce an appropriate sentence for a

variety of social functions (e.g., requesting, turn-taking, repairing conversational breakdowns) when given moderate prompting (e.g., verbal and/or visual prompts) with 80% accuracy.across 10 trials as measured by recorded data.

MOTOR SPEECH

Target Area: Voice

Objective 1: The patient will demonstrate controlled exhalation by sustaining phonation of the vowel /a/ for 10 seconds or longer, in 80% of trials, across two consecutive therapy sessions.

Objective 2: The patient will demonstrate controlled exhalation by sustaining phonation of the vowel /a/ for 20 seconds or longer, in 80% of trials, across two consecutive therapy sessions.

Target Area: Fluency 2

Goal: The client will increase fluency in response to token reinforcement (response cost) in structured play therapy.

Objective 1: The client will demonstrate increased fluency in response to token reinforcement (response cost) with no more than 30 dysfluencies during 5 minutes of structured play therapy.

Objective 2: The client will demonstrate increased fluency in response to token reinforcement (response cost) with no more than 20 dysfluencies during 5 minutes of structured play therapy.

Objective 3: The client will demonstrate increased fluency in response to token reinforcement (response cost) with no more than 10 dysfluencies during 5 minutes of structured play therapy.

PHONOLOGY

Target Area: Phonological Awareness 3

Goal: The client will demonstrate phonological awareness skills by identifying initial and final sounds in CVC, CV, and VC words.

Objective 1: Given a visual cue and verbal prompts, the client will match the beginning sounds of words with 70% accuracy as measured by clinician observation, other informal assessments, and data collection.

Objective 2: Given a visual cue and verbal prompts, the client will identify the beginning sounds of words with 70% accuracy as measured by clinician observation, other informal assessments, and data collection.

Objective 3: Given a visual cue and verbal prompts, the client will match the ending sounds of words with 70% accuracy as measured by clinician observation, other informal assessments, and data collection.

Objective 4: Given a visual cue and verbal prompts, the client will match the ending sounds of words with 70% accuracy as measured by clinician observation, other informal assessments, and data collection.

Target Area: Articulation

Goal: XXX will produce /s/ in the initial and final position at the word level 50% of the time.

Objective 1: Given pictures, a model, and a verbal prompt, XXX will produce /s/ in the initial and final position, at the word level, with 20% accuracy.

Objective 2: Given pictures, a model, and a verbal prompt, XXX will produce /s/ in the initial and final position at the word level with 40% accuracy.

Target Area: Articulation

Goal: The student will produce the phonemes /r/, /l/, /s/, and /z/ in all positions in one-syllable words.

Objective 1: With no more than one prompt, the student will produce the phonemes /r/, /l/, /s/, and /z/ in CV and VC syllables with 80% accuracy.

Objective 2: The student will produce the phonemes /r/, /l/, /s/, and /z/ in the initial position of one-syllable words with 70% accuracy.

Objective 3: The student will produce the phonemes /r/, /l/, /s/, and /z/ in the final position of one-syllable words with 70% accuracy.

CHAPTER 8
Data Collection

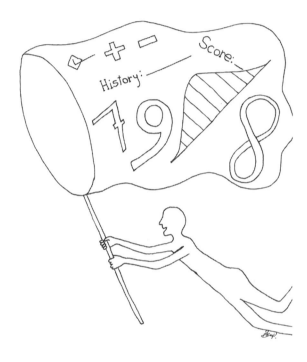

Accuracy of observation is the equivalent of accuracy of thinking.
Wallace Stevens (Pulitzer Prize–winning poet)

The terms *data* (plural) and *datum* (singular) refer to "factual information (as measurements or statistics) used as a basis for reasoning, discussion, or calculation" (Merriam-Webster, 2003). Hence, data collection is the process of obtaining this information. In the field of speech-language pathology, collecting, analyzing, and summarizing data is a vital part of decision-making and documentation.

As a speech-language pathology assistant (SLPA), you will learn about evidence-based practice (EBP), which is the "integration of clinical expertise, best current evidence, and client values to provide high-quality services reflecting the interests, values, needs, and choices of those we serve" (Rao, 2011, para. 4). Data collection is an integral part of EBP (Boswell, 2005; Epstein, 2008; Lemoncello &

Fanning, 2011) and as such is a very important aspect of what speech-language pathologists (SLPs) and, in turn, SLPAs do. Box 8–1 contains some of the job responsibilities of an SLPA that may involve data collection.

Clinically, data collection begins during assessment when the SLP analyzes information about communicative or swallowing behaviors. Although an SLPA does not conduct assessment or interpret any data collected (ASHA, 2013), as an SLPA you may be asked to *assist* during screening or assessment. This could include data collection, such as tallying or recording specific behaviors, transcribing a language sample, making phonetic notations, calculating percentages, transferring data onto standardized protocols, or displaying assessment or screening data in graphs or charts.

Data collection about a client continues during and after treatment. This type of data is also critical and allows the SLP to monitor the client's progress from session to session and to document the efficacy of a given treatment strategy (Mowrer, 1982; Roth & Worthington, 2001). This, too, may be an area where an SLPA can assist, performing tasks such as tallying or recording specific behaviors, making phonetic notations, calculating percentages, or preparing charts or graphs about treatment data. As discussed in Chapter 7, treatment objectives include information about the types of data needed in establishing if a client has met a given objective. This information is present in the "criterion" portion of behavioral objectives.

As an SLPA, your role in accurately collecting data is crucial, since inaccurate data will negatively influence clinical decisions. The sections that follow will discuss methods for observing and recording data, including ideas for ways to record specific types of data. Chapter 9 discusses ways to summarize these data in note format. The CD associated with this book contains samples of score sheets, which can be used for charting data.

Box 8–1. Examples of SLPA Duties Involving Data[1]

a. Assist the SLP with speech, language, and hearing screenings **without** clinical interpretation.
b. Assist the SLP during assessment of students, patients, and clients exclusive of administration and/or interpretation.
c. Follow documented treatment plans or protocols developed by the supervising SLP.
d. Provide guidance and treatment via telepractice to students, patients, and clients who are selected by the supervising SLP as appropriate for this service delivery model.
e. Document student, patient, and client performance (e.g., tallying data for the SLP to use; preparing charts, records, and graphs) and report this information to the supervising SLP.

RECORDING AND DESCRIBING BEHAVIOR

There are many different methods for observing and recording/describing communication behaviors. At the heart of each, however, is careful observation, meaning that you actively and directly "see" and "listen" to the client, taking care to accurately record what you observe (Kawulich, 2005; Taylor-Powell & Steele, n.d.). This careful observation requires understanding the behaviors to be observed, the type of data to be collected, and the method for summarizing this information.

Some methods for recording data in the field of speech-language pathology include frequency count/tally, response analysis, and transcription/narration.

Frequency Counts/Tally

Frequency counts or tallies determine if a behavior is present (and at what rate) in a specific period (Moore & Pearson, 2003; Mowrer, 1982; Roth & Paul, 2007). This method is also referred to as simple enumeration (Mowrer, 1982). In this technique, the objective is to record the presence of a specific behavior, such as a client interacting with a peer, asking a question, saying a specific sound or type of word, and so forth. To record this type of data, you must know the length of time to observe for this behavior and during what activity, as well as what specific behavior you are to observe. You would then record the number of times that behavior occurred in that specified period (e.g., two times in 1 minute, 10 times in 2 minutes, etc.). Tallies, hash marks, checks, or other symbols could be used to record this information. Figure 8–1 contains an example of a chart that could be used to record this type of information.

Response Rate

Response rate is a variant of frequency count/tally whereby a specific behavior is counted, similar to frequency count/tally, but this number is then converted to a value that denotes responses per unit of time. Words per minute (WPM) is a common measurement that uses this technique (Shipley & McAfee, 2009). In this instance, the behavior is the number of words produced. To record WPM you would count the number of words produced. This amount is then divided by a unit of time you observed the person speaking (typically in minutes). Syllables per minute (SPM) is also calculated in this fashion but, of course, the count would consist of the number of syllables produced (Mowrer, 1982).

Checklists

A checklist is also a variant of frequency count/tally. This technique is used to denote the presence of a list of behaviors (Moore & Pearson, 2003; Roth & Paul, 2007). This could be a checklist specifically created by your supervising SLP for a specific client (or group of clients), or it may be a modified version of an already existing checklist. Figure 8–2 contains an example of a checklist specifically created to track behaviors in a group setting.

The important thing about recording behaviors using frequency count/tally, response rate, or checklist is that you are very clear about the behavior to be counted. For instance, in the example

Client: Scott Smith (Mrs. Smith's Classroom)

Behavior/Time/Activity	Count
Behavior: Whole-word repetition	√ √ √ √ √
Length of Time: 10 minutes	
Activity: Story retell	(5 in 12 min.)
Date: 12/15/12	
Clinician: Sarah S. Assistant	
Behavior: Final Consonant deletion	~~IIII~~ II
Length of Time: 10 minutes	
Activity: Story retell	(7 in 12 min.)
Date: 12/15/12	
Clinician: Sarah S. Assistant	

Figure 8–1. Sample Frequency Count/Tally Data Sheet.

Client: John Jones

Activity: Aphasia Support Group – Thursday Session

SLPA: Sarah S. Assistant

Date: 1/3/13

Behavior	Note Y for *Yes* or N for *No*
Greets fellow group members upon entering room	Y
Finds name tag	N – located table, but needs assistance from group facilitator in locating name tag.
Finds designated seat	Y
Initiates small talk with a fellow group member	Y
Responds to a question posed by group facilitator	N
Comments during group discussion	Y – states "Like pizza" when discussing favorite foods

Figure 8–2. Sample Checklist Data Sheet.

above relative to frequency count/tally, if you did not know what a whole-word repetition was or how it differs from a part-word repetition, you would not accurately record its occurrence and, in turn, would be sharing inaccurate information about the frequency of this behavior with your supervising SLP. As such, you should always confirm that you understand the exact parameters of the behavior to be counted. You can ask your supervising SLP if you have any questions.

Screening. In some settings, you may be asked to assist with speech, language, or hearing screenings (ASHA, 2013). A screening "involves the collection of data to decide whether there is a strong likelihood that an individual does or does not have a problem that will require more in-depth assessment" (Kennedy, 2007, p. 42). Screenings are not diagnostic in nature. Rather, they are used to determine if further testing is needed. Screenings use a predetermined cutoff or expected performance level to determine if a client either *passes* or *fails* the screening. Your supervising SLP may use a setting-specific instrument or one of many commercially available screening tools.

In some cases, screenings used are similar to checklists (above) in that specific behaviors are listed and the screener's job is to denote the presence or absence of each behavior in a specific context. In other cases, screenings involve a specific task given by the screener, followed by the screener denoting the presence or absence of a required response. For example, in a hearing screening, the client is told to raise her or his hand in response to a series of tones, presented at different frequencies and loudness levels. The screener presents the tones and then notes whether the client raised her hand (presence of required response) or did not raise her or his hand (absence of required response) in the presence of each tone. Similarly, in a kindergarten speech and language screening, a student may be asked to count from 1 to 10. The screener then notes whether the student counted from 1 to 10 (presence of required response) or did not count from 1 to 10 (absence of required response). In these instances, the screener uses a fully correct response as the criterion for the presence of a behavior. Any other response is noted as the absence of the required behavior. No interpretation of the meaning behind why the student did not count from 1 to 10 or raise her hand in response to a specific tone is made.

In most cases, screeners require the use a binary score, such as yes/no, absent/present, correct/incorrect, and so forth. In addition, some speech and language screeners require errors to be transcribed using the International Phonetic Alphabet (IPA) or written verbatim. A list of IPA symbols is available in Appendix 4–B in Chapter 4. The comments section of many screeners often ask the screener to note any special circumstances related to the screening that may have influenced the results, such as if the client was not paying attention during the task or did not appear to understand the directions. This additional information can be used by the SLP (in the case of speech and language screenings) to interpret the results of the screening.

Conducting screenings will require specific training on the screening tool to be used. Administration of hearing screenings will also require that you learn how to operate an audiometer.

SLPA Roles: Caution. A word of caution is in order as well about checklists and screenings and their use by an SLPA. Many checklists and, in some cases, commercially available screeners are used by SLPs to *assess* specific behaviors. These should not be confused with checklists and screenings designed for implementation by an SLPA. In cases where *interpretation or diagnosis* is required or implied, that is the sole domain of an SLP. For example, a common assessment tool utilized by an SLP is an oral peripheral examination, used to "identify or rule out structural or functional factors that relate to a communicative disorder or dysphagia" (Shipley & McAfee, 2009, p. 158). There are a number of "checklists" or forms available for use by SLPs for this purpose. In most cases, however, these forms include some interpretative or diagnostic aspect. For example, Figure 8–3 contains an excerpt from the Oral-Facial Examination Form (Shipley & McAfee, 2009). In addition, some checklists contain rating scales that require the respondent to classify or rate the severity of a behavior, which is also diagnostic and interpretative in nature. For example, Figure 8–4 contains an excerpt from the Checklist for the Assessment of Clients with Clefts (Shipley & McAfee, 2009).

A diagnosis is "a concise technical description" (Merriam-Webster, 2003). The examples from Figures 8–3 and 8–4 both require interpretation and precise description. ASHA (2013) states that SLPAs may not "perform standardized or nonstandardized diagnostic tests, formal or informal evaluations, or swallow-

---

Evaluation of tongue

_____ Surface color: normal/abnormal (specify)_____
_____ Abnormal movements: absent/jerky/spasms/writhing/fasiculations_____
_____ Size: normal/small/large_____
_____ Frenum: normal/short _____

Tell the client to protrude the tongue.
_____ Excursion: normal/deviates to right/deviates to left _____
_____ Range of motion: normal/reduced_____
_____ Speed of motion: normal/reduced_____

(Shipley & McAfee, 2009, p. 196)

Figure 8–3. Excerpt from Oral-Facial Examination Form.

Assessment of Voice

Instructions: Evaluate the client's voice, paying particular attend to possible cleft-related problems. Check the deficits that are present and indicate severity. Record additional notes in the right-hand margin.

1 = Mild
2 = Moderate
3 = Severe

____ Pitch variation is reduced_____
____ Vocal intensity is reduced_____
____ Vocal quality is hoarse/harsh/breathy (circle)_____

(Shipley & McAfee, 2009, p. 574)

Figure 8–4. Excerpt from Checklist for the Assessment of Clients with Clefts.

ing screenings/checklists" (Responsibilities Outside the Scope of an SLPA, para. 1). In addition, ASHA also specifically highlights the use of checklists for dysphagia (interpretative or otherwise) to be outside the scope of responsibilities of an SLPA, stating that SLPAs "may not use a checklist or tabulate results of feeding or swallowing evaluations" (Responsibilities Outside the Scope of an SLPA, para. 1). As an SLPA, it is important that you maintain these boundaries for the benefit and safety of the clients you serve. There could be legal and ethical ramifications as well if you go beyond your scope of responsibilities as an SLPA.

Response Analysis

Response analysis is an additional type of data analysis beyond counting it or denoting the presence of a behavior. Response analysis techniques look at the dimensions of correctness (response accuracy), delay (response latency), and assistance needed (response independence) to further quantify a behavior. Appendix 7–D in Chapter 7 contains samples of treatment goals and objectives across a variety of response categories. After you read the sections that follow, see if you can identify what type of response analysis is utilized and what data collection methods you might use to record these behaviors.

Response Accuracy

In recording response accuracy, you would be told about a behavior and given details about what constitutes an accurate response (Mowrer, 1982). You would then count the number of correct responses as well as the total number of opportunities for that behavior to occur. An example of

this is percent correct (Mowrer, 1982). In this method, you would divide the total number of correct responses by the total number of opportunities. This could then be converted to a percentage of correct responses, which is helpful as it denotes if the behavior occurred, but also what portion of the time it was accurate. For example, in charting accuracy in producing /s/ in the initial position of words, you would count the number of times the client produced the /s/ correctly in the initial position of words (total correct) and divide by the total number of opportunities the client had to say words with /s/ in the initial position (total opportunities). To convert this number to a percentage, you would then multiple by 100, as follows:

$$5 \div 10 \times 100 = 50\%$$

5	10	50%
Total Correct	*Total Opportunities*	*Percent Correct*

An example data collection sheet for this task may look similar to the one listed in Figure 8–5. Figure 8–6 contains a similar way to record these same data. You can see in both of these examples, the client had 10 opportunities to say a word with /s/ in the initial position and did so accurately five times, resulting in a percent correct of 50%.

In Figure 8–5, the opportunities, as well as the words themselves, are recorded as a reference, and the score sheet includes a key to denote that a "+" indicates times when the client produced /s/ in the initial position correctly, while a "−" indicates times when /s/ in the initial position of a word was not produced accurately. In Figure 8–6, no individual words are recorded, but an accurate production is noted with an X and an inaccurate production is noted with a /.

Client: Tina Thomas

SLPA: Sarah S. Assistant

Date: 1/15/12

Target: /s/ initial/single words   Key: + = correct/− = incorrect

Word	Response
Sew	−
Say	+
Soup	+
Suit	−
Sock	−
Sub	−
Soap	+
Set	+
Sun	−
Sit	+

Score: 5/10 = 50%

Figure 8–5. Sample Percent Correct Data Sheet (Targets Noted).

Client: Tina Thomas   SLPA: Sarah S. Assistant

Date: 1/15/12   Objective: /s/ initial/single words

										Score
/	/	/	X	X	/	X	X	X	/	50%

Key: X = correct   / = incorrect

Figure 8–6. Sample Percent Correct Data Sheet (No Targets).

Another common technique that uses the concept of percent correct is a dysfluency index (Shipley & McAfee, 2009). This method counts the total number of syllables (total opportunities) and the total number of disfluencies. A percentage is then calculated, either as a measure of all types of disfluencies (e.g., % Total Disfluency) or for certain types of disfluencies (e.g., % Repetitions, % Prolongations, etc.). A similar calculation is also used in determining Percent Syllables Stuttered (%SS) as follows (Jones, Onslow, Packman, & Gebski, 2006):

$$\frac{Syllables\ Stuttered}{Total\ Syllables} \times 100 = SS\%$$

Response accuracy can also be described using an opportunity statement. In this method, correct response and total opportunities are recorded, but the information is not displayed as a percentage. Rather, this information is summarized in a written statement, such as, *3 of 4 opportunities*, *in 8 of 10 instances*, or *given 20 of 25 attempts*. The following objectives have criteria that use response accuracy

- Given a verbal label of a category, the client will name three items that belong to that category in 8 of 10 opportunities.
- With a visual cue or gesture prompt, Johnny will respond to a teacher-directed question by touching an appropriate symbol on his AAC device, in three of four opportunities, over three consecutive sessions.
- The student will correctly use present progressive tense to describe 15 of 20 pictures not visible to the clinician.

Response accuracy can be used for almost any type of behavior, using either percent correct or an opportunity statement. In fact, response accuracy is a common measure used by SLPs in the criterion portion of treatment objectives.

The key to collecting response accuracy is understanding what constitutes a correct or an accurate response and also in noting how many opportunities the individual had to produce a correct

response. Keep in mind as well that a correct response may not necessarily be synonymous with a perfect response. There are instances when a close approximation or a partly correct response may be determined by your supervising SLP as correct. This information may be noted in the client's goal. If not, you can check with your supervising SLP to confirm that you understand the parameters of her or his expectations of "correct."

Response Latency

Response latency is a method for analyzing a response, given how long it took to produce a behavior (Mowrer, 1982). Use of this type of data collection is less common than response accuracy in the field of speech-language pathology. To calculate response latency, you would need to count the length of time between when a "stimulus" is presented and when the client responded. This is typically calculated in seconds and measured with a stopwatch. A stimulus is basically an opportunity to respond. For example, when you ask a client to name something, like a picture of a train, a line drawing of a bed, or a real object like a cup, each of these items (the train, the line drawing, and the cup) is a stimulus. Response latency would be measured from the time the item is presented until when the client responds. A question or command, such as, "Is grass green?" "What sound does a cow make?" or "Give me your hand," are also each a stimulus, since they are each an opportunity for the client to respond. Figure 8–7 is an example of a data collection sheet for recording response latency. As you can see, in this instance, the task is for the client to point to a picture described by the clinician in less than 5 seconds. Data collection sheets can be very basic in this

Client: Tim Thomas

SLPA: Sarah S. Assistant

Target: Point to picture described by clinician in <5 seconds

Measurement: Start – End of Questions/Stop – Points to a Picture

											Average Time
Items in field: 2 Date: 2/7/12	5.3 –	4.3 –	2.5 +	3.6 +	6.7 –	3.3 –	11.9 –	3.1 +	4.5 +	3.4 +	
Items in field: Date:											
Items in field: Date:											

Figure 8–7. Sample Response Latency Data Sheet (Timed).

case, but the key in collecting this type of data is precision in timing. In most cases, the timer would be started at the end of stimulus presentation, such as at the end of a question or command or once the picture or object stimulus was in full view. The timer would then be stopped at the *onset* of a response, although in some cases, time may be stopped once the response is completed. When collecting data on response latency, you should familiarize yourself with the timer to be used and also confirm with your supervising SLP the intended start and stop times.

In some instances, a rating scale may also be used to denote an immediate or delayed response. This may eliminate the need for a stopwatch, but it still requires you to monitor if the client responded right away after the stimulus was presented (immediate) or if there was a delay in responding (delayed). An example of a score sheet that uses this type of rating scale for charting response latency is in Figure 8–8.

You will note for both the score sheets discussed above (see Figures 8–7 and 8–8), each also has a mechanism for recording response accuracy (in addition to response latency). For example, in Figure 8–7, response accuracy is represented with a "+" under items that were correct and produced within the required length of time (less than 5 seconds) and a "–" for items that were either incorrect or were correct but not produced in less than 5 seconds. In Figure 8–8, response accuracy is noted with a "+" next to items named correctly. Often this potential exists to collect more than one form of data simultaneously. This can add important details to your data collection.

Response Independence

Response independence is another version of response analysis, fairly common

Client: Jessica Jones

SLPA: Sarah S. Assistant

Date: 8/14/12

Target: Name familiar, real objects

Key: 1 = Immediate response
      2 = Delayed response (greater than 3 seconds)
      NR = no response

Object	Response
Comb	1
Key	NR
Knife	1+
Cup	1+
Phone	1+
Fork	1
Pen	2
Shoe	NR
Sock	1
Book	2+

Figure 8–8. Sample Response Latency Data Sheet (Rating Scale).

in the field of speech-language pathology, particularly when clinicians use some type of assistance or "prompt" to achieve a desired response. Chapter 10 provides an overview of common prompts used in treatment.

In measuring response independence, you would be given details about a desired or accurate response, as well as the levels/types of assistance you can provide to help the client produce this response. You would then record if assistance was needed and, if so, what type of assistance was provided. For example, in targeting the production of prepositions, the desired/correct behavior may be for the client to say one of four types of prepositions (e.g., *in, on, over,* or *under*) in response to a question such as, "Where is the kitten?" In this case, the desired response could be a short phrase (e.g., *in the box*) or a single word (e.g., *in*). An example of a task may be to use a stuffed toy kitten and a basket, eliciting different descriptions as the client moves the toy kitten to different locations (e.g., kitten in the basket, under the basket, etc.).

In terms of assistance, some potential options may be to give the client a gestural cue, such as a hand motion representing the preposition; a phoneme cue, such as the initial sound of the appropriate

Client: Florence Flower   **SLPA:** Sarah S. Assistant
Objective: Produce prepositions in, on, over and under

										Date/Score
0	0	√	√	0	√	√	√	√	√	Date: 7/22/12
GPM	GPM	G	G	GPM		GPM	G	GP	GPM	No Cue = 10%
										G =30%
										GP = 10%
										GPM = 20%
										Date:
										Date:

Key: √ = correct 0 = incorrect   CUES: G = Gesture   P = Phoneme Cue   M = Model

Figure 8–9. Sample Response Independence Score Sheet (Key Code).

preposition; or even a verbal model. Figure 8–9 contains a sample data collection sheet representing this task. As you can see, there is a code that represents three dimensions of assistance: gestural assistance, represented by a *G*; a phoneme cue, represented by a *P*; verbal model, represented by an *M*. In this example, there is also notation for accurate production represented with a √. Inaccurate production is represented with a 0, which would denote that despite assistance, the client was not able to produce the desired response. In the example provided, consistent cues were needed to obtain an accurate response. There are, of course, a variety of other ways to record this same task in terms of response independence, including the data collection sample evident in Figure 8–10, which represents the same data in a different format.

The key to recording response independence is to understand what consti-

tutes an accurate response, to know the types of assistance that are appropriate, and to have a method for recording when assistance is provided. Of note as well, as with response latency (above), in both the samples provided you can also determine response accuracy. This combination of response accuracy and response independence within a single data collection method can be highly valuable in providing very detailed information to your supervising SLP. Furthermore, collecting data with this level of detail means that, if needed, you can categorize or summarize the client's performance based on what your supervising SLP indicates is an acceptable level of cues. For instance, in the example above, if the supervising SLP indicated that an accurate response was only a correct response produced with *no additional assistance or cues*, then the client's accuracy is 10% since in only 1 of 10 attempts was a preposition accurately produced without

Client: Florence Flower   SLPA: Sarah S. Assistant
Date: 5/18/12   Objective: Produce prepositions in,
                                         on, over and under

No Assist	Gesture	Phoneme Cue	Model	Preposition
–	–	–	–	Over
–	–	–	–	Under
–	+			In
–	+			On
–	–	–	–	Over
+				In
–	–	–	+	Under
–	+			In
–	–	+		On
–	–	–	+	Under

Figure 8–10. Sample Response Independence Score Sheet (Column Tally).

any assistance. However, if the supervising SLP deemed that an accurate response could include the provision of a gestural cue, then the client's response accuracy would be 40% since she was successful in accurately producing a preposition one time without assistance and three times with only a gestural cue.

Narration/Transcription— Speech and Language Sample

The last area of data collection to be discussed is a speech and language sample. Speech and language samples are commonly used in the field of speech-language pathology (Haynes & Pindzola, 1998; Owens, 2004). Box 8–2 lists several potential uses for a speech and language sample (Shipley & McAfee, 2009).

Research has noted many potential advantages of speech and language samples, including ecological validity (e.g., how well it relates to real-life skills), its use in outcome and intervention measures, and sensitivity in assessment, particularly for individuals who find standardized assessment difficult (Costanza-Smith, 2010). The disadvantage, however, is that a speech and language sample is only as good as the sample collected and the skill of the person transcribing and summarizing the sample. In addition, speech and language samples can be time-consuming to record, transcribe, and analyze (Costanza-Smith, 2010). SLPAs can play an important role in collecting a speech and language sample and performing initial calculations of this sample for their supervising SLP. As such, what follows is a discussion of ways to collect and analyze a speech and language sample.

Box 8–2. Potential Uses of a Speech and Language Sample[2]

- Identify speech sound errors.
- Evaluate rate of speech, fluency, and voice.
- Determine speech intelligibility.
- Compare errors in structured tasks with those of connected speech.
- Analyze language, including skills in the areas of semantics, phonology, morphology, syntax, and pragmatics.
- Determine mean length of utterance (MLU) and type token ratio (TTR).
- Identify dysarthria and apraxia.

Collecting the Sample

If your supervising SLP asks you to collect a speech and language sample, it is important that you do so in a way that is both reliable and valid. Reliable means the sample can be replicated (e.g., someone else could obtain a similar sample), whereas valid means the sample is a reasonable reflection of the client's actual speech and language abilities (Shipley & McAfee, 2009).

The first step in collecting a speech and language sample is asking your supervisor where, when, and what type of sample will be needed. Audio recording is required for in-depth analysis and transcription. Videotaping is possible, but only if good audio quality is also available. Generally, the use of digital audio files that can be stored and viewed on a computer-based program is preferred (Bunta, Ingram, & Ingram, 2003). The advantage of this method is that specific segments of the sample (e.g., sounds, words, phrases) can be reviewed more easily than with a traditional analog recording, such as a tape recorder. Samples of the digital audio files can also be embedded within a transcription for future reference.

A word of caution is in order regarding audio or video recordings. First, this will require consent from the client or the client's guardian, typically in writing. Never audio- or videotape a client without his or her knowledge and expressed consent. Second, if audio or visual information is collected, this information becomes part of the client's official records and is protected by the same confidentiality regulations discussed in Chapter 3.

In general, a sample of at least 50 words is needed, but 100 to 200 words are recommended (Constanza-Smith, 2010; Shipley & McAfee, 2009). Samples should be collected in a variety of communication contexts (e.g., a variety of communication activities). A general rule is to collect both a conversational sample and a narrative sample (Price, Hendricks, & Cook, 2010), but of course this will depend on the instruction of your SLP supervisor. When collecting a sample, it is important that you help the client become comfortable in interacting with you. This is particularly true with children, as the sample collected may not be a good reflection of their skills if you dominate the conversation or the client feels shy or nervous about communicating with you. As such, establishing a positive relationship before you collect the sample is very important (Shipley & McAfee, 2009). For young children, this may mean engaging in play before you begin collecting the sample; for older children or adults, this may mean engaging in small talk on a topic of interest. Box 8–3 contains additional recommendations in collecting a reliable and valid sample.

Conversation Sample. If you are working with adult clients or older children, you can collect a conversation sample by asking open-ended questions, such as, "Tell me about . . . " (Shipley & McAfee, 2009). Box 8–4 contains a list of additional conversation starters. For young children, incorporating pictures that depict the topic starter or pictures showing a scene with a variety of activities, such as a carnival or playground scene, may also be a good topic starter (Shipley & McAfee, 2009). Try to avoid, though, having the client name items in the picture. Rather,

---

Box 8–3. Recommendation in Collecting a Sample and Language Sample[3]

- Minimize interruptions and distractions.
- Be willing to wait for the client to talk.
- Do not talk to fill silence.
- Preselect materials and topics of interest.
- Follow the client's lead.
- Vary the subject matter.
- Limit the use of yes/no questions.
- Ask questions that elicit a longer response (e.g., Tell me about _____, What happened then? Why?).
- Make natural contributions to the conversation.

Box 8–4. Sample Conversation Starters[4]

- Tell me about what you would do if you won a million dollars (you had super-powers, or you _____)?
- Have you ever been to a hospital (airport, or _____)? Tell me about it.
- Do you like video games (movies, or _____)? Tell me about your favorite one.
- Pretend I've never had a pizza (ice cream, or _____) before. Describe it to me.
- What is your dream vacation (home, or _____)? Describe it to me.
- Do you have a pet (brother/sister, or children)? Tell me about him/her/them.

attempt to engage the client in natural conversation, with open-ended and topic-continuing statements, such as, "Tell me more about that" (Costanza-Smith, 2010; Shipley & McAfee, 2009).

Narrative Sample. A narration is a story (Merriam-Webster, 2003). Producing a narrative requires more planning and organization than a conversation (Price et al., 2010; Shipley & McAfee, 2009). One common method for collecting a narrative sample is story retell (Price et al., 2010; Shipley & McAfee, 2009). For example, you could read the client a story and then ask him or her to retell the story to you after you are done. You could also ask if they can recall a familiar story, such as *Goldilocks and the Three Bears* or *Little Red Riding Hood*, and ask them to tell it to you. Alternatively, you could show them a wordless storybook and ask them to tell you the story depicted or give them several pictures depicting the elements of a story and then ask them to place them in order and tell you the story it depicts.

Sample Transcription/Analysis

To transcribe something is to make a written copy (Merriam-Webster, 2003). The first step in transcribing a speech and language sample is to listen to the audio recording and write (or type) *everything* said by the client and any conversation partners.

You should label who is speaking (e.g., P: _____ (Partner), C: _____ (Child), Cl: _____ (Clinician), etc.). The acronyms you assign to each person should be something easily recognized. Start a new line each time a new person speaks. Number the utterances and place a / at the end of an utterance. IPA symbols can be used to transcribe errors; how-ever, for the sake of time, use IPA symbols only with errors in production (Shipley & McAfee, 2009). Unintelligible utterances can be marked with a – (e.g., I like to play –). Be sure to record everything said, including repeated words and phrases (e.g., "because he (he) doesn't like me"), filler (e.g., "the girl likes (um) strawberry ice cream with (uh) sprinkles"), and revisions ("the cat has (had) a string on her tail") (Price et al., 2010). Listen carefully. Remember that our minds are specifically tuned to make sense of what we hear. As such, although a word may make sense, you need to write down what was actually produced. For example, in the sentence, "I go to bed," you may understand in the context of the conversation that the client meant that he "went" to bed. You should write *go,* though, as this is exactly what was said. Similarly, if a client produced a distorted production of the /r/ in the word *rabbit,* you would note the distorted production, even though you may have understood the word to be *rabbit,* despite this distortion. In fact, that is a perfect example of an opportunity to use IPA symbols so that you are able to note exactly what was said.

Once you have transcribed the sample accurately, the next step is to perform an analysis of the content. Your supervising SLP will instruct you on the type of analysis to be performed. As discussed, there are many ways that a speech and language sample can be used, crossing the areas of phonology, morphology, syntax, semantics, and pragmatics. Although an extensive review of these methods is beyond the scope of this textbook, calculating mean length of utterance (MLU), as a measure of morphological complexity, and calculating lexical diversity, using TTR, are discussed in the sections that follow as these are fairly common analyses.

Last, as technology advances, computer-aided language sample analysis (CLSA) is also available and may be used by your supervising SLP. Using CLSA, information from a client's language sample is entered into specialized software, designed to perform a wide variety of in-depth analyses. The use of CLSA requires specialized training. For readers interested in learning more about CLSA, Price et al. (2010) provide a helpful tutorial on the topic of CLSA in clinical practice.

Mean Length of Utterance (MLU). MLU is the average number of morphemes (or words) produced per utterance (Shipley & McAfee, 2009). A morpheme is "a minimal meaningful unit of language" (Paul, Tentnowski, & Reuler, 2007, p. 121). For example, in the sentence, "The cats are brown," there are five morphemes, as follows:

1. the
2. cat
3. -s (to denote the meaning of more than one)
4. are
5. brown

To calculate the MLU based on morphemes (MLUm), you would first count the total number of morphemes (total morphemes) and then divide by the total number of utterances (total utterances). For example:

$$\frac{200 \text{ morphemes (total morphemes)}}{43 \text{ utterances (total utterances)}}$$
$$= 4.6 \text{ MLUm}$$

SLPs use MLU as a general indicator of language development, which corresponds to a child's chronological age in young children (Brown, 1973; Klee, Schaffer, May, Membrino, & Mougey, 1989; Miller & Chapman, 1981). SLPAs do not interpret the MLUs, but as a general reference, Appendix 8–A contains information about MLUs relative to chronological age and the age of acquisition of common morphological features. Box 8–5 contains additional recommendations for counting morphemes.

Some SLPs prefer to calculate MLU using words (MLUw). In this case, you would count the total number of words (total words) and divide by the total number of utterances (total utterances, as follows:

$$\frac{115 \text{ words (total words)}}{41 \text{ utterances (total utterances)}}$$
$$= 2.8 \text{ MLUw}$$

Type Token Ratio (TTR). TTR, developed by Johnson (1944), is a ratio of the different words (or *types*) compared with the total words produced (or *tokens*). In children, SLPs use this information to assess the semantic aspects of a speech and language sample (Hess, Haug, & Landry, 1989; Owen & Leonard, 2002). In the sentence, "Me go go go dance" there are three types (me, go, and dance), whereas in the sentence, "I like to go dancing" there are five types (I, like, to, go, dancing). Both sentences have the same number of tokens (five). TTRs closer to one represent a sample with a greater number of word types. To calculate TTR, count the total number of different words (types) and divide by the total number of words (tokens). For example:

$$\frac{32 \text{ different words (types)}}{65 \text{ total words (tokens)}} = .49 \text{ TTR}$$

Box 8–5. Recommendations for Counting Morphemes
(Lund & Duchan, 1993; Paul et al., 2007)

1. Only use intelligible utterances.
2. Count the morphemes in the first 50 consecutive utterances.
3. Do not count:
   a. Imitations
   b. Rote passages, such as nursery rhymes, songs, and so on, which have been memorized
   c. Noises (unless they are integrated into meaningful verbal utterances)
   d. Identical utterances to those already said by the client. In this case, the utterance is counted only on its first occurrence and not on subsequent attempts.
   e. Counting or other sequences of enumeration (e.g., "blue, green, yellow, red, purple")
   f. Fillers (e.g., um, well, oh)
4. Count each of the following as one morpheme:
   a. Compound words (e.g., birthday, somebody, etc.)
   b. Proper names (e.g., Mickey Mouse, etc.)
   c. Ritualized reduplication (e.g., choo-choo, night-night, etc.)
   d. Diminutive forms (doggie, daddy, etc.)
   e. Catenatives (e.g., gonna, wanna, etc.)
   f. Auxiliary verbs (contracted and noncontracted forms; e.g., He is = 2, He's = 2)
   g. Inflections (e.g., possessives, plural s, regular past –ed)

EFFICIENCY/ACCURACY IN DATA COLLECTION

Each of the above sections on data collection has stressed the importance of accuracy in data collection and things that you can do to ensure you understand and can implement data collection that meets the needs of your supervising SLP. One additional factor, which applies to all types of data collection, is efficiency—that is, your ability to quickly (and accurately) collect data under a variety of circumstances.

Hopefully, as you read about these techniques, they make sense to you and seem manageable; however, remember that you will be collecting data while you are implementing treatment and performing other tasks. In other words, you will need to multitask! You may also be collecting data in a variety of positions/locations and, in some cases, as discussed in Chapter 11, on more than one client at a time. Depending on the client, you may have only a small window of time between tasks to record data. In addition, in some cases, your data collection may be a distraction or negatively affect your client's performance. With time, you will refine your methods for collecting data and you will improve, but this is an area that will always benefit from refinement. Data collection is not easy, but as the introduction to this chapter suggests, it is critical. The following are additional tips for enhancing the efficiency of your data collection, regardless of the situation:

1. *Plan in advance:* Review what is needed in advance. Make sure you have a data collection sheet ready in advance of data collection. Fill in any details you can in advance, including things like the client's name, date, goals, and so on.

2. *Make notes or cheat sheets:* If you are using different symbols or notations to represent levels of cues (e.g., S = semantic cue, P = phoneme cue), record these symbols either at the top of your data collection sheet or in a location you can easily reference. Similarly, if you are addressing more than one goal/objective or collecting different types of data, make a note or two in a convenient location to remind you of these important details.

3. *Do not wait to summarize:* As much as possible, summarize your data and make important notes right after the session ends.

4. *Be discrete:* Use symbols or coded scoring, such as O/Xs or A/B for correct/incorrect instead of +/−; this may be needed for some clients, particularly if you are working with a client who may be distracted by your data collection or concerned about errors in performance. Chapter 10 also discusses additional techniques for positioning your data collection

sheets so that they are accessible to you but out of view of your clients.

5. *Get creative:* Sometimes it will be necessary to get creative with where you place your score sheet and what type of data collection sheet you use. For example, while engaging in a play activity on the floor with a group of preschoolers, it is not convenient to have a full sheet of paper located on a table in the room. Instead, try making tally makes or notes on a sticky note placed in a strategic location among the clients and the toys. Each client will be different, but think creatively about the circumstances and ways that you can improve efficiency with alternate solutions.

6. *Employ continuous quality improvement:* Data collection is not easy. It takes time to develop skills. Take every opportunity to learn from your mistakes. Talk to your supervising SLP about the quality of your data collection. If data collection is an area to improve, use the techniques suggested in Chapter 4, in the area of self-assessment, to evaluate your skills and look for ways to improve.

REFERENCES

American Speech-Language-Hearing Association (ASHA). (2013). *Speech-language pathology assistant scope of practice*. Retrieved from http://www.asha.org/policy

Boswell, S. (2005, September 27). Show me the data: Finding the evidence for school-based clinical decision making. *ASHA Leader.*

Brown, R. (1973). *A first language*. Cambridge, MA: Harvard University Press.

Bunta, F., Ingram, K., & Ingram, D. (2003). Bridging the digital divide: aspects of computerized data collection and analysis for language professionals. *Clinical Linguistics and Phonetics, 17*(3), 217–240.

Costanza-Smith, A. (2010). The clinical utility of language samples. *Perspectives on Language Learning and Education, 17*(1), 9–15.

Epstein, L. (2008). Clinical therapy data as learning process: The first year of clinical training and beyond. *Topic in Language Disorders, 28*(3), 274–285.

Haynes, W. O., & Pindzola, R. H. (1998). *Diagnosis and evaluation in speech pathology* (5th ed.). Boston, MA: Allyn & Bacon.

Hess, C. W., Haug, H. T., & Landry, R. G. (1989). The reliability of type-token ratios for the oral language of school-age children. *Journal of Speech and Hearing Research, 32,* 536–540.

Johnson, W. (1944). A program of research: Studies in language behavior. *Psychological Monographs, 56,* 1–15.

Jones, M., Onslow, M., Packman, A., & Gebski, V. (2006). Guidelines for statistical analysis of percentage of syllables stuttered data. *Journal of Speech, Language, and Hearing Research, 49,* 867–878.

Kawulich, B. B. (2005). Participant observation as a data collection method. *Forum: Qualitative Social Research, 6*(2). Retrieved from http://www.qualitative-research.net/index.php/fqs/article/view/466/996

Kennedy, M. (2007). Communication intervention. In R. Paul & P. Cascella (Eds.), *Introduction to clinical methods in communication disorders* (pp. 157–178). Baltimore, MD: Paul H. Brookes.

Klee, T., Schaffer, M., May, S., Membrino, I., & Mougey, K. (1989). A comparison of the age-MLU relation in normal and specifically language impaired preschool children. *Journal of Speech and Hearing Disorders, 54,* 226–233.

Lemoncello, R., & Fanning, J. L. (2011, November). *Practice-based evidence: Strategies for generating your own evidence.* Presented at the 2011 ASHA Convention, San Diego, CA.

Lund, N. J., & Dunchan, J. F. (1993). *Assessing children's language in naturalistic contexts.* (3rd ed.). Englewood Cliffs, NJ: Prentice-Hall.

Merriam-Webster. (2003). *Merriam-Webster's collegiate dictionary* (11th ed.). Springfield, MA: Author.

Miller, J., & Chapman, R. (1981). The relation between age and mean length of utterance in morphemes. *Journal of Speech and Hearing Research, 24,* 154–161.

Moore, S. M., & Pearson, L. (2003). Intervention. In, *Speech-language pathology assistants* (pp. 449–461). Clifton Park, NY: Thomson Delmar Learning.

Mowrer, D. E. (1982). *Methods of modifying speech behaviors: Learning theory in speech pathology.* Prospect Heights, IL: Waveland.

Owen, A. J., & Leonard, L. B. (2002). Lexical diversity in the spontaneous speech of children with specific language impairment: Application of D. *Journal of Speech Language and Hearing Research, 45,* 927–937.

Owens, R. E., Jr. (2004). *Language disorders: A functional approach to assessment and intervention* (4th ed.). Boston, MA: Allyn & Bacon.

Paul, R., Tentnowski, J., & Reuler, E. (2007). Communication sampling procedures. In R. Paul & P. Cascella (Eds.), *Introduction to clinical methods in communication disorders* (pp. 111–156). Baltimore, MD: Paul H. Brookes.

Price, L. H., Hendricks, S., & Cook, C. (2010). Incorporating computer-aided language sample analysis into clinical practice. *Language, Speech, and Hearing Services in Schools, 41,* 206–222.

Rao, P. R. (2011, June 7). From the president: Evidence-based practice: The coin of the realm in CSD. *ASHA Leader.*

Roth, F., & Paul, R. (2007). Communication intervention. In R. Paul & P. Cascella (Eds.), *Introduction to clinical methods in communication disorders* (pp. 1–18). Baltimore, MD: Paul H. Brookes.

Roth, F. R., & Worthington, C. K. (2001). *Treatment resource manual for speech-language pathology.* Albany, NY: Delmar.

Shipley, K. G., & McAfee, J. G. (2009). *Assessment in speech-language pathology: A resource manual.* Clifton Park, NY: Delmar Cengage Learning.

Taylor-Powell, E., & Steele, S. (n.d.). *Collecting evaluation date: Direct observation.* Program Development and Evaluation: University of Washington, Cooperative Learning. Retrieved from http://learningstore.uwex.edu/assets/pdfs/G3658-5.PDF

Williamson, G. (2009). *Mean length of utterance.* Retrieved August 18, 2013, from http://www.sltinfo.com/downloads/mean-length-of-utterance.pdf

CHAPTER ENDNOTES

1. American Speech-Language-Hearing Association (ASHA, 2013, Service Delivery, para. 1)

2. Adapted from Shipley and McAfee (2009).

3. Adapted from Shipley and McAfee (2009, pp. 161–162).

4. Adapted from Shipley and McAfee (2009, p. 163).

APPENDIX 8–A

Mean Length of Utterance (MLU) and Age Equivalent

MLU	Age Equivalent (Within 1 Month)
1.31	18 months
1.62	21 months
1.92	24 months
2.54	30 months
2.85	33 months
3.16	36 months
3.47	39 months
3.78	42 months
4.09	45 months
4.40	48 months
4.71	51 months
5.02	54 months
5.32	57 months
5.63	60 months

Source: Miller, 1981, as cited in Williamson, 2009.

APPENDIX 8–B

Common Morphological Features and Age of Mastery

Rank	Morphological Feature	Example	Age of Mastery
1	present progressive -*ing*	daddy sing<u>ing</u>, mummy play<u>ing</u>	19–28
2	in	key <u>in</u> cup, ball <u>in</u> box	27–30
3	on	ball <u>on</u> bed, cup <u>on</u> table	27–33
4	regular plural -*s*	two cat<u>s</u>, three dog<u>s</u>	27–33
5	irregular past tense	mummy <u>fell</u>, daddy <u>went</u>	25–46
6	possessive -*'s*	mummy<u>'s</u> hat, daddy<u>'s</u> car	26–40
7	uncontractible copula	she <u>is</u> (response to who is happy?)	28–46
8	articles	mummy got <u>a</u> dog, <u>the</u> ball	28–46
9	regular past tense -*ed*	daddy walk<u>ed</u>, a car crash<u>ed</u>	26–48
10	regular third person -*s*	mummy walk<u>s</u>, daddy play<u>s</u>	28–50
11	irregular third person	mummy <u>does</u>, daddy <u>has</u> a ball	28–50
12	uncontractible auxiliary	she <u>is</u> (response to *who is coming?*)	29–48
13	contractible copula	he<u>'s</u> happy (cf. *he is happy*)	29–49
14	contractible auxiliary	mummy<u>'s</u> playing (cf. *mummy is playing*)	30–50

Source: Brown, 1973; Miller, 1981, as cited in Williamson, 2009.

CHAPTER 9
Note Writing

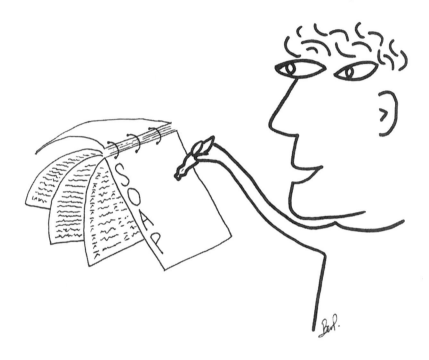

Observe, record, tabulate, communicate. Use your five senses. Learn to see, learn to hear, learn to feel, learn to smell, and know that by practice alone you can become expert.
William Osler (one of the fathers of modern medicine)

As mentioned in Chapter 1, speech-language pathology assistants (SLPAs) may be asked to assist their supervising speech-language pathologist (SLP) in providing treatment or screening and data collection on individuals with communication disorders (American Speech-Language-Hearing Association [ASHA], 2013). In some cases, this may be with your supervisor present. In other cases, you may provide these services when your supervising SLP is not physically present in the room but given her specific instructions. In either case, as Chapters 7 and 8 suggest, it is critical that you perform these tasks as instructed and that you accurately record important aspects of the client's performance. It is equally important that you are able to effectively summarize and consolidate this information, both as formal documentation of the services you provided and as a means of conveying important information to other professionals, including your supervisor. Writing a clinical note is often used for this purpose. The format of these notes can vary across settings and given the mechanism(s) for reimbursement of services (ASHA, n.d.-a, n.d.-b; Sutherland Cornett, 2006). In addition, as an SLPA, how often you write a note on a client will be directed by your supervisor. Notes in some settings are written after every encounter with the client, whereas in other settings, they are written on a weekly basis, or as needed, given a specific type of interaction.

A common format in the field of speech-language pathology for writing notes is an SOAP note (Moon-Meyer, 2004; Roth & Worthington, 2001; Shipley & McAfee, 2009). SOAP is an acronym for the following: subjective (S), objective (O), assessment (A), and plan (P) (Shipley & McAfee, 2009). SOAP notes are often used in medical settings (Roth & Worthington, 2001) but can be modified in form and content to fit the needs of an educational setting. Understanding the SOAP format, as well as the ways to effectively convey information in a clinical note in your setting, is an important skill for an SLPA. However, as will be discussed, specific aspects of the SOAP note format are not consistently applicable to an SLPA's role or scope of services. The sections that follow discuss each aspect of a SOAP note from the perspective of an SLPA. The CD of this textbook contains a blank version of an SLPA applicable SOAP note for your use.

SUBJECTIVE (S)

The subjective (S) portion of an SOAP note contains "nonmeasurable and historical information" important in understanding the client's performance (Shipley & McAfee, 2009, p. 138). A good way to think about this portion of the note is that it provides context to help the reader interpret what will follow in the remaining portions of the note. The dictionary defines *subjective* as "arising out of or identified by means of one's perception" (Merriam-Webster, 2003). This fits well with the language of this section as it contains your opinions, observations, or information reported to you by others.

Key areas to include in the subjective section of an SOAP note (Moon-Meyer, 2004; Roth & Worthington, 2001; Shipley & McAfee, 2009) and corresponding examples are as follows:

Your observations about the client's mood:

- The client smiled and laughed frequently throughout the session.
- The patient was tearful today.
- Melissa greeted the clinician in the waiting area with a hug and was eager to begin the session.

Statements about the client's behavior or his or her current status, from the perspective of the client or family member(s) or others involved in the client's care (e.g., teachers, nurses, aides):

- Johnny's mother indicated that he has been remembering to close his mouth while breathing.
- The client indicated that he was successful with his homework

and felt it helped his recall of the relaxation techniques, which he used during his classroom science fair presentation.
- The patient's wife indicated that the patient is talking more at home and is regaining movement of his right arm.
- Mrs. Smith reported that Susan experienced three seizures this week, with one resulting in admittance to the emergency room on 10/20/13.

A description of the client's level of cooperation and participation:

- Rebecca appeared reluctant to engage with her peers during the group reading activity, often averting her eyes or looking away when asked questions by her peers.
- The client was cooperative and participated fully with all tasks.
- The client refused to participate in the oral reading task.
- Steven appeared distracted by the noise from the playground during screening. He frequently turned to look at the window and asked several times to be excused from the session.

A description of any factors in the environment, or other relevant conditions, that may have influenced the client's performance:

- Due to a fire drill, screening was interrupted for 10 minutes while the SLPA and the client evacuated the building. Screening resumed after the drill.

- The client's wife, Susan, was present during treatment.
- Henry arrived 15 minutes late for the session, due to an assembly in home period.

Keep in mind in this section of the note, you should describe what you see and not simply label the behavior. For example, if the client appeared happy to you, rather than saying, "Johnny was *happy*," describe the behaviors that you think lead you to that opinion, such as, "Johnny smiled and laughed frequently during the session." Similarly, when you are reporting information shared with you, be sure to identify the source of this information in your statement. For example, instead of saying, "The patient was tired as he did not sleep well last night," report instead, "The nurse on duty indicated that the patient did not sleep well last night," or "The patient reported that he felt tired from not sleeping well the night prior." Remember, too, that your verb choice in this section and the objective (O) section (below) should be past tense, as you are describing something that already occurred.

Last, you will note that in the examples provided, the client is sometimes referred to by first name and other times by "the client" or "the patient." This will apply to all other sections of the note as well and will depend on the setting. In most hospital and clinical settings, the client's name is not used within the body of the medical records, such as in an SOAP note, and other reports. As such, in those settings, "the client" or "the patient" is the preferred term. In most educational settings, however, the client is referred to by first name. You should check with your supervising SLP to confirm which form is appropriate in your setting.

OBJECTIVE (O)

The objective (O) section of the SOAP note contains facts and measurable findings about the session (Moon-Meyer, 2004; Roth & Worthington, 2001; Shipley & McAfee, 2009). Typically, the "data" collected during the session (see Chapter 8) are reported in this section. As the definition of *objective* suggests, this section contains observable and measurable information about the client's performance during that session (in contrast to opinion or reports from others).

This section typically begins with a brief summary of what was done during the session. If screening was performed, state the name of the screener used or describe the methods of screening or other forms of data collection, as instructed by your supervising SLP. If this was a treatment session, state the goal(s)/objective(s) targeted that session. This is then followed by the actual data regarding the client's performance. Examples from objective (O) sections of SOAP notes are as follows:

- John's AAC goals were targeted today. For Objective 3 (requesting an activity using eye gaze), Johnny requested Bingo and Candy Land using eye gaze when the SLPA presented a field of two icons choices. For Objective 5 (switch activation), Johnny answered 10 yes/no questions accurately using his yes/no voice output device.
- Objective 1a (word opposites): 15 of 20 (75%) using picture cards.
- Fluency count performed during morning story time in David's classroom (Figure 9–1).

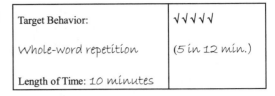

Figure 9–1. Sample frequency count table for objective (O) section of a SOAP note.

- Goal: *The client will correctly produce the /r/ phoneme in all positions of a word with 100% accuracy.* Performance: The client was 75% accurate for this task, during a Go Fish activity requiring the client to request cards containing one- and two-syllable words with /r/ in the initial, medial, and final position of the word.
- Prepositions (Objective 5) (Figure 9–2).

In some of the examples provided, the information is very brief, and in others, more detail is provided. In some instances, the information is provided in text format, and in others, tables and charts are used. The level of detail needed, and the actual format of this section, will vary from setting to setting and depend on your supervisor's needs and her or his instructions in this area. In some settings, the content of an SOAP note is incorporated within the actual data collection sheets used to record client performance (Appendix 9–A). In that case, an additional SOAP note may not be required. The CD of this textbook contains a blank version of this form for your use. In preparation for writing an SOAP note, you should review typical notes in your setting, as well as discuss with your supervisor the depth, format, and type of

No Assistance	Gestural Cue	Sound Cue	Modeled Production	Preposition
−	−	−	−	Over
−	−	−	−	Under
−	+			In
−	+			On
−	−	−	−	Over
+				In
−	−	−	+	Under
−	+			In
−	−	+		On
−	−	−	+	Under
TOTALS: 1/10 (10%)	3/10 (30%)	1/10 (10%)	2/10 (20%)	

Figure 9–2. Sample cue record table for objective (O) section of a SOAP note.

information she or he needs in this (and the other sections) of the note.

Note that in some of the examples provided, a third-person personal pronoun is used to describe the SLPA's actions (e.g., "when *the SLPA* presented a field of two icons to choose from" as in the first example). Third-person pronoun use is common in professional writing in the field of speech-language pathology and may be the preferred form in your setting. If that is the case, instead of saying, "*I* gave the client paragraphs to read," which used a first-person pronoun (I), you would reword the note and refer to yourself as "the SLPA," as in "*The SLPA* gave the client paragraphs to read." You should model your style of writing to match acceptable standards in your setting.

ANALYZE (AZ)

This section of the SOAP note and the one that follows (P) are sections that require modification for SLPA use as they differ substantively from the forms suggested for use by SLPs. In most references about SOAP notes, written for SLPs, the "A" portion of the SOAP note is referred to as "assessment" (Moon-Meyer, 2004; Roth & Worthington, 2001; Shipley & McAfee, 2009). As discussed in Chapters 1 and 2, SLPAs are not to perform any type of assessment, whether formal or informal (ASHA, 2013). As such, changes in content and wording of this section are required to align with the duties and responsibilities of an SLPA. A plausible change in this area would be to revise this section to consist of *analyze* (Az), meaning that it is appropriate, and within the scope of an SLPA, to *analyze* one of two aspects of the session itself: (1) an objective summary of the client's current performance compared with a previous session(s) (Statement of Performance) and (2) a description of the prescribed task, stimulus, or reinforcement that was easy or difficult to implement during that session (Description of Task, Stimulus, Reinforcement).

In terms of a Statement of Performance, Table 9–1 contains a comparison of an A that an SLP may write assessing the client's performance versus an Az, appropriate for an SLPA.

As you can see in this table, for the SLPA Az section, there is no *interpretation* of this information in terms of progress made to achieving goals or in relation to the client's current status. Rather, appropriate SLPA format in this section would be to limit the discussion to a summary of objective information from today's session as it relates to a previous session(s).

Also in the Az section, it is appropriate for the SLPA to comment on the tasks, materials, and reinforcement that were easy or difficult for the SLPA to implement (Description of Task, Stimulus, Reinforcement). This may be helpful to your supervising SLP in planning future sessions or understanding the objective data in more detail. Relative to a description of tasks, stimulus, or reinforcement, Table 9–2 contains a comparison of an A that an SLP

Table 9–1. Assessment Versus Analyze (Statement of Performance)

Assessment (A) Appropriate for an SLP	Analyze (Az) Appropriate for an SLPA
Susan has made good progress in achieving Goal 2 (Objective 5). Her production for /s/ initial sounds has increased in accuracy from initial sessions, with some generalization noted for nontarget positions (e.g., /s/ final production). She is stimulable for /s/ final position sounds and was noted on one occasion during today's session to produce an /s/ initial word accurately in a conversational context.	Susan's performance on Goal 2 (Objective 5—/s/ in initial position of words) was 70%. During the previous session, her performance was 50% on this same objective.
The client remains with significant aphasia and significant difficulty verbally naming pictured items; however, he has improved in his use of multiple modalities, such as gestures, drawing, and writing. His performance on Objective 3 (use of gestures) indicates an increase in performance from the previous sessions.	This session, the client's scores on Objective 3 (use of gestures) increased from a score of 1 of 10 during last week's session to a score of 5 of 10 during today's session.

Note Writing **277**

Table 9–2. Assessment Versus Analyze (Description of Task, Stimulus, Reinforcement)

Assessment (A) Appropriate for an SLP	Analyze (Az) Appropriate for an SLPA
The client continues to need cues to employ communication strategies during a group context and may benefit from a written reminder or one-on-one training in the scripted language needed to initiate questions or ask for clarification/assistance in group contexts.	During the barrier communication task (Objective 5), the client needed several reminders (5) to *describe* the picture to fellow group members and to ask group members for questions if he did not understand their descriptions. (*Task*)
Jane's participation during speech sessions has increased with the use of personally relevant stimulus and given treatment activities using social structure and reinforcement. She may also benefit from treatment during small group sessions with peers.	Jane appeared to enjoy using the Sponge Bob cartoons to elicit the /s/ sound. She requested additional turns in making sentences with these cards. (*Stimulus*)
Steven benefits from the use of token reinforcement to increase on-task behaviors during speech sessions. This may be an area to discuss with his classroom teacher in increasing on-task participation during classroom activities as well.	Steven began following directions and participating more fully when tokens were provided for on-task behaviors. (*Reinforcement*)

may write versus an Az, appropriate for an SLPA, for this type of information.

Note that for each of the examples in Table 9–2, the information under Az for an SLPA is limited to a *description* of some aspect of the task itself, the stimulus or materials used, or the reinforcement. It does not extend to interpreting what this information means or generalizing what was observed to a statement about the client's overall performance or status. That is limited to the scope of an SLP (ASHA, 2013).

MY PLAN (PM)

The final section of a SOAP note is that of the "P." Similar to the A portion of a SOAP, this is a section that requires modification compared with the version that would be written by an SLP. Traditional textbooks on the topic of SOAP, written for SLPs, state that the "P" portion of an SOAP consist of the plan for the future course of treatment (Moon-Meyer, 2004; Paul & Cascella, 2007; Roth & Worthington, 2001; Shipley & McAfee, 2009). Developing, modifying, or altering a client's plan of treatment from that specifically prescribed by the SLP is not within the scope of an SLPA (ASHA, 2013). As such, discussing the future course of treatment for a client in the "P" section of a note is outside the scope of practice for an SLPA. A reasonable modification, however, would be to include a plan of action specific to the needs of the SLPA herself or himself, or a "Pm," meaning "my" plan as an SLPA.

An excellent use of the Pm section of an SLPA note is to relay any specific concerns or requests conveyed to you by the client, family members, or other team members involved in the client's case. Counseling or the provision of "interpretative information to the student/patient/client, family, or others regarding the patient/client status or service" is outside the scope of duties of an SLPA (ASHA, 2013, Responsibilities Outside the Scope of an SLPA, para. 2). As such, if, for example, a client or family member expresses a concern or request for information about services, the SLPA should first inform the client or family member that she or he will relay this information directly to her or his supervising SLP. In most cases, this information should be given verbally, and immediately, to your supervising SLP. The Pm portion of your note is *also* a place to document this information, such as the following:

- The client requested additional information about options for additional days of services.
- Alice's mothers asked to speak with the supervising SLP about Alice's performance in the classroom and impending IEP meeting.
- Stephen's teacher (Mr. Collings) requested information about the client's treatment goals and progress.
- The client indicated he is concerned that his speech is not improving with treatment. He indicated that he fears he will not improve further.
- Mrs. Smith asked about developmental milestones and if Susan has met those in the areas of language and speech.

You should also check with your supervising SLP to confirm her or his preference as to the location of this information. Some supervisors may prefer this information go in the S section of the note. Remember in this section, similar to the S section, when you are reporting information shared with you, be sure to identify the source of this information in your statement. Be sure as well to indicate how you responded to this request or concern, such as, "The SLPA indicated she would ask her supervising SLP to contact the client's mother immediately with these details," "The SLPA informed the client that this information was not within her scope of duties to discuss but that she would convey his concerns directly to her supervisor," or "The SLPA provided Mr. Collings with the SLP's direct phone number and indicated that she would relay this request directly to her as well."

The Pm section is also an area to request additional information, assistance, or resources from your supervising SLP. In this respect, most of these types of statements in the Pm section would start with, "Plan to discuss with supervisor . . . ," or "Plan to . . . " such as the following:

- Plan to discuss with supervisor Johnny's distraction during treatment tasks and ways to increase his participation during group activities.
- Plan to discuss with supervisor how the client's AAC system should be used during reading activities.
- Plan to clarify what would be classified as a whole-word repetition during Stephen's conversational speech.
- Plan to request additional information about facilitating techniques referenced in Scott's treatment plan.
- Plan to review with supervisor current data collection methods to ensure accuracy in recording information requested.

Last, the Pm section of an SLPA note can be used to detail any specific preparation you as an SLPA will need to take, before the next session with this client, such as the following:

- Plan to place game choices under the table before beginning session so they are not a source of distraction during the group treatment session.
- Plan to presort stimulus cards into three piles (sounds, words, phrases) to facilitate easy access while targeting Objective 5.
- Plan to code data collection sheet ahead of time with required scoring parameters to make data collection more efficient and effective during the treatment session.
- Plan to use timer to ensure treatment activities end with enough time to review assigned homework activities.
- Plan to start next treatment with a review of "good listening" rules.

These statements would most likely begin with the statement, "Plan to . . . " They may be items you have already identified as applicable to a future session. If not, you can list them as an area to discuss with your supervising SLP. However, importantly, consistent with an SLPA scope of practice, any plan of action outlined by an SLPA must *not* be related to the client's course of treatment, such as, "Plan to target short-term Goal 5," "Plan to discharge Goal 3 due to achievement," "Plan to modify literacy objective to include sound letter correspondence training," and so on. Each of these statements is the specific domain of the supervising SLP (ASHA, 2013).

As discussed in Chapter 4, the use of a reflection journal documenting your performance in a clinical session may be a good source of information to include in the Pm section of an SLPA note. The CD of this textbook contains a blank reflection journal sheet for your use. Box 9–1 contains a sample of a reflection journal entry provided in Chapter 4. The sections highlighted in bold are examples of items that may carry over into a Pm note for that particular session, such as the following:

- **Plan to discuss with supervisor methods for effective data collection.**
- **Plan to rearrange position of table in treatment room, facing away from the window to ensure students are not distracted during treatment.**
- **Plan to change instruction and procedures for group activity, including preselecting order of activities and assigning turns for who goes first in each activity.**

TIPS FOR EFFECTIVE NOTE WRITING

Appendix 9–B contains samples of SLPA notes written following the format described above. You will note that they vary in length and complexity, but all roughly follow an S, O, Az, Pm format. It is valuable to review examples of notes in your setting to ensure your notes are consistent with setting-specific expectations. In addition, keep in mind as well that many of the tips on professional writing discussed in Chapter 4 still apply in writing a clinical note. Specific to clinical notes, Figure 9–3 contains a checklist of tips to employ in effective note writing in any setting. This information is also available in a checklist on the CD of this chapter.

Box 9–1. Reflection Journal Entry

Date: 2/14/2013
Task: *10:00 a.m. Small Group Session (JL, AS, TM)*

Successes:
JL and AS participated fully and had high levels of accuracy for target sounds. The session ended on time. The students appeared to enjoy the session and were eager to begin. I felt relaxed and was able to stay focused on each student's targets during the session.

Difficulties:
TM was distracted during the session. He left the table several times to look out the window. I wasn't sure how to shape this behavior, other than reminding him that he needed to participate. I had difficulty keeping track of errors and the number and type of cues I gave for sound production. When I listened to the audio recording of the session, I provided many more models than I had noted on my data sheet. I also said "okay" twice when JL's target sound was not correct. The time spent on preparing for the session's activities took too long (10 minutes). The students argued about which activity to do first and who would start in each activity.

Areas to Improve:
1. *Increase structure of the session at the onset.* **Make sure to briefly instruct the students in the rules of the activity. Don't allow them to choose the order of the activities. Rotate who goes first per session or have them draw from a deck of cards and whoever gets the highest card goes first.**
2. *Improve data collection methods. Collect additional examples of data collection sheets used for group sessions.* **Check with supervisor about her methods for effectively and quickly noting both errors and cues in group settings.** *Possibly rearrange data collection sheet in advance with a column to place an X under each type of cue. Place a sticky note reminder on my data collection sheet for next time reminding me not to say "okay." Listen to the audio recording from next week's session to record the number of "okays."*
3. *Close the blinds in the room or* **move the table so the students aren't distracted by the things happening outside the window.**

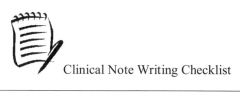 Clinical Note Writing Checklist

___ Note is dated.

___ Note is free of spelling errors.

___ Note is free of grammatical errors.

___ Note is free of any interpretation, assessment, or recommendation about a specific course of treatment.

___ Note is free of slang and colloquialism

___ Note uses standard forms of medical abbreviation and phonetic notation

___ As applicable, third person personal pronoun is used to describe your actions (e.g., "The SLPA . . . ")

___ Setting specific terms are used to reference the client (e.g., referring to the client by his first name, full name, or by using the terms "the client" or "the patient").

___ Information conveyed to you by others is referenced as such (e.g., The client's family reports . . . , Susan stated . . . , etc.)

___ Note uses language that describes a behavior observed and does not label or diagnosis the behavior.

___ Note contains a description of what was done.

    ___ Note states specific treatment goals and objective targeted

    ___ Note states specific tools or procedures used

___ Note contains a summary of the client's performance in objective terms (e.g., percentages, frequency counts, etc.).

___ Note uses past tense in applicable sections (typically O and S, and sometimes Az section)

___ Note uses future tense in the Pm section.

Figure 9–3. Clinical Note Writing Checklist.

281

REFERENCES

American Speech-Language-Hearing Association (ASHA). (n.d.-a). *Documentation in school settings: Frequently asked questions.* Retrieved February 12, 2013, from http://www.asha.org/SLP/Documentation-in-Schools-FAQs

American Speech-Language-Hearing Association (ASHA). (n.d.-b). *Private health plans frequently asked questions: Speech-language pathology.* Retrieved February 12, 2013, from http://www.asha.org/practice/reimbursement/private-plans/php_faqs_slp.htm#7

American Speech-Language-Hearing Association (ASHA). (2013). *Speech-language pathology assistant scope of practice.* Retrieved from http://www.asha.org/policy

Merriam-Webster. (2003). *Merriam-Webster's collegiate dictionary* (11th ed.). Springfield, MA: Author.

Moon-Meyer, S. (2004). *Survival guide for the beginning speech-language clinician.* Austin, TX: Pro-Ed.

Paul, R., & Cascella, P.W. (2007). *Introduction to clinical methods in communication disorders* (2nd ed.). Baltimore, MD: Paul H. Brookes.

Roth, F. R., & Worthington, C. K. (2001). *Treatment resource manual for speech-language pathology.* Albany, NY: Delmar.

Shipley, K. G., & McAfee, J. G. (2009). *Assessment in speech-language pathology: A resource manual.* Clifton Park, NY: Delmar Cengage Learning.

Sutherland Cornett, B. (2006, September 5). Clinical documentation in speech-language pathology: Essential information for successful practice. *ASHA Leader.* Retrieved from http://www.asha.org/Publications/leader/2006/060905/f060905b/#1

Data Sheet Incorporating SOAP Format

Student: _____ **Teacher:** _____/**Room #:** _____

Date: _____ (Length of Session: _____)

Session goal(s)	Comments (S)	Data (O) Results (A)	Plan

Date: _____ (Length of Session: _____)

Session goal(s)	Comments (S)	Data (O) Results (A)	Plan

Date: _____ (Length of Session: _____)

Session goal(s)	Comments (S)	Data (O) Results (A)	Plan

APPENDIX 9–B

Sample SOAP Notes

SOAP NOTE EXAMPLE 1

S:/ The patient's wife indicated that the patient is talking more at home and is regaining movement of his right arm. The patient greeted group members with a smile as he entered the treatment room.

O:/ Target Goal 2a (in response to word-finding difficulties during group conversation, the patient will independently use a related gesture in three of five opportunities):

Word Retrieval Difficulty	Spontaneous Gesture	Gesture With Cue (# of Cues)
1.	+	
2.	+	
3.	–	+ (cues: 2)
4.	–	–
5.	+	

Az:/ This session, the client's scores on Objective 2a (spontaneous gestures) increased from a score of 1 of 5 during last week's session to a score of 3 of 5 (criteria) during today's session. Spontaneous gestures included swinging his arms to represent "home run," a motion to his head to represent "baseball cap," and a thumbs-up letting the group know his dinner last night was good.

Pm:/ Plan to discuss with supervisor how to change procedures for initiating the group's conversation activity, including potentially preselecting the order of activities prior to the session or assigning turns for who goes first in each activity. This may decrease time spent organizing these aspects of the conversation during the session. The patient's wife asked to speak with the supervising SLP about additional community resources in the area of physical therapy. The SLPA notified her that she would share this request with her supervisor. The SLPA also gave the patient's wife her supervisor's direct phone line.

Note Writing **285**

SOAP NOTE EXAMPLE 2

The client smiled and laughed frequently throughout the session. He indicated he was successful with his homework and felt it helped him recall relaxation techniques, which he indicated he used during his classroom science fair presentation. Stutter-free speech in 2-minute narratives (Goal 4) was targeted during today's session. The client completed 10 of 13 2-minute narratives, with zero (0) disfluency (76% accuracy). The use of narratives about NASCAR (describing features of favorite teams) elicited amble client narration. Plan to review with supervisor current data collection methods for noting number and type of disfluency.

SOAP NOTE EXAMPLE 3

Subjective: Jill was tearful today and reluctant to leave her mom to participate in treatment. Jill's mom attended the first 15 minutes of treatment.

Objective:

Goal 1 (phonologic awareness—syllable identification)
Jill was 100% accurate (20/20) for clapping once per syllable for words read by the SLPA.

Goal 2 (phonologic awareness—identification of initial sound)
Jill was 75% accurate (15/20) for pointing to the initial sound of words read by the SLPA, given a choice of five printed letters.

Goal 3 (phonologic awareness—sound blending)
Jill was 90% accurate (18/20) for blending and producing the correct target word from syllable segments read to her by the SLPA.

Analysis: Jill appeared to enjoy the use of Sponge Bob–related vocabulary during sound blending and initial letter identification tasks. Her scores across all goals have improved from the previous session when accuracy for Goals 1, 2, and 3 were all less than 50%.

Plan: Plan to identify additional topic areas to incorporate into future sessions. Plan to discuss with supervisor the potential use of crayons and drawing during treatment tasks. During the first portion of the session, when Jill experienced difficulty separating from her mom, a drawing activity was initiated by Jill's mom. Jill's mom indicated that Jill enjoys drawing at home and has started writing the letters of her name within drawn images.

CHAPTER 10

Implementing Treatment

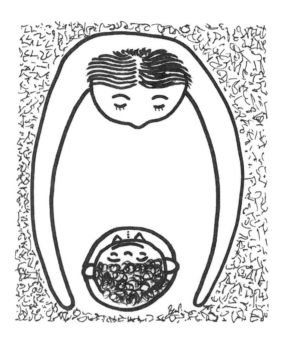

To do something, however small, to make others happier and better, is the highest ambition, the most elevating hope, which can inspire a human being.

John Lubbock

As has been mentioned, as a speech-language pathology assistant (SLPA), you may be called upon to implement treatment services with individuals with communicative disorders (American Speech-Language-Hearing Association [ASHA], 2013). This, of course, will be under the direct supervision and instruction of your supervising speech-language pathologist (SLP) (ASHA, 2013). Often, the thought of this is both exciting and intimidating to a new SLPA. When you see an experienced and effective SLP implementing services, it may seem effortless and easy, but in fact it requires very careful planning, specific training, and, in many cases, years of experience.

The term *service delivery model* is used to describe "where, when, and with whom" clinical services in speech-language pathology are provided (Cascella, Purdy, & Dempsey, 2007, p. 259). In terms of *where* treatment is provided, this can vary greatly with the population you primarily serve and the setting in which you are employed. Treatment could be provided within the client's environment, such as in his or her classroom, community, home, or work setting. In some settings, this is referred to as a "push-in" (Cirrin et al., 2010) or an "integrated" (Buysse & Bailey, 1993) service delivery model. This is in contrast to treatment services provided outside the client's environment, such as within a clinical space designated for these purposes. This is often referred to as a "pull-out" (McGinty & Justice, 2006) or a "clinical" (Cascella et al., 2007) service delivery model.

In recent years, a new venue in the location of treatment services has also emerged in an area known as telepractice. Telepractice refers to "the application of telecommunications technology to the delivery of speech-language pathology and audiology professional services at a distance by linking clinician to client/patient or clinician to clinician for assessment, intervention, and/or consultation" (ASHA, n.d., Telepratice: Overview, para. 1). ASHA's scope-of-practice document states that provided training, supervision, and planning are appropriate, SLPAs may "provide guidance and treatment via telepractice to students, patients, and clients who are selected by the supervising SLP as appropriate for this service delivery model" (ASHA, 2013, Service Delivery, para. 1). If you are asked to provide treatment services via telepratice, many of the concepts discussed in this chapter relative to treatment implementation are applicable to telepractice, but specialized training, beyond these principles, will also be required for the implementation of telepractice (ASHA, n.d.). As an SLPA, you may also be asked to serve as a "facilitator" for treatment services provided by the SLP via telepractice (ASHA, n.d., Telepractice: Key Issues, Facilitators in Telepractice for Audiology and Speech-Language Services, para. 1). In these instances, you are not the one providing treatment but rather are present, at the client's location, to assist the client while the SLP provides treatment remotely via telecommunication technology. Specialized training is also required to serve as a facilitator for telepractice. A helpful overview for school-based clinicians on this topic is available from Garcia (2013).

When treatment is provided addresses the frequency and duration of services, such as the amount of time per session, the number or sessions per week or month, and the total duration of treatment. The *whom* in service delivery refers to which professional is most appropriate for providing these services. In the case of an SLPA, this may mean a decision of whether services are provided solely by the SLP or with the assistance of an SLPA.

Your supervising SLP will determine the optimum delivery model for each individual client, including where, when, and with whom treatment services are to be provided. You should familiarize yourself with each of these aspects of your client's service delivery format. *How* treatment is implemented is also highly variable and determined by your supervising SLP. Treatment may be provided to an individual or to a small group of individuals, using a wide array of methods and intervention models (Cascella et al., 2007). How treatment is provided can generally be described given the two extremes of clinician-directed or client-centered approaches (Roth & Paul, 2007).

Clinician-directed approaches are highly structured and directed by the clinician. The most common forms of clinician-directed approaches are either "drill" or "drill and play" (Roth & Paul, 2007, p. 164). In drill activities, a very specific chain of events occurs. First, the clinician presents a stimulus, such a picture, a written word, a question, or some other method of eliciting a desired response from the client. This is known as the antecedent. The client then produces the required/requested response. This is referred to as the behavior. The clinician then responds to this behavior with reinforcement or corrective feedback (also known as the consequence). Generally, this same procedure of *antecedent-behavior-consequence* is then repeated multiple times, in a very similar fashion, until a required level of accuracy is obtained. A similar procedure is implemented with "drill and play," except the sequence of *antecedent-behavior-consequence* is embedded within some type of motivating activity. For children, this is typically some type of game or play activity, as in the case of eliciting target words using a series of bags labeled with a target word and a small sponge (Roth & Paul, 2007). The client is given the small sponge and allowed to select the word to be produced by throwing the sponge into one of the bags (the antecedent). The client then produces the corresponding word labeled on the bag (the behavior). This is then followed by the clinician reinforcing or providing feedback about the client's production (the consequence).

In client-centered approaches, less clinician direction is provided. The emphasis in this type of approach is on eliciting a desired behavior in a natural context and then on responding in a communicative way (Roth & Paul, 2007). The sequence of *antecedent-behavior-consequence* is modified at the level of the antecedent and consequence. In client-centered approaches, the clinician waits for the client to initiate a behavior spontaneously, instead of directly eliciting it. Generally, this is done by structuring the environment to facilitate meaningful and enjoyable communication attempts in a naturally occurring context. For children, this usually means engaging in play activities that are rewarding and motivating and then encouraging communication during play. For adults, this may mean engaging in conversation regarding topics that are meaningful and interesting to the client. In terms of consequences, rather than providing specific corrective feedback or reinforcements such as "good" or "correct" (as is typical in clinician-directed approaches), in client-centered approaches, the clinician responds in a communicative way back to the client's behavior. For example, if while engaging in a play activity with trains, the client spontaneously uses a targeted behavior, such as "my train is going *under* the bridge" (behavior), the clinician would then respond as would be typical in a communicative context, such as, "I see your train is going under the bridge. My train is traveling *over* the bridge" (the consequence).

In real-world settings, SLPs and SLPAs will engage in a blended approach, incorporating elements of both clinician-directed and client-centered approaches, as applicable to the service delivery model, goals of intervention, and the client's needs and preferences. Using either approach requires careful planning and consideration relative to the client, the environment, and your actions as the clinician. The sections that follow highlight some general concepts and things to consider in each of these areas.

THINGS TO CONSIDER: THE CLIENT

When it comes to thinking about the client in the scope of successful treatment sessions, there are many avenues to explore, such as things like the client's age, goals, interests, strengths, and weaknesses, and so forth. Many of these details will be discussed in the client's assessment report and treatment plans, compiled by your supervising SLP. One of the most important things in addition to these core features is, "Is the client ready to participate in the treatment session?" This seems simplistic, but it is the most basic and minimal requirement for *any* successful treatment session.

Cognitive researchers describe two important principles related to client readiness—namely, low road processing and high road processing (Cox, 2007; Meltzer, 2010; Ward, 2009). *Low-road processing* entails attention to basic biologic and physiologic need states, such as hunger, thrist, fatigue, pain, fear, and so forth. In contrast, *high-road processing* is a set of mental processes that allow us to regulate our thinking and learning. Collectively, high-road processes are referred to as executive control. These include skills such as the ability to pay attention, plan, prioritize, organize, shift between tasks, access working memory, and monitor our performance (Cox, 2007; Meltzer, 2010; Ward, 2007). Regardless of the task, these are all important skills in fully participating in treatment sessions and are a key component of learning. The level of complexity needed in each of these areas will of course be tailored to the client's abilities, but the important point in understanding these principles is that if the client's resources are diverted to low-road processing, he or she will have

limited ability to engage in high-road processing (Ward, 2007). For example, if a client is hungry, in pain, tired, angry, upset, scared, frustrated, and so forth, this makes high-road processing challenging and will dramatically reduce the client's ability to learn. As such, a key first step in a successful treatment session is ensuring the client's basic needs are met so that she or he can focus on high-road (and not low-road) processing.

Developing a strong clinician-client relationship (as discussed below) will address some of the emotional aspects of low-road processing, such as anxiety, frustration, fear, and so forth. In terms of biologic needs, such as hunger, fatigue, pain, the need to use the restroom, and so forth, if these are things you can address in the moment of a specific session, do so. If not, work with your supervising SLP, the client, the client's family, and related professionals to see how these needs can be met *before* attending the treatment session.

Another important factor related to if a client is ready to participate in treatment pertains to motivation. Motivation plays a key part in successful treatment sessions. Two important elements in motivation are: (1) understanding the purpose of treatment and (2) seeing a benefit in participation (Larson, 2010; Moon-Meyer, 2004; Ragan, 2011). As an SLPA, it is outside your scope of practice to discuss the outcomes of treatment *overall*, but this does not preclude you from explaining the tasks and intended activities of a specific session (ASHA, 2013). Taking time in treatment to explain what is planned for that session is valuable in helping the client to understand what to expect from the session. This, in turn, may carry over to helping the client understand the purpose of treatment and, hopefully, seeing the benefit in participation. This will be particularly true if the client can see the connection between the treatment task in a specific session and her or his overall personal goals (Larson, 2010; Thomas & Storey, 2000).

Another important element in motivation is interest and engagement in the task (Grubbs & Paradise, 2010; Larson, 2010; Ragan, 2011). Often with young children, we say this means *make it fun*. This relates not simply for children, though, but adults as well. Beyond knowing why you are there and seeing the benefits of participation, participating in something that is interesting and engaging *to you* will have a positive impact on motivation. Think about the example of physical fitness. Many of us may understand the purpose of exercising on a regular basis and, with some effort, we may see the benefits of doing so; however, we may only continue to participate in physical fitness activities if we enjoy them as well. Hence, your job as an SLPA is to get to know the client and understand what aspects of treatment you can tailor to improve interest and thereby motivation in your session.

THINGS TO CONSIDER: THE ENVIRONMENT

Your environment is your stage, and as such, it must be carefully arranged to support the services you provide. If arranged effectively, it will aid in the implementation of treatment. If not, it can detract from your effectiveness as a clinician.

First, all environments where treatment is provided should be clean and safe. Chapter 6 discusses procedures and requirements for disinfecting surfaces and materials. Your employer will also have additional and specific requirements in this area as well. Most employers are required to establish minimal environmental safety standards, such as maximum occupancy in a given space, rules about exit accessibility, and procedures for evacuation in case of an emergency. You should familiarize yourself with all applicable rules in these areas. In addition, when arranging the environment for treatment services, you should also consider the nature of the sensory environment present during treatment, the furniture and seating arrangements of the treatment setting, and your materials and stimulus presentation methods.

Sensory Environment

The two senses of sight and hearing are important things to consider when arranging your environment for treatment services. In the area of vision, the environment should be well lit to allow for adequate visual processing of treatment materials. You should also minimize the level of visual distraction in the treatment environment. If there are additional items, such as toys or equipment, not used during a particular session, it is generally best to remove them or place them in an area of the room where they will not be a source of distraction for your client. In the area of hearing and auditory attributes of the environment, you will want to provide treatment services in an environment that is conducive to adequate hearing. This means a quiet enough environment for comfortable, conversational-level speech. Similar to vision, you should also arrange the environment to eliminate sources of auditory distraction, such as excessive background noise. This may mean closing a door or window to eliminate noise from the outside or moving to a location that is less noisy overall. Last, in some instances, you may work with clients with specific and additional needs in the area of vision and/or hearing. If so, you should consult with your supervising SLP, the client and his or her family, or related professionals, such as an audiologist (for hearing issues), to establish an optimum visual and/or hearing environment for that particular client.

Furniture Choice and Seating Arrangement

A big portion of the environment will include the furniture and seating arrangements. These can enhance or detract from the overall effectiveness of the clinical environment. First, make sure to select furniture that is suited to the size of your client (Moon-Meyer, 2004). You do not want an adult client seated in a child-size chair, nor do you want a child client seated in an adult-size chair. Generally, when tabletop activities are performed, you should select furniture that allows for comfort and free mobility of the upper extremities (e.g., arms and hands). The concept of "proximal stability = distal mobility" (Costigan, n.d., slide 27) can be used to ensure the client is in a position that is optimum. This means that if the client's trunk is supported and comfortable, he or she will have maximum use of the upper extremities. An easy way to remember this is "90-90-90" when it comes to seating (Costigan, n.d., slide 40), meaning the hips, knees, and ankles should be in neutral positions at roughly 90-degree angles (Figure 10–1). In some cases, no furniture at all is appropriate, as in the case of young children engaged in play activities. In any seating position, if a client has unique motor and/or physical needs, you should consult with your

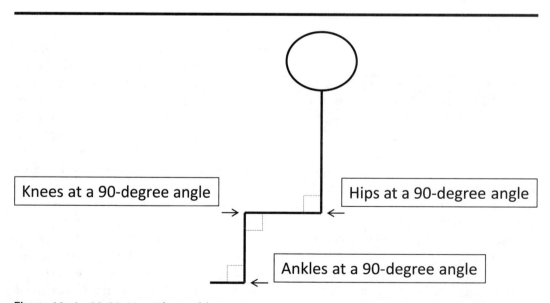

Figure 10–1. 90-90-90 seating position.

supervising SLP, client and his or her family, and related professionals, such as an occupational therapist, to ensure the client's seating and positioning allow for maximum participation. Remember, too, in terms of seating, you do not want to be dominant by, for example, seating yourself in a tall chair while the client is seated on the floor (Moon-Meyer, 2004). In general, maintaining an eye-level position with your clients will optimize communication between you and your client.

Where you place yourself in relation to the door is also important. It is generally best to position yourself with your back to the exit (Figure 10–2). In cases where a client, such as a young child, tries to exit the session abruptly, this gives the clinician control of the exit, if needed (Moon-Meyer, 2004). In addition, there may be situations when, for example, the clinician needs to exit the session quickly to obtain assistance. Placing yourself closest to the exit, with your back to the door, ensures you will have a clear path to do so (Moon-Meyer, 2004).

Your position for data collection is also something to consider when arranging furniture and seating. Data collection sheets should be placed to the side of the hand you use to write (Moon-Meyer, 2004) (Figure 10–3). This can occur in any location, such as seated at a table or seated on the floor. This allows you to easily record information and leaves your nondominant hand for manipulating materials, as needed. In addition, the client should be positioned furthest from the data collection sheet so that what you are writing is out of view of the client (Moon-Meyer, 2004). In cases where you are seated at a table and the client is positioned directly across from you, positioning a clipboard at a slight angle may be appropriate. Figure 10–3 represents a variety of possible options for positioning the client in relation to your data sheet, in both individual and group treatment. Of course, these positions would be adjusted for other seating arrangements, such as on the floor. The key is to arrange your data collection sheet so that it is easily accessible to you but not in view or a distraction to your client.

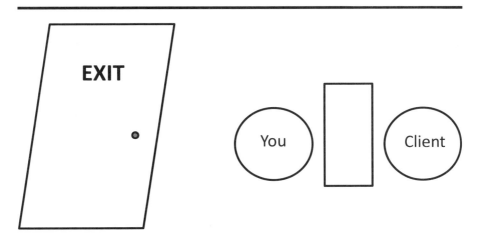

Figure 10–2. Positioning relative to the exit.

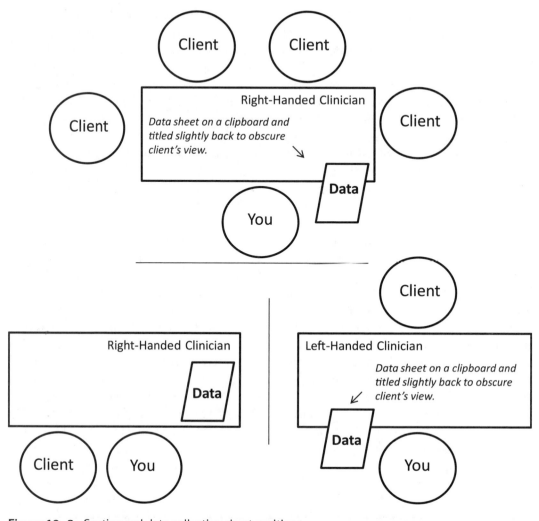

Figure 10–3. Seating and data collection sheet positions.

Materials and Stimulus Presentation Methods

Treatment often involves the use of props, such as pictured items, written material, real objects, a variety of games/toys, and so forth (Hegde, 1998). These are often referred to as stimuli (plural) or a stimulus (singular). As discussed in Chapter 7, these items are carefully selected with the guidance of your supervising SLP, based on the unique aspects of your client and her or his goals (Hegde, 1998).

Examples of "pictured" stimuli could be things like a picture of a dog to elicit verbal production of the word *dog*, a line drawing of a summer scene to elicit conversation about a recent vacation or favored summer activity, or a set of cartoon images the client places in order and then uses to verbally tell a story. Pictured stimuli may also display important concepts, such as a line drawing of the placement of the tongue when producing a specific sound. Pictured stimuli can be line drawings (black and white or color), real color photographs, or a combination of the two. Pictured stimuli can also be combined with written text, as applicable. The images used can be obtained from commercially available sets, magazines, or online sources such as Microsoft Clip Art, Getty Images, or Google Images.

Generally, pictured stimuli should be, "clear, simple, direct, and unambiguous" (Hegde, 1998, p. 154). This means that when a client views the stimulus, it should be obvious to her or him what is intended. Furthermore, pictured stimuli should be attractive and motivating for the client (Hegde, 1998). For example, if a young child is interested in a specific cartoon character, incorporating that character into pictured stimuli may be motivating for that client. Similarly, if a client has a specific interest or hobby, using pictured stimuli with these themes may be particularly rewarding. In this respect, whenever possible, using images and pictured stimuli from the client's environment is highly effective. Pictured stimuli should also match the client's age and level of development. For adults, you should avoid selecting stimuli that are child-like in nature. Similarly, for young children, you should select pictured stimuli that are appropriate to the client's specific developmental level.

In some cases, real-object stimuli may be preferred, such as balls, dolls, toys, or real or simulated daily items, such as kitchen utensils and food items. For young children engaged in play during treatment activities, Chapter 12 discusses ideas for selecting toys and stimuli used for play. Remember, too, in the case of objects used by different clients, as discussed in Chapter 6, these items should be cleaned and disinfected between uses.

Written stimuli may also be used. Examples of written stimuli could be things like a textbook from the client's science class to be read by the client to target reading comprehension or to elicit description and conversation; written words, sentences, or paragraphs to be read aloud; or a worksheet with written directions targeting certain grammatical elements. Similar to pictured stimuli, written stimuli should be direct and specifically designed to effectively meet their intended purpose. They should also match the client's reading abilities and his or her interests. If you are not sure what level of reading material is appropriate for a specific client, speak with your supervising SLP to gain additional details about the client's skills and needs in this area. In addition, you should make sure the size of written text is most appropriate for use with a particular client. In some cases, clients may have visual impairments that necessitate larger print than would be typical in traditional reading materials. Remember, too, that even if you have a young child who is not literate, presenting pictured or written stimuli in a sequence consistent with his or her future literacy lays a good foundation for literacy development (Moon-Meyer, 2004). For English speakers, this is a left-to-right, top-to-bottom position.

Importantly, all stimuli, in any form, should be "ethnoculturally appropriate" (Hegde, 1998, p. 154). Chapter 5 provides additional explanation and instruction in this area. Furthermore, you should prepare your stimuli in advance of a clinical session, making sure they are presorted in the appropriate order. This saves time during the session and presents a professional and organized impression. For some individuals, you will want to keep the work area clear and have only the stimuli needed for one activity at a time in view. In that case, you should have the next set of stimuli easily accessible so that you can transition between activities quickly. Last, if you are presenting stimuli that require the client to choose a specific target from an array of choices, as in a receptive task where the client points to a specific pictured item named by you, you should consider carefully the number of choices (Moon-Meyer, 2004). For example, Figure 10–4 displays a scenario in which the client is asked to point to an item described by the clinician. You can see that in the first attempt (#1), the clinician has presented four cards (also known as a "field" of four) and then given the client a command to point to one of them. After the client points to one of the cards, in theory the field of choices is now narrowed to three cards that the client has not selected. If the clinician does not replace the card for "dog" in the second trial (#2) and gives the next command, the client is now selecting not from a field of four, as in the first attempt, but from a field of three choices. Similarly, in the third attempt (#3), the choices have narrowed

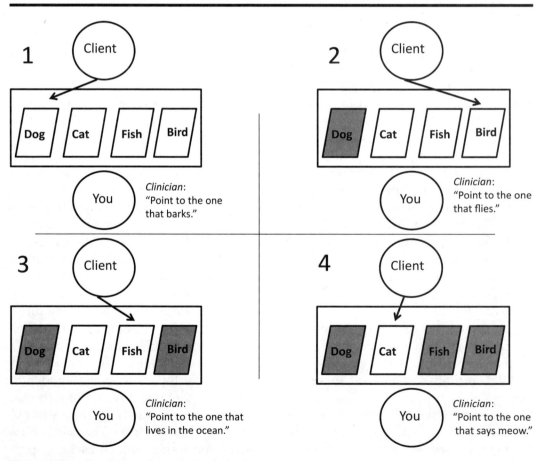

Figure 10–4. Consistency in response choices.

even further to only two possibilities, followed finally by the fourth trial (#4), which is effectively a field of one, because the client has already pointed to all but one item on the table. This decreasing field of choices actually makes the task easier with each successful attempt. The best method for countering this occurrence is to replace items selected/identified after each attempt or present a new set of cards for each attempt.

THINGS TO CONSIDER: THE CLINICIAN

Much of the outcome of a positive treatment session rests with the clinician and her or his behavior. When a session has not gone as anticipated or did not have a positive outcome, the best course of action is to look to your own behaviors and interactions *first* as the primary source of variance. Often, when you do this, you will find that there are elements of your performance that negatively affected the outcome. The good news is that if your behaviors can negatively affect the outcome, they can also positively affect it as well. You will want to consider developing a good clinical rapport, as well as a refining your clinical interactions, including things like how you give instructions, model behaviors, provide hints (also known as prompts), and use effective reinforcement techniques. Each of these areas will be discussed in the sections that follow.

Clinical Rapport

Developing a positive rapport with the clients you serve can have a dramatic impact on treatment services. Rapport is not simply if your clients "like" you (Pattison & Powell, 1990). Rather, rapport is "the establishment and maintenance of an interactive, harmonious, and communicative relationship" (p. 77). Important to note as well is that rapport can change over time (Pattison & Powell, 1990). This means that you must work first to develop a positive clinician-client rapport and then to *maintain* this positive relationship over time. Chapter 4 discusses tips for effective communication. These will be very helpful in establishing a strong communicative relationship with your clients.

In addition, an important element of establishing and maintaining a positive rapport is to be sensitive to the client's *physical* and *emotional* needs (Pattison & Powell, 1990). The sections above on the environment and the client discuss things to consider in the areas of a client's *physical* needs, such as a supportive and comfortable environment and making sure the client's basic needs are met and so forth. In terms of *emotional* needs, keep in mind that clients vary in their feelings and emotions about treatment. Some individuals are excited to attend treatment and view it positively, whereas others feel anxious about treatment activities and communicative tasks (Brumfitt, 2010; Flasher & Fogle, 2004; Holland, 2007). In addition, some individuals may be depressed or have strong emotional reactions to their communicative impairment (Brumfitt, 2010; Flasher & Fogle, 2004; Holland, 2007). The provision of counseling to individuals with communicative disorders is outside the scope of an SLPA (ASHA, 2013). If you are concerned about the psychological well-being of any of the clients you serve, you should *immediately* notify your supervising SLP. Two important ways SLPAs can support their client's emotional needs, while further establishing a positive rapport, are as follows:

1. *Show that you are attentive and focused on your client's needs.* This means, first, limiting discussion about yourself and personal topics. It is appropriate on a limited basis to share personal stories and experiences with your clients, but the focus of treatment sessions should not be on you. In fact, you should limit that total amount of time you spend talking in general (Moon-Meyers, 2004; Pattison & Powell, 1990). You can encourage a client who is shy to interact with you during a clinical session by: (a) allowing for a brief period of small talk at the beginning or end of each session (tailored to the his or her age and abilities), (b) showing a genuine interest in the client's well-being, and (c) speaking slowly, asking open-ended questions, and offering periods of silence to encourage the client to talk (Pattison & Powell, 1990). This is particularly true when you first get to know a client. You should also be conscious of your nonverbal behaviors to ensure you are welcoming. For example, you do not want to inadvertently convey the wrong messages nonverbally, such as fidgeting (e.g., tapping your pencil, twirling your hair, shaking your legs, etc.) or resting your hands on your chin, since these can make you appear nervous or bored (Moon-Meyer, 2004). In addition, you should silence your cell phone and other sources of personal electronic distraction, such as e-mail and text message notifications on your electronic devices. In this respect, it is also professional to place these items out of view of the client since it may give the impression that you are waiting for a call or other contact not related to the client's session. Starting and ending your clinical sessions on time also gives the impression that you are focused on the client's needs and are conscious that her or his time is valuable.

2. *Structure the session to decrease negative emotions.* Start each session with a brief description of the tasks/activities for that particular session (Moon-Meyer, 2004). Letting the clients know what is planned will allow those clients who are anxious to prepare for the session's activities. It also reinforces the purpose of the session and helps to facilitate shared responsibility for session goals, which in turn helps to build positive client-clinician rapport (Roth & Worthington, 2001). The section that follows on positive behavioral support (PBS) provides additional details on how visual schedules can be used for this purpose. In addition, consult with your supervising SLP to ensure you are pacing sessions so that activities are not too fast or too slow for each individual client (Roth & Worthington, 2004). This will decrease any undue frustration for tasks that are either too easy or boring or tasks that are too difficult. In addition, follow a general pattern of targeting tasks that are easier at the beginning and ending of the session (Moon-Meyer, 2004; Roth & Worthington, 2001). This allows treatment to begin and end on a positive note. Last, remember to leave time at the end of the session to:
   a. Provide a warning shortly before the session ends, especially for

clients who may feel frustrated with ending the session or anxious in transitioning to the next activity (Moon-Meyer, 2004).

b. Provide a recap of the client's performance (Roth & Worthington, 2001). This is also an opportunity to highlight any positive accomplishments made that session (Moon-Meyer, 2004).

c. Provide a summary of any home activities or additional outside assignments (Roth & Worthington, 2001). These, of course, are those recommended and assigned by your supervising SLP, applicable to your client's course of treatment.

d. Offer an opportunity for the client to ask questions.

One additional avenue for improving your clinical effectiveness and establishing a positive client-clinician rapport is to give the clients an opportunity to provide feedback about the services provided. In allied health fields, this is often referred to as customer-oriented care (Reisberg, 1996). One important aspect of customer-oriented care is an opportunity for the customer to give feedback, both positive and negative, about the services provided (Frattali, 1991; Reisberg, 1996). In the case of speech-language pathology, our clients (and their families) are our customers. Obtaining feedback from clients can be done in a formalized fashion through written or online client satisfaction surveys (Frattali, 1991). Often these measures will be developed and administered by your employer (or your supervisor). If your setting uses a client satisfaction survey, you should familiarize yourself with the questions on this survey.

Informal mechanisms of feedback can also be used during individual clinical sessions to obtain client feedback (Frattali, 1991). The use of a rating scale, such as the ones in Figure 10–5, can be helpful for receiving feedback during clinical interaction (Brumfitt, 2010; Wewers & Lowe, 1990). These are examples of visual analog scales (VAS).

A VAS is "a straight line, the end anchors of which are labeled as the extreme boundaries of the sensation, feeling, or response to be measured" (Wewers & Lowe, 1990, p. 13). VAS can be modified and used with any sensation or feeling. VAS have been frequently used as a way for clients to report their pain or mood in clinical settings (Wewers & Lowe, 1990). They have also been used with pictorial representations at the ends of lines to represent applicable extremes (Brumfitt, 2010). Clarifying words, numbers, and/or additional written descriptors can also be added (Wewers & Lowe, 1990). Some advantages of VAS, particularly those with pictorial representations, are that they are less tied to the more complex language or speech skills needed, for example, to describe a specific sensation or feeling or to understand a complex verbal or written question about a sensation or feeling (Brumfitt, 2010). This makes them potentially applicable for use with many clients with communicative disorders of varying ages and abilities.

Some ways that SLPAs can incorporate VAS into their sessions could be by asking the client to give feedback in general or about a specific treatment task. Some areas that could be used include the following:

■ Frustration (frustrated to not frustrated)

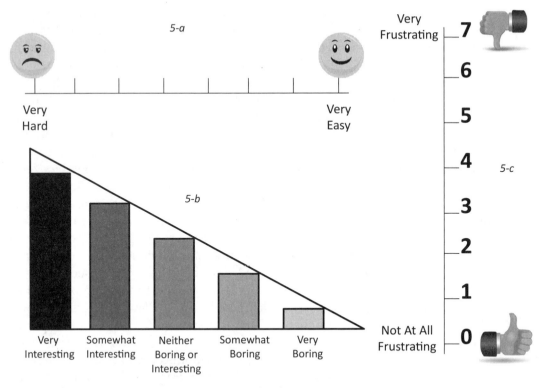

Figure 10–5. Examples of Visual Analog Scales (VAS).

- Pain (not painful to painful)
- Difficulty (easy to hard)
- Interest level (boring to interesting)
- Comfort level (comfortable to uncomfortable).

Traditionally, VAS are measured using very specific numeric procedures, but for use as above, they can simply serve as a qualitative (e.g., nonnumeric) and subjective form of feedback from the client about his or her experience, feelings, or attitude related to something about the clinical session. For example, if you employed the scale represented in Figure 10–5c during a treatment task and the client indicated by pointing closest to the 6, which is close to "very frustrated," this would suggest that she or he is becoming frustrated with the task and a break may be needed. Similarly, if the VAS in Figure 10–5a was used and the client pointed close to the "very easy" symbol, this could be information to share with your supervising SLP, so that she or he could review the task to see if a potential modification is needed in a future session.

As with all clinical interfaces, the use of these scales should first be discussed with your supervising SLP to ensure they are appropriate for a specific client. You should obtain her or his guidance in developing both an applicable VAS and in establishing how and when to request this type of feedback from the client. Generally, VAS used in this way are most effective when they are combined with careful instructions (Wewers & Lowe, 1990). Being given a similar VAS more than once allows the client to become comfortable with offering opinions in this fashion. It also provides an opportunity to track the client's opinions over time and across tasks. Of course, remember, too, that a VAS is not the only way to ask a client's opinion about some aspect of your clinical services. You can also do so simply with direct questions and verbal replies (e.g., Are you feeling frustrated? Is this task boring? Am I going too fast?). The key here is to offer an opportunity, appropriate to the client's abilities, for the client to express opinions about the clinical session.

Clinical Interactions

Directions

Your verbal and written directions about a treatment task will have a positive or negative impact on if that task is performed accurately (and as you intended). Your directions to the client should be short and to the point. You should also allow sufficient time for the client to respond before repeating directions (Roth & Worthington, 2001). The form of your direction is important as well. In general, your directions should be in declarative form (Roth & Worthington, 2001), such as the following:

Name this picture

Say the word _____

Write these words in sentences

Let's begin

Tell me what happened this weekend

Repeat after me

Place the picture in the box

Take a card from the stack of cards.

You should avoid combining a command and a question, such as, "*Can you name this picture?*" and "*Can you repeat after me?*" In these instances, the appropriate response is for the client to answer yes or no, not for the individual to perform the requested task. Similarly, note that when some commands are converted to questions, such as, "Are you ready to begin?" (and not "Let's begin."), the question form allows the client an opportunity to say no and in that case not begin the task. In some situations, it is perfectly appropriate and acceptable to request information about a client's readiness to begin, while in others, it may be an opportunity for the client to avoid or escape a nondesired task. In those instances, it is better to avoid asking such a question and stick to a command (Roth & Worthington, 2001).

Demonstration/Modeling

Beyond clinical directions, treatment interface typically requires a clinician to provide demonstration and modeling (Hegde, 1998). The distinction between these two behaviors is that in demonstration, there is not an expectation that the client immediately repeat the behavior demonstrated, whereas in modeling, the client is expected to imitate the behavior after it is modeled. Clinicians may provide frequent demonstrations of a desired response to help reinforce a concept or behavior (Roth & Worthington, 2001). For example, the clinician speaking at a slow rate demonstrates slow, controlled speech for an individual who stutters, or a clinician frequently using a specific grammatical form in her conversation offers repeated exposure to this form for an individual with a language impairment.

In the case of modeling, knowing when and how to model is an important skill (Hegde, 1998). Modeling is used when a client is able to imitate a behavior and when a question, prompt, or physical stimulus is not sufficient to elicit the desired response. Modeling occurs most frequently in the initial stages of developing a behavior (Hegde, 1998; Roth & Worthington, 2001). Box 10–1 contains helpful tips for providing effective models.

Rarely do we use imitation in our daily conversational tasks. As such, when using modeling to elicit a behavior, generally the client's goals will gradually transition to less and less clinician support in eliciting a desired response. This is known as fading (Hegde, 1998). A related technique to fading is shaping (Hegde, 1998). Shaping occurs when a client is not able to imitate a behavior from a model or when the behavior is complex. Shaping breaks a behavior into small, progressively more complex steps (starting from easy to hard) until the final level of performance is obtained (Hegde, 1998).

Prompts/Scaffolding

A prompt is assistance provided by the clinician to facilitate a desired response from the client (Hegde, 1998; Roth & Worthington, 2001). Prompts are generally what we think of as hints. Some clinicians also refer

---

Box 10–1. Providing an Effective Model

1. *Make sure the stage is set for the client to receive and imitate your model.* Model the behavior only when you have the client's attention and when he or she knows an imitation of the model is to follow. Giving a model when the client is not paying attention or when he or she is not ready to imitate will just require a repetition of the model.
2. *Avoid unnatural models.* Model the behavior as you would like it imitated. This means not, for example, overly exaggerating or slowing certain elements to such an extent that they become distorted or inaccurate (Moon-Meyer, 2004).
3. *Avoid ungrammatical utterances in your models* (Moon-Meyer, 2004).
4. *Model language at a level appropriate to the client's abilities* (Moon-Meyer, 2004).
5. *As needed, emphasize target behaviors with vocal changes.* When you are modeling a behavior that is embedded, for example, in a sentence or phrase, emphasizing the model using an increased vocal pitch or loudness may be appropriate, as in the sentence, "the boy *is* runn*ing*," when the auxiliary verb + present progressive is the target behavior (Hegde, 1998). Remember Principle 2 (above), though, and do not emphasize this to such an extent that the model becomes unnatural.

to prompts as "cues," but generally speaking, a cue comprises a behavior from the clinician (whether verbal, nonverbal, or physical) that instructs the client *when* to respond versus a prompt (whether visual, auditory, or tactile), which offers assistance to the client on *how* to respond (Roth & Paul, 2007). For example, a clinician tapping the client's hand to signal it is the client's turn to respond could be classified as a cue (as it denotes *when* to respond), whereas a clinician using vocal emphasis to highlight a helpful feature of the required production, such as, "The boy is runn*ing*. What is the girl doing?" is a type of prompt (as it offers information about *how* to respond).

Prompts are used when the a stimulus alone is not sufficient to elicit the desired responses but when more direct elicitation, such as modeling, is not preferred. The term *scaffolding* is also used to describe the use of prompts (or other assistance) from a listener (or clinician) to enable an individual to communicate a message that would not be possible otherwise (Norris & Hoffman, 1990). As the name denotes, scaffolding is thought of as a bridge of support provided to the speaker until she or he is able to obtain similarly complex messages, without the support of prompts. Chapter 12 provides additional information and examples of the use of scaffolding in treatment with young children during play activities. Typically, prompts can be classified as visual, auditory, or tactile (Box 10–2). Remember, too, that in some cases, you may provide more than one prompt simultaneously or present them successively, until a desired response is obtained.

The purposeful and, importantly, documented use of prompts is an important part of clinical interaction. New clinicians often are not aware of the level of prompting needed by a particular client or in some cases even that they are providing prompts to a client. This is problematic since prompts can influence how independent a client is in performing a task. As discussed in Chapter 8, accurate data collection about the client's performance is critical. If you are providing assistance to the client in the form of prompts but not denoting this assistance in your data about the client, this will negatively affect the accuracy of that data. These faulty data may then be used by your supervising SLP to make decisions about the client's care. In Chapter 7, lesson plans are described, including the column for "Prompts/Modifications" or "Make It Easier/Make It More Difficult," which are used to describe suggested prompts and/or modifications that may be recommended for a specific task. Before you implement any treatment, you should discuss with your supervising SLP the types of appropriate prompts and/or modifications applicable for a specific client, as well as how these prompts should be reflected in your data collection methods. Chapter 8, particularly the section on "Response Independence," offers additional suggestions in this area.

Equally important is presenting prompts systematically, using some form of hierarchy individualized to the client. There are two general approaches to hierarchies of prompting: effortful learning and errorless learning (Abel et al., 2005; Mosall, Choe, Cronin, & Massery, 2012; Sohlberg, Ehlardt, & Kennedy, 2005). In *effortful learning* approaches, prompts are ordered from the least assistance to most assistance, allowing a client to respond with the greatest level of independence first. If the client is not successful, then additional prompts provide greater assistance until the desired response is

Box 10–2. Examples of Visual, Auditory, and Tactile Prompts

Auditory prompts: Prompts *heard* by the client

- Using a modulation in your pitch/loudness to vocally emphasize an important concept ("The *girl* is sad.")
- A verbal question that provides details about an important feature (e.g., "Where do you find these?" "The lion is hungry. What does he want to eat?")*
- A verbally presented cloze sentence (e.g., "You bounce a _____." "The baby is tired. She wants to go to _____.")*
- Verbally saying the first sound or syllable of a word, the first portion of a sentence, or any part of the required response*

Note. Many of the items highlighted with an *, can also be presented in written form and in that case would be considered visual prompts.

Visual prompts: Prompts *seen* by the client

- Positioning your mouth in the shape of a target phoneme (e.g., placing you lips together to demonstrate /m/)
- A pictured representation of a particular concept (e.g., a diagram showing the position of the tongue)
- A *written* cue, reminder, or question (e.g., "Remember to _____." "This animal lives in the jungle." "When do we eat these?")
- Gesturing your hand above your head to indicate a high(er) pitch
- Pantomiming an action related to a targeted response (e.g., yawning when "sleep" is the target response)

Tactile prompts: Prompts *felt* by the client

- Tapping out the syllabus of a word on the client's hand
- Placing your hand on the client's throat to indicate voiced production
- Running your finger gently down the client's forearm to represent continuous sound (as in the production of /z/)
- A tactile real object that aids in production or comprehension (e.g., a piece of sand paper and silk to contrast soft versus harsh vocal production)

obtained. Take, for example, a client-centered approach in which the clinician is playing with a doll and related items with a young client. To elicit production of the word *bottle* in response to a question, the clinician says, "Oh the baby is so hungry. What should we give her?" If the client does not respond, two potential prompts at ends of the spectrum are possible. The clinician could say, "The baby needs a bottle. Say bottle." (greatest level of assistance and least level of independence), or preferably, the clinician could give a minimal visual prompt such as looking at the bottle (least assistance and greatest level of independence). In the latter example of using a minimal visual prompt, if the client then responds, saying "a bottle," she or he has done so with minimal assistance and with greater independence than imitating the response "bottle" after it has been modeled by the clinician.

In *errorless learning* approaches, prompts are presented from the greatest assistance to the least assistance. For example, in a clinician-directed approach such as teaching a client to use a memory device, the clinician may present the steps of accessing the device (e.g., opening the device, finding the applicable page, identifying information on that page) first by modeling each step and having the client copy her. Then, the clinician may provide a model for all but the final step. In that case, the greatest level of assistance (and thereby prompts) was provided because rather than independently recalling and performing *all* the steps, the client only needs to perform a minimal step (the final one after all previous steps are modeled). Gradually, then, less and less prompts are provided, until the client is successful in performing all the steps independently. As an SLPA, you should confirm with your supervising SLP which approach is most applicable to a specific treatment target and given each client's individualized goals.

Operant Conditioning

How an SLPA responds to a client's communication, whether elicited (as in the case of clinician-directed treatment) or produced spontaneously (as with client-centered treatment), plays an important role in the treatment process. Clinical interactions that are positive and motivating are equally important.

At a very basic level, the job of the SLP is to design treatment that creates, increases, and in some cases decreases specific behaviors (Hegde, 1998). Behaviors targeted are typically those of communication (Roth & Worthington, 2001), although in recent years, the scope of an SLP has extended to behaviors outside of communication, such as swallowing (ASHA, 2007). Operant conditioning is a theory used to explain how human behaviors can be influenced (either positively or negatively) by the consequences that follow a behavior (Mowrer, 1982). Clinician-directed treatments rely heavily on this theory and the principles of *reinforcement* and *punishment* (Roth & Paul, 2007), but these concepts are also applicable to client-centered treatment approaches. As discussed above, a framework of antecedent-behavior-consequence is used in both types of approaches. The principles of reinforcement and punishment explain how the consequence of a behavior will affect its occurrence and frequency.

Reinforcement. Reinforcement has the impact of increasing the frequency of a behavior (Hegde, 1998). There are two types of reinforcement: positive reinforcement and negative reinforcement. A *positive* reinforcer is a rewarding item, event, or action that is presented in response to a desired behavior, whereas a *negative* reinforcer is an unpleasant item, event, or action that is removed in response to a desired behavior. Although both positive and negative reinforcement increase the frequency of a desired behavior, negative reinforcement is not commonly used in clinical settings in the field of speech-language pathology (Roth & Worthington, 2001).

Positive reinforcement (and thereby positive reinforcers) are common in the field of speech-language pathology and are classified as primary or secondary. Primary reinforcement is physiologically or biologically driven. Food is one of the most common examples of a primary reinforcer (Roth & Worthington, 2001). The use of food as reinforcement, however, should be used with caution (Hegde, 1998) and only under the direction of your supervising SLP. Given the potential for food allergies/sensitivities, specific parental preferences, and religious and/or cultural considerations, parental consent is typically sought for the use of food as a reinforcement during treatment sessions.

Secondary reinforcers are items, events, or actions that a client learns are rewarding. Secondary reinforcers are commonly used in the field of speech-language pathology and include social rewards, tokens, and performance feedback (Box 10–3).

Punishment. In contrast to reinforcement, punishment has the impact of decreasing the frequency of a behavior. Punishment generally consists of two types, Type I and Type II (Roth & Worthington, 2001).

Type I punishment involves an averse consequence to an undesired behavior. Corrective feedback is a common form of Type I punishment used in the field of speech-language pathology, including verbal, nonverbal, and mechanical corrective feedback (Hegde, 1998) (Box 10–4). As with reinforcement, punishment may be deployed in relation to the communicative behaviors targeted in treatment and/or those behaviors that interfere with treatment, such as aggressive or uncooperative behaviors (Hegde, 1998).

Type II punishment consists of removing a pleasant condition in response to an undesired behavior (Roth & Worthington, 2001). The two most common types of Type II punishment used in the field of speech-language pathology are timeout and response costs (Hegde, 1998; Roth & Worthington, 2001) (Box 10–5).

New clinicians may be reluctant to provide punishment, given the negative connotation associated with the word *punishment* (Hegde, 1998). It is correct to be cautious about the use of punishment. However, as you can see from the examples provided, some forms of punishment, such as corrective feedback, can be minimally aversive and serve the important purpose of providing feedback about an inaccurate response. Generally, though, only very minimally aversive forms of punishment should be employed. Punishment (particularly Type II punishment) should be employed only with the guidance of your supervising SLP and only after reinforcement of a desired behavior has been ineffective (Bopp, Brown, & Mirenda, 2004). Working closely with your supervising SLP to ensure you have adequate knowledge and skills in the use of reinforcement and punishment is critical.

Box 10–3. Examples of Secondary Reinforcers

Social Rewards

A social reward is an action, such as smiling, eye contact, or verbal praise, given in response to a desired behavior (Roth & Worthington, 2001). This serves the purpose of giving the client immediate positive feedback about the accuracy of a desired response. This type of reinforcement is frequently used in the field of speech-language pathology (Roth & Worthington, 2001). Social rewards of a communicative nature (such as those that would naturally occur with a successful communication exchange) are commonly used in client-centered treatment approaches.

Tokens

A token is an item given in response to a desired behavior that alone is not particularly rewarding but can be accrued and exchanged for a specific reward. Examples of tokens commonly used in the field of speech-language pathology are points, checkmarks, stickers, chips, and so forth. The use of token systems is more common in clinician-directed approaches to treatment and is frequently utilized in some settings, particularly with children, in response to both communicative behaviors targeted in treatment and those behaviors related to participation in treatment, such as attention, participation, and so forth (Hegde, 1998).

Performance Feedback

Performance feedback is information provided to the client about a desired behavior(s). This type of feedback is also called *informative feedback* because it provides information about the client's performance (Hegde, 1998). It can include information such as percent correct, frequency of occurrence, biofeedback, or numerical ratings of the client's performance. It can be presented verbally or in written form. It is not necessarily intended to be praise but can be combined with either tokens or social rewards. Responding with the phrase, "Excellent work, you kept your rate slow that time," is an example of the use of social reward ("excellent work") + performance feedback ("you kept your rate slow that time"). Combination of this nature can be highly effective (Moon-Meyer, 2004).

Box 10–4. Examples of Corrective Feedback

Verbal Corrective Feedback

Verbal corrective feedback is typically a minimally aversive verbal response to a behavior that is judged by the clinician to be inadequate or inaccurate for some reason (Hegde, 1998), such as "no," "try again," "incorrect," and so forth. This gives the client immediate feedback about the inaccuracy or inappropriateness of a specific response. As with combining social reward and performance feedback (reinforcement), verbal corrective feedback can also provide the client with specific information about the inaccuracy of a response, such as "no, remember to place your tongue between your teeth."

Nonverbal Corrective Feedback

Nonverbal corrective feedback is similar to verbal corrective feedback but delivered in a gesture or other nonverbal signal, such as a hand single to denote the need to slow speech rate for an individual who stutters (Hegde, 1998). Generally, nonverbal feedback is best used in combination with verbal feedback, such as saying "slow down" (verbal feedback) while providing a hand motion to represent slowed rate (Hegde, 1998).

Mechanical Corrective Feedback

Mechanical corrective feedback includes visual and/or auditory signals in response to an inaccurate, inadequate, or inappropriate response, *given by an external device such as a computer* (Hegde, 1998). Increasingly, computer programs are used to give this type of feedback in response to a variety of related behaviors. Commonly, they combine mechanical corrective feedback with reinforcement (Hegde, 1998), such as a low pitch tone or flashing signal to indicate inaccurate and the word *correct* combined with a visual image of a happy face to indicate accurate production.

Effective Use of Operant Principles. The key to using both reinforcement or punishment is to do so specifically and with an understanding of its purpose and impact. What makes something a "reinforcement" versus a "punishment" depends on the individual. As such, the use of these techniques first requires an understanding of what will serve as an effective reinforcement (increase a desired behavior) or punishment (decrease an undesired behavior). A classic example of this comes in the area of punishment, when a novice clinician, for example, inaccurately believes that a

Box 10–5. Timeout and Response Cost

Timeout

Timeout involves "temporary isolation or removal of a client to an environment with limited opportunity to receive positive reinforcement" (Roth & Worthington, 2001, p. 15). An example of this with a young client might be turning his or her chair to a blank wall in the treatment room for a brief period.

Response Cost

Response cost involves removing a previously earned positive reinforcer (Hegde, 1998; Roth & Worthington, 2001). This is commonly employed with the use of tokens, by removing a token earned in response to an undesired behavior.

---

timeout from participating in treatment will be a form of punishment for an undesired behavior (e.g., a loud aggressive comment) only to find that in fact the incidence of that behavior increases. In that case, the brief and temporary removal from the treatment session was actually a reward for the client, and as such, the behavior increased. Similar effects can also be seen, for example, when a clinician responds by giving attention to an undesired behavior, only to find that behavior increases. In that case, the attention from the clinician was reinforcing for the client, and as such, the undesired behavior increased in frequency in an attempt to get additional clinician attention. This is why training and practical application is imperative to ensure you are implementing these techniques effectively. Specific instruction from your supervising SLP, as well as having her or him evaluate your effectiveness in deploying these techniques, is a top priority. Several additional tips in deploying effective operant principles are as follows:

1. *Emphasize the positive.* Use positive reinforcement first and most readily. Positive praise, particularly descriptive praise, is very powerful in shaping behaviors but also in building self-esteem.
2. *Use descriptive praise and avoid evaluative praise.* In terms of reinforcement, use descriptive praise and not evaluative praise (Soclof, 2010). Descriptive praise tells the client specifically why she or he has earned praise/reinforcement (e.g., "Great focus. That time you kept your tongue tip up" or "Good, you corrected all the spelling errors in this sentence"), whereas evaluative praise provides only a generic comment about performance, not linked to the behavior itself (e.g., "good girl," "nice work," etc.) (Soclof, 2010). Table 10–1 contains several examples of descriptive and evaluative praise.
3. *Establish a behavior code.* A behavior code consists of the rules of participation in treatment. These will vary but may be things like waiting for

Table 10–1. Examples of Evaluative Versus Descriptive Praise

Evaluative Praise	Descriptive Praise
"Good job"	"You worked hard on this reading comprehension sheet. You were able to determine the main point and the conclusion."
"You are so strong"	"You pushed that finger right into the playdoh, you made a pancake—that is using those fingers muscles and making them strong."
"Good girl"	"You said the 's' sound clearly, you put your tongue right behind your teeth and that 's' sound came right out."
"You are so smart"	"You got a match! They are the same—two horses!" or "You got two pegs into the pegboard—two more to go."
"You are a great artist"	"I like the way you used the black border around the pink. It really makes the pink color pop out."
"You are the best at coloring"	"I love to look at this picture. All the rainbow colors make me smile."
"You are so nice"	"You picked up Mark's scarf after it fell on the floor. That is a kind thing to do."
"I am so proud of you, you got all A's"	"This report card shows a lot of effort and hard work, you should be proud of yourself."

Source: Copyright Soclof (2010). Reprinted with permission.

the clinician to explain a task before the client begins, staying seated in the chair during the treatment session, not interrupting someone when they are speaking, and so forth. For some clients, this code may need to be written and/or visually displayed and explained each session. Chapter 11 discusses group treatment. Behavior codes in group treatment can be highly valuable since they establish a uniform code of conduct and expectations across all group members.

4. *Combine corrective feedback with descriptive praise.* Corrective feedback (and in particular *verbal* corrective feedback) can shape the nature of production and offer suggestions for improvement (e.g., correct feedback + descriptive praise) (Soclof, 2010). However, corrective feedback that is generic in nature can be perceived as criticism,

which is associated with negative emotions (Soclof, 2010). Table 10–2 offers suggestions for shaping feedback from criticism to corrective feedback and combining it with descriptive praise.

5. *Avoid the OK syndrome (Moon-Meyer, 2004).* The "OK" syndrome is when the clinician frequently says "OK," for things such as a conversational filler (e.g., "OK, let's begin"), tagging questions (e.g., "Read this paragraph, OK?"), and in response to a client's behavior (e.g., "OK." or "OK, not quite, let's try again") (Moon-Meyer, 2004). As you can see, in each of these examples, removing the "OK" actually adds clarity and specificity to the clinician's verbal statements. In particular, the use of OK in response to a client's behavior is problematic since it is a vague comment that does not assist the client in understanding whether

Table 10–2. Criticism Versus Corrective Feedback + Descriptive Praise

Criticism	Corrective Feedback + Descriptive Praise
"This is a sloppy paper!"	"This word here and this letter here are on the line. Here is a good amount of space between the words. Can you try that with the rest of the line?"
"Stop saying you can't do this, you can if you try!"	"You are halfway through the maze, only a little more to go."
"It is not enough times!"	"You said the 'r' sound five times correctly, five more to go!"
"Stop fidgeting, sit down and finish."	"You knew baby and mommy, now show me the dog."
"Stop running and yelling."	"You walked all the way from your class to the steps using a quiet voice—only a few more steps to go using a quiet voice and steady feet."
"You won't be able to play any of the games you like if you don't hurry up and finish your work."	"You did a whole worksheet. One more to go before we play 'Operation.'"

Source: Copyright Soclof (2010). Reprinted with permission.

her or his response was accurate/inaccurate, desired/undesired, and so on.

6. *Place your emphasis on the target behavior, not the activity.* Often, in treatment with young children, games are used as a vehicle for eliciting target behaviors. This may create the "mirage" that the game is the emphasis of treatment and not the target behaviors (Moon-Meyer, 2004, p. 313). To ensure this does not occur, clinicians must tie reinforcement to treatment targets. This can be done, for example, by having the reinforcer be some aspect of game performance but only provided when a target behavior meets a criterion (e.g., saying /r/ five times correctly and moving five spaces, using the past-tense verb to collect a certain score or move a given number of spaces).

Positive Behavioral Supports (PBS). Thus far, the discussion of operant conditioning has focused mainly on the *consequences* of a behavior to either increase or decrease the frequency of that behavior. Increasingly, SLPs also employ an approach known as positive behavior supports (PBS) for understanding and changing behaviors that interfere with successful participation in meaningful and productive activities, including the presence of problem behavior such as withdrawal, screaming, repetitive behaviors, aggression, tantrums, and self-injury (Bopp et al., 2004; Dunlap, 2005). PBS has been widely studied for use with individuals with severe developmental disabilities, particularly individuals with autism spectrum disorder (ASD), but it has also been applied to adults with challenging behaviors and individuals without disabilities as well (Bopp et al., 2004; Dunlap, 2005). PBS addresses all three aspects of the *antecedent-behavior-consequence* chain but with the important underlying assumption that problem behaviors are "not just a response that should be reduced or eliminated; rather, they represent an individual's best attempt to transmit a message or meet a need" (Bopp et al., 2004, p. 5). For example, perhaps an individual who is screaming or acting aggressively toward a classmate is attempting to say, "I want X," "I don't want X," or "I need X," and so forth (p. 5). As such, PBS focuses on the following:

1. Modifying specific aspects of the environment to prevent problems from occurring (antecedent)
2. Teaching new skills to replace problem behavior (behavior)
3. Using functional consequences to encourage positive behavior (consequence).

Two important treatment approaches used in the field of speech-language pathology, related to PBS, are functional communication training (FCT) and visual schedules.

Functional Communication Training. FCT is designed to "teach socially acceptable communication alternatives to problem behavior" (Bopp et al., 2004, p. 6). The first step in this process is a careful assessment of the meaning or "message(s)" conveyed by a problem behavior and antecedents in the environment related to that behavior (Beukelman & Mirenda, 2013). This is achieved through a detailed and comprehensive assessment, undertaken collaboratively with the client, his or her family, individuals in the client's environment, and related professionals such as the SLP, psychologist, teacher, and so forth (Bopp et al., 2004). When applicable, changes to the environment (e.g., antecedents) are undertaken that remove the need for the behavior. Once the messages (or meanings of a behavior) are deciphered, the next step is to establish a new means of conveying this information. This new method must be equivalent in meaning and one that can be conveyed by the client effectively and efficiently in his or her environment. Often, FCT is used with individuals with severely limited or no expressive communication abilities, and as such, the use of augmentative and alternative communication (AAC) is employed, such that messages are conveyed through words or short phrases, manual signs, gestures, pictured symbols, or written words. Chapter 14 discusses the use of AAC in greater detail, including elements of AAC systems that may be applicable within FCT. Once a suitable alternative to a problem behavior is identified, an intervention plan is established. This plan addresses instruction in the use of this new behavior, as well as training and collaboration with individuals in the client's environment to ensure socially meaningful and appropriate consequences are in place to generalize this new behavior to the client's environment. Typically, this intervention plan is systematic in nature, employing many of the principles described above, such as modeling, shaping, prompts, and the principles of operant conditioning. As an SLPA, you may be asked to assist in providing FCT or to employ specific consequences in response to desired and undesired behaviors (as outlined in a specific FCT plan). In both cases, familiarity with the client's assessment and intervention plan for FCT is critical.

Visual Schedules. Visual schedules are visual displays of activities, steps, or rules applicable to a specific individual and routine(s) (Beukelman & Mirenda, 2013; Bopp et al., 2004). Visual schedules can display routines across days, weeks, hours, or at a high level of detail for a very specific routine (e.g., using the bathroom, doing the laundry, baking a cake). The purpose of a visual schedule is to "provide the individual with a way to predict or understand upcoming events in order to reduce problem behaviors and increase independence" (Bopp et al., 2004, p. 14). The use of visual schedules is based on the knowledge that many individuals of all ages, particularly individuals with developmental disabilities, benefit from highly structured environments (Beukelman & Mirenda, 2013; Bopp et al., 2004). Visual schedules are often augmented with verbal input provided to the individual, which allow the individual to comprehend information about upcoming events and task requirements. Visual schedules commonly include aided symbols, such as real objects, photographs, line drawings, or written words, common to AAC systems. Figures 10–6, 10–7, and 10–8 contain examples of visual schedules. Several additional examples can be

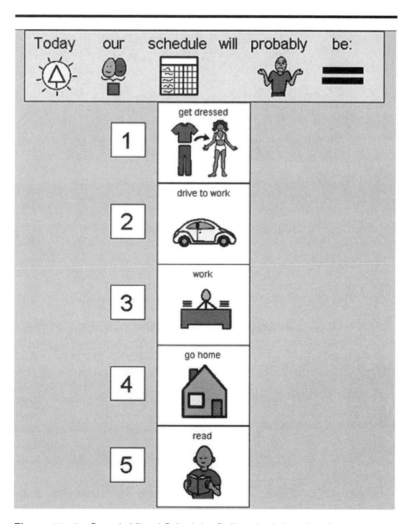

Figure 10–6. Sample Visual Schedule: Daily schedule, using line drawings. Copyright © 2013 DynaVox Mayer-Johnson. Reprinted with permission.

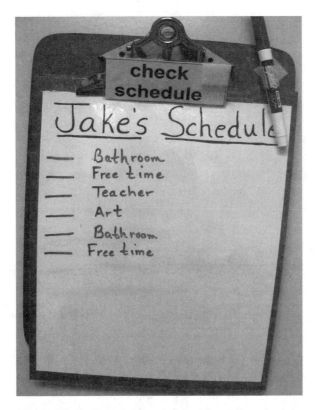

Figure 10–7. Sample Visual Schedule: Daily schedule, using written words, with space to note task completion. Copyright © 2013 Indiana University: Indiana Resource Center for Autism. Used with Permission.

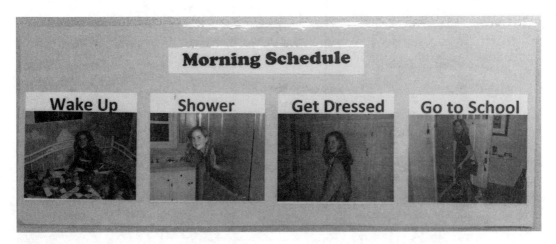

Figure 10–8. Sample Visual Schedule: Daily schedule, using real color photographs.

found on the Indiana Resource Center for Autism website (under Visual Supports: http://www.iidc.indiana.edu/). As is evident in Figure 10–7, in some cases, visual schedules will contain opportunities to denote when a specific step in the routine has been completed (e.g., moving a symbol to the "done" column, crossing off the task after completion, assigning a token such as a happy face). Similar to FCT, the use of visual schedules is preceded by a careful assessment and a systematic intervention plan for implementing visual schedules in the client's environment. As an SLPA, you may be asked to assist your supervising SLP in creating a visual schedule to be used in a client's intervention plan or to deploy the use of a visual schedule while providing services to a specific client. As such, familiarity with their use and purpose is highly valuable. A helpful resource in the creation of visual supports is available from Vanderbilt University (http://csefel.vanderbilt.edu/modules/module3b/handout2.pdf).

REFERENCES

Abel, S., Schultz, A., Radermacher, R., Willmes, K., & Huber, W. (2005). Decreasing and increasing cues in naming therapy for aphasia. *Aphasiology, 19*(9), 831–848.

American Speech-Language-Hearing Association (ASHA). (n.d.). *Telepractice.* Retrieved from http://www.asha.org/Practice-Portal/Professional-Issues/Telepractice/

American Speech-Language-Hearing Association (ASHA). (2007). *Scope of practice in speech-language pathology.* Retrieved from http://www.asha.org/policy

American Speech-Language-Hearing Association (ASHA). (2013). *Speech-language pathology assistant scope of practice.* Retrieved from http://www.asha.org/policy

Beukelman, D., & Mirenda, P. (2013). *Augmentative and alternative communication: Supporting children and adults with complex communication needs* (4th ed.). Baltimore, MD: Brookes.

Bopp, K. D., Brown, K. E., & Mirenda, P. (2004). Speech-language pathologists' roles in the delivery of positive behavior supports for individuals with developmental disabilities. *American Journal of Speech-Language Pathology, 13,* 5–19.

Brumfitt, S. (2010). *Psychological well-being and acquired communication impairments.* San Francisco, CA: John Wiley.

Buysse, V., & Bailey, D. B. (1993). Behavioral and developmental outcomes in young children with disabilities in integrated and segregated settings: A review of comparative studies. *Journal of Special Education, 26,* 434–461.

Cascella, R., Purdy, M. H., & Dempsey, J. J. (2007). Clinical service delivery and work settings. In R. Paul & P. Cascella (Eds.), *Introduction to clinical methods in communication disorders* (pp. 259–282). Baltimore, MD: Paul H. Brookes.

Cirrin, F. M., Schooling, T. L., Nelson, N. W., Diehl, S. F., Flynn, P. F., Staskowski, M., . . . Adamczyk, D. F. (2010). Evidence-based systematic review: Effects of different service delivery models on communication outcomes for elementary school–age children. *Language, Speech, and Hearing Services in Schools, 41*(3), 233–264.

Costigan, A. (n.d.). *An introduction to seating and positioning for individuals who use assistive technology* [Video webcast]. Retrieved from http://mcn.educ.psu.edu/dbm/S_P_AT_pt1/S_P_AT_HO.pdf

Cox, A. (2007). *No mind left behind: Understanding and fostering executive control—The eight essential brain skills every child needs to thrive.* New York, NY: Penguin.

Dunlap, G. (2005, March). Positive behavior supports: An overview. *Language Learning and Education,* pp. 3–5.

Flasher, L.V., & Fogle, P.T. (2004). *Counseling skills for speech-language pathologists and audiologists.* Clifton Park, NY: Thomson Delmar Learning.

Frattali, C. (1991, Winter). Measuring client satisfaction. *ASHA Quality Improvement Digest.* Retrieved from http://www.asha.org/SLP/healthcare/Measuring-Client-Satisfaction/

Garcia, C. (2013). *Online manual for the school-based telepractice paraprofessional.* Unpublished manuscript. Retrieved August 12, 2013, from http://schooltelepracticeparaprofessional manual.webs.com/SchoolBasedTelepractice ParaprofessionalManual.pdf

Grubbs, C., & Paradise, D. (2010). *Making speech therapy fun: Motivating children with autism to speak.* Retrieved from http://www.asha.org/ Events/convention/handouts/2010/1446-Grubbs-Christine/

Hegde, M. N. (1998). *Treatment procedures in communicative disorders* (3rd ed.). Austin, TX: Pro-Ed.

Holland, A. (2007). *Counseling in communication disorders: A wellness perspective.* San Diego, CA: Plural.

Larson, V. (2010). *Empowering adolescents to be partners in the learning process: Motivational strategies.* Retrieved from http://www.Speech Pathology.com

McGinty, A. S., & Justice, L. M. (2006). Classroom-based versus pull-out interventions: A review of the experimental evidence. *EBP Briefs, 1*(1), 1–25.

Meltzer, L. (2010). *Promoting executive function in the classroom.* New York, NY: Guilford.

Moon-Meyer, S. (2004). *Survival guide for the beginning speech-language clinician.* Austin, TX: Pro-Ed.

Mosall, A., Choe, Y., Cronin, M., & Massery, M. (2012). *Effortful vs. errorless learning in computer-mediated home practice.* Retrieved from http:// www.asha.org/Events/convention/hand outs/2012/5082-Effortful-vs-Errorless-Learn ing-in-Computer-Mediated-Home-Treatment/

Mowrer, D. E. (1982). *Methods of modifying speech behaviors: Learning theory in speech pathology.* Prospect Heights, IL: Waveland.

Norris, J. A., & Hoffman, P.R. (1990). Language intervention within naturalistic environments. *Language, Speech, and Hearing Services in Schools, 21,* 72–84.

Pattison, G. A., & Powell, T.W. (1990). Establishing rapport with young children during speech and language diagnostic evaluations. *National Student Speech Language and Hearing Association, 17,* 77–80.

Ragan, T. (2011). 10 ways to motivate the unmotivated student [Web blog]. Retrieved from http://blog.asha.org/2011/04/05/10-ways-to-motivate-the-unmotivated-student/

Reisberg, M. (1996). Customer satisfaction in health care. *Perspectives on Administration and Supervision, 6*(2), 12–15.

Roth, F., & Paul, R. (2007).Communication intervention. In R. Paul & P. Cascella (Eds.), *Introduction to clinical methods in communication disorders* (pp. 157–178). Baltimore, MD: Paul H. Brookes.

Roth, F. R., & Worthington, C.K. (2001). *Treatment resource manual for speech-language pathology.* Albany, NY: Delmar.

Soclof, A. (2010). *The absolute best way to motivate your clients.* Retrieved from http://www .SpeechPathology.com

Sohlberg, M. M., Ehlardt, L., & Kennedy, M. (2005). Instructional techniques in cognitive rehabilitation: A preliminary report. *Seminars in Speech and Language, 26,* 268–279.

Thomas, B., & Storey, E. (2000, April). Motivating the elderly client in long-term care. *Advance for Physical Therapy and Rehab Medicine.* Retrieved from http://physical-therapy .advanceweb.com/

Ward, S. (2009). *Executive function skills for the SLP.* Retrieved from http://www.asha.org/ Events/convention/handouts/2009/1718_ Ward_Sarah_2/

Wewers, M. E., & Lowe, N. K. (1990). A critical review of visual analogue scales in the measurement of clinical phoneme. *Residential Nursing Health, 13*(4), 227–236.

CHAPTER 11

Group Therapy

Jennifer A. Ostergren and Sarah Guzzino

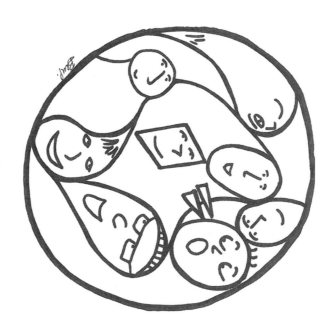

Unity is strength . . . when there is teamwork and collaboration, wonderful things can be achieved.

Mattie Stepanek (nationally recognized poet and peace advocate. Mattie died at age 13 of complications related to dysautonomic mitochondrial myopathy, a rare form of muscular dystrophy)

As has been mentioned, you may be asked to provide treatment services under the supervision and guidance of your supervising speech-language pathologist (SLP) (American Speech-Language-Hearing Association [ASHA], 2013). These services may be delivered to a single individual or to a small group of individuals (Cascella, Purdy, & Dempsey, 2007). Provision of treatment services to small groups of individuals is common in a variety of settings, including school settings for children (Mire, 2007) and medical and community settings for adults (Elman, 2007). Chapter 10 shares ideas for implementing treatment services that are applicable to both individual and group treatment models. The sections that follow focus on the unique aspects of group models of treatment that warrant additional consideration.

The purpose of group treatment varies (Roth & Worthington, 2001) but can include the following:

1. Teaching participants a new communication skill at an introductory level
2. Providing participants with practice in skills established in an individual session
3. Providing participants with socialization, self-help, and/or counseling

Not all groups are appropriate for a speech-language pathology assistant (SLPA) to lead. For example, groups in which counseling and adjustment is the primarily (or secondary) purpose would not be appropriate for implementation by an SLPA. Group intervention can occur concurrent with individual sessions or as the sole source of intervention (Roth & Worthington, 2001). It may be provided early, late, or throughout the client's course of treatment. In some cases, group sessions will comprise individuals with similar skills, abilities, and intervention goals, whereas in other instances, group members will be individuals with diverse skills, abilities, and intervention goals (Elman, 2007; Luterman, 2008; Moon-Meyer, 2004). Groups can range in size from as small as two individuals to as large as an entire classroom, as may be the case in community-based groups or in the case of a self-contained classroom in a school setting (Cascella et al., 2007; Elman, 2007). A self-contained classroom is common for students with special needs. Self-contained classrooms place a small group of pupils with special needs with generally one instructor (often assisted by paraprofessionals) for most of the day (Mattinson, 2011; Schubert & Baxter, 1982; Walker, 2009).

The role of the clinician during group treatment can be directive or nondirective (Roth & Worthington, 2001), based on the purpose of the group. In the case of a directive model, the clinician "sets the agenda, chooses the materials and activities, provides specific instruction, and gives corrective feedback (Roth & Worthington, 2001, p. 25). In a nondirective role, the group members participate in these activities and the clinician serves as a facilitator in helping group members to accomplish the group's goal(s). An example of a nondirective group model is that of peer-mediated groups. According to Carter and Kennedy (2006), peer-mediated support interventions involve equipping one or more peers, without disabilities, to provide ongoing social and/or academic support to special needs peers of a similar age, under the guidance of educators, paraprofessionals, or other school staff. This intervention is thought to promote independence, due to the students involved becoming more acquainted with working together and leading their own progress. This support arrangement consists of the following: identifying students with a disability and their peers who would benefit from involvement, equipping peers to provide support, arranging opportunities for students to interact and support one another, and monitoring and offering guidance when needed (McCauley & Prelock, 2013).

In any form, clinicians working with groups maintain responsibility for ensuring that group dynamics and communication among group members support a positive learning and social environment for all members. Similar to individual sessions, group treatment activities should be driven by a specific set of goals, applicable to either individual group members or a collective group goal, shared by all members.

Table 11–1 contains a list of several advantages and disadvantages of group treatment. As with any aspect of treatment, your supervising SLP will weigh the advantages and disadvantages of group treatment in deciding when and if it is applicable to a client's needs (ASHA, 2013). She or he will also be responsible for establishing the size, composition, and purpose of group intervention, as well as recommending group activities to target treatment goals.

Moon-Meyer (2004) coined an important term: "therapy in a group" (p. 262). This warrants additional consideration, in contrast with group therapy. According to Moon-Meyer, therapy in a group is not the same as group therapy. Rather, therapy in a group employs the same tenets of an individual session but with multiple clients present. As an example, consider a small group of third graders in a school setting with the following treatment goals:

- John has a treatment goal targeting /r/ sounds in the final position of words.
- Sue has a treatment goal targeting the reduction of disfluencies in conversational speech.
- Bill has a social interaction and pragmatic treatment goal.

Using a *therapy in a group* model, time is split between each individual in targeting treatment goals. When John is practicing /r/ sounds in words, the clinician

Table 11–1. Advantages and Disadvantages of Group Therapy

Advantages of Group Therapy	Disadvantages of Group Therapy
• Group participants may motivate each other or offer insight and assistance that a clinician cannot readily provide.	• Individual participants may receive less direct attention from the clinician.
• More opportunities exist for natural speaking situations, socialization, and peer interactions. This may enhance carryover and generalization of a target behavior.	• Some participants may be reluctant to participate fully in group interactions, particularly those who are shy or self-conscious.
• Participants have an opportunity to observe group members and may recognize that others have problems similar to their own.	• Some participants may monopolize group interactions.
• Group interactions, especially when the clinician takes a nondirective role, may decrease dependence of the clinician and thereby increase client independence.	• Generally there are fewer opportunities per participant, per increment of time, to engage in a specific behavior (compared with individual sessions). This may mean fewer opportunities to address specific weaknesses and less direct practice of a specific skill.
	• The pace of the group (or the rate of progress) may not be exactly matched with each participant.

Source: Roth & Worthington, 2007, p. 26.

interacts with him, providing feedback and correction to shape accurate production of target words. While this occurs, Sue and Bill wait for their turn. Next, Sue receives the clinician's attention, practicing fluent speech in short narratives. Again, the clinician focuses her attention on Sue, while John and Bill now wait. Finally, it is Bill's turn, and the clinician turns her efforts to discussing sample scenarios of appropriate and inappropriate personal space diagrams, while group members John and Sue now wait. As you can see from this interaction, there is very little interaction *between* the group members themselves, as well as a reduction in the total amount of interaction each group member has with the clinician. This is problematic, particularly when you consider the amount of treatment received per the amount of participation. If this were, for example, a 30-minute session, each participant would have received roughly 10 minutes of *treatment* and 20 minutes of *waiting*. This is not group therapy. None of the advantages of group therapy (described above) could be realized with this model (e.g., group participants motivated by each other, group participants engaging in natural speaking situations), but all of the disadvantages are magnified (e.g., less direct attention from the clinician, fewer opportunities to practice). In this instance, a group member's time is better spent engaging in other activities and attending only an individual session with the clinician for 10 minutes.

As this example shows, the main distinguishing feature of group therapy and that of therapy in a group is interaction, both between the clients and with the clinician. In terms of client interactions, Moon-Meyer (2004) outlines two types of interaction that should be considered: non-goal-related interaction and goal-related interaction. With non-goal-related interaction, as the name suggests, the interaction between clients does not target the treatment goal, as in the case of waiting their turn or performing tasks not related to their treatment goal. In contrast, goal-directed interactions target each of the client's treatment goals. Maximizing the amount of goal-directed interaction should always be your primary goal during group sessions. This, of course, is easiest when individuals share a similar goal, but with careful planning, group therapy and maximum goal-directed interaction can also be achieved when individuals do not share similar goals.

CHARACTERISTICS OF EFFECTIVE GROUP DYNAMICS

The term *effectiveness* refers to "the extent to which a specific intervention, regimen, or service, when deployed in routine practice, does what it is intended to do" (Baum, 1998, p. 237, cited in Last, 1983). Travis (1957) outlined five characteristics that aid in effective group dynamics, including creating a positive atmosphere, facilitating observation, making tools available, providing opportunities for repeated experiences, and helping to reduce barriers. Each is a factor to consider in designing and/or modifying the dynamics of a group treatment session.

In *creating a positive atmosphere*, as an SLPA, you must demonstrate acceptance, respect, and belonging for each individual. This process may be implemented through your behaviors of speech, facial expressions, postures, and so forth, which should all communicate a positive and welcoming attitude toward group members. This will set the foundation for group interaction. In addition, you must be conscious of the fact that the world is viewed differently by others. Therefore, not projecting your own attitudes on the group will benefit the group atmosphere. Furthermore, allowing group members to participate in selecting and planning activities will influence this as well and create a sense of belonging within that group.

By exhibiting these behaviors and attitudes, you also promote the next characteristic of an effective group dynamic: *facilitating observation*. This means that you assume that group members will be influenced by the behavior(s) they observe, both your behavior and those of the other group members. One issue in this area is placing undue pressure on a group member to respond. You can be mindful of how you introduce group activities and what will be required of group members. You want to ensure the group dynamic is such that group members can participate with ease and pleasure. In addition, as much as possible, use naturally occurring, intrinsic rewards over artificial rewards (such as tokens or "good work"). In educational settings, it is common for students to become influenced by their group members, especially if those members seem to be doing better than them (Travis, 1957). For example, when a student struggles to produce a target utterance, this may create anxiety within the student, especially when she observes overt and artificial praise given to other students. This may decrease future participation in group activities.

The third characteristic of effective group therapy dynamics is *making tools available*. Use of the proper tools to complement the group and individual goal(s) is critical. You can plan in advance of group sessions by listing the materials needed to implement group treatment. This information can be listed on the lesson plan for that session (see Chapter 7). You should make sure all materials are modified to meet each group member's abilities and that there are ample materials, accessible to all members. You will want to ensure, however, that emphasis is on the interactions of group members and the goals of the group session. Chapter 10 discusses the concept of the "game mirage" (Moon-Meyer, 2004). This applies to groups as well. You can avoid the game mirage and reinforce goals of group treatment by providing an introduction to the session, stating the goals to be targeted, elaborating on them during the session, and then concluding with a summary of the group session (Vinson, 2009, p. 310).

Opportunities for repeated experience is also a characteristic of effective group dynamics. This does not mean learning will take place solely through repetition of an activity, as discussed in Chapter 10 relative to clinician-directed treatment that employs drill activities. It does mean, though, that group dynamics and learning are enhanced through opportunities to practice skills with diverse peers who may differ in gender, age, and status (e.g., authority figure vs. peer).

Reducing barriers is the final factor to consider in ensuring a positive group dynamic. This can vary greatly but would include the group leader analyzing factors that impeded the effectiveness of the group, the group dynamics, or group learning. In the field of augmentative and alternative communication (AAC), researchers describe barriers that may impede the use of AAC. These principles can also be applied to group dynamics as well and include opportunity barriers and access barriers (Beukelman & Mirenda, 2005). Opportunity barriers are factors outside the individual that may affect the individual or group dynamics. Three opportunity barriers that may be particularly relevant to your work as an SLPA in group sessions are skills, attitude, and knowledge barriers. These pertain to having the skills and knowledge needed to be effective in a group situation and your attitude toward group situations. If any of these are areas of concern, you can work with your supervising SLP to ensure you have the adequate skills, abilities, and attitudes to successfully run a group session. Access barriers relate to "the capacities, attitudes, and resources" of the individual, including "a lack of ability or difficulty with manipulation and management of objects, problems with cognitive function and decision making, literacy problems, and/or sensory-perceptual impairments (i.e., vision or hearing impairments)" (Roth & Worthington, 2001, p. 116). Here, too, you can work with your supervising SLP to identify any barriers in these areas applicable to group members and their participation in group treatment.

SAMPLE GROUP ACTIVITIES

The activities used in group sessions are a vehicle for obtaining specific goals and can vary greatly, per the group's purpose. As discussed in Chapter 7, lesson plans serve the purpose of directing specific elements of a given session, such as the goals to be targeted, materials to be used, potential prompts or assistance, and data collection methods. Carefully prepared and detailed lesson plans for group treatment sessions will serve a similar purpose.

Although an extensive review of all applicable activities used within group treatment sessions, across the multitude of settings and clients an SLPA may serve, is beyond the scope of this chapter, Table 11–2 contains a sampling of activities for children. Box 11–1 contains a list of suggested activities for adults.

In addition, Chapters 12 and 13 also contain additional examples of treatment activities that can be adapted to group dynamics. Ideas for activities can also be found in resources devoted to group approaches for specific age groups or disorders. For example, *Group Treatment of Neurogenic Communication Disorders: The Expert Clinician's Approach* (Elman, 2007) provides a comprehensive review of group treatment approaches for individuals with neurogenic disorders, such as aphasia, traumatic brain injury, and dementia. Similarly, *Group Treatment for Asperger Syndrome: A Social Skills Curriculum* (Adams, 2006) provides a valuable resource in the area of group treatment for Asperger syndrome. A sample of activities suggested by Adams (2006) for social skills is listed in Appendix 11–A.

Table 11–2. Sample Group Activities for Children

Activity	Suggested Target Area(s)
Shared book reading, card games such as Go Fish, board games, and Tic-Tac-Toe (Figure 11–1) using target sounds	Articulation
Shared reading activities, story retelling rope (Figure 11–2), and comic strips (Figure 11–3)	Language comprehension, verbal expression, writing, WH-questions
Venn diagrams (Figure 11–4) and visual aids, comparing and contrasting topics like sports, foods, presidents, holidays, and so forth	Curriculum-based information, language comprehension, language expression, vocabulary, same/different, narrative writing
Theme-based art and creative endeavors, such as coloring, crafts, building projects, and so forth	Following directions, sequencing, vocabulary, and verbal expression
Obstacle course and building activities	Prepositions
Hangman	Spelling
Treasure or scavenger hunts, conversational ladder (Figure 11–5), conversational starter cards (e.g., If you could have any superhero powers, what would they be? What would you buy if you won a million dollars? If you could invent a video game, what would it be like?), off-campus outings, and role-play (e.g., student becomes the teacher)	Verbal expression, stuttering/disfluency, and social skills

Tic-Tac-Toe

Figure 11–1. Sample group activity: Tic-Tac-Toe with target words.

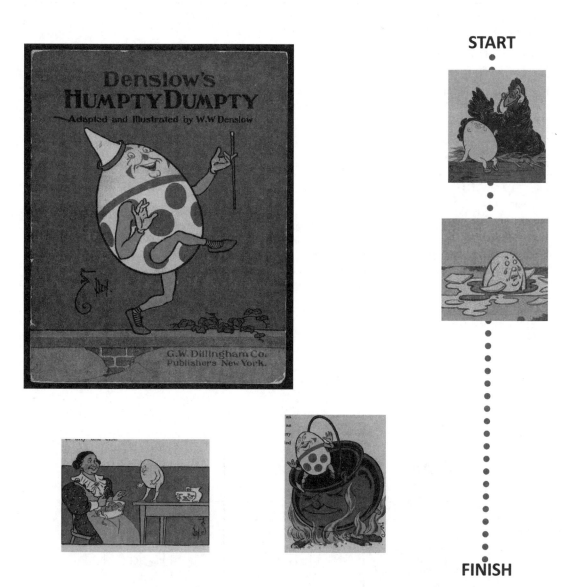

Figure 11–2. Sample group activity: Story retelling rope, using Denslow's *Humpty Dumpty*. *Note.* Group members engage in a shared book reading and then retell the story, placing images from the book along a rope to guide retelling. Images in the public domain. Courtesy of U.S. Library of Congress Rare Book and Special Collections Division.

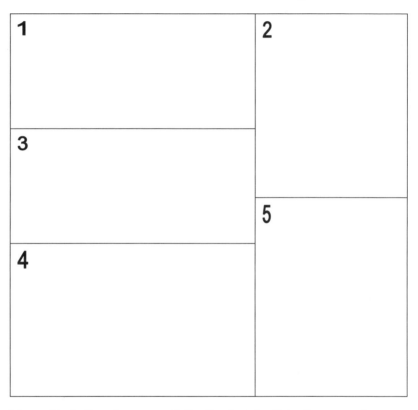

Figure 11–3. Sample group activity: Comic strip. *Note.* Group members create and tell a story by drawing images in the comic strip boxes or using the provided images, arranged and placed in the boxes.

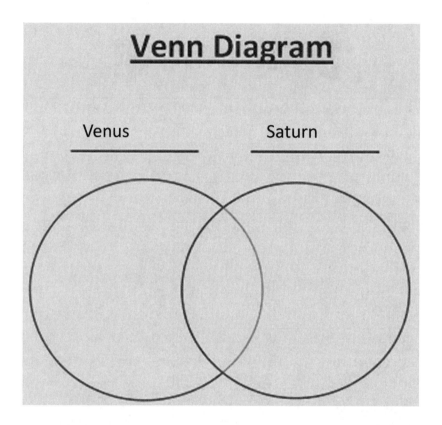

1. How many moons does each planet have?
2. What is the planet made of?
3. How many rings does the planet have?

Figure 11–4. Sample group activity: Venn diagram. *Note.* Group members discuss attributes of related/unrelated items.

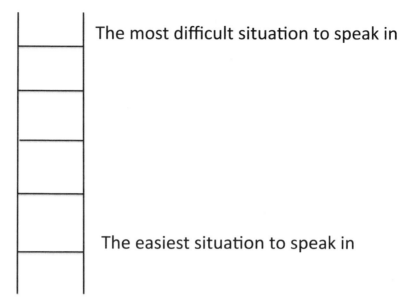

Figure 11–5. Sample group activity: Conversation ladder. *Note.* Group members rank and discuss contrasting concepts (e.g., easiest/most difficult speaking situations, most/least favored activity in school, etc.).

Box 11–1. Suggested Activities for Adult Groups

- Role-play real-life activities, using communication strategies, conflict resolution, self-advocacy techniques, and so forth.
- Charades-based activities using gestures, drawing, writing, and description
- Facilitated discussion centered on favorite activities/hobbies, recent events, strategy use, problem solving, and so forth.
- Performance, either impromptu (e.g., group script reading) or group activities centered on a specific performance (e.g., putting on a play for family, friends, community members)
- Poem reading, either impromptu or planned
- Community outings to practice daily living skills (e.g., money use, conversations with strangers, map reading, effective medical visits)
- Team activities, such as scavenger hunts, building activities, board or card games, cooking activities, and so forth
- A movie club centered on having facilitated discussion about selected movies watched by group members
- A book club centered on reading a book and facilitated discussion about its content

APPLYING CLASSROOM MANAGEMENT PRINCIPLES TO GROUP TREATMENT

In the field of education, teachers commonly work with groups of students, using techniques known as classroom management techniques. These are a set of principles that involve the actions of the teacher "to create a learning environment that encourages positive social interaction, active engagement in learning, and self-motivation" (Burden, 2006, p. 4). Many of these principles are also applicable to the services SLPs and SLPAs provide during group treatment. Research in this area suggests that several key factors underlie effective teaching and positively functioning classroom environments (Parsonson, 2012, p. 17), as follows:

1. Clear, simple rules and expectations that are consistently and fairly applied.
As an SLPA, it will be important for you to establish the rules of the group session. An example of applicable rules for children may be the following (Adams, 2006, p. 9):

- Raise your hands before you talk.
- Keep good eye contact.
- Listen when others are talking.
- Take turns talking about topics of interest.
- Use your inside voice.

These can be modified for adults as well. It is important to inform members of the rules at a level appropriate to the age, abilities, and purpose of the group. For young children, this may mean posting something in the group environment, similar to Figure 11–6, and then reviewing this information at the beginning of each session and as needed, given any potential rule violations.

2. Predictable events and routines, including cues and signals about upcoming activities.
Chapter 10 discusses similar concepts in the area of visual schedules. The samples of visual schedules provided in Chapter 10 can be adapted to represent the agenda of activities planned for a group session. For adult, literate clients, this can be accomplished by providing a written agenda for group sessions, similar to those used in business meetings. You can also maintain consistency in the design of group sessions by starting each session with a consistent opening activity, such as greetings and updates, followed by a core activity (that changes on a regular basis) and then a consistent closing activity. After a few sessions, as applicable, clients can begin to actively participate (or even lead) these opening and closing activities.

3. Frequent use of specific and descriptive praise, including verbal and nonverbal praise.
Chapter 10 provides a thorough discussion of operant conditioning and positive behavioral supports, both of which are applicable to the use of reinforcement and praise. The section on the effective use of operant principles provides several helpful examples of descriptive versus evaluative praise and effective reinforcement techniques. In the area of classroom management, Bradley, Pauley, and Pauley (2006) also suggest that teachers *know their students* and their personalities, motives, and desires as an important factor in the use of praise and reinforcement. This is good advice for SLPAs as well.

Relative to disruptive behaviors, researchers in the area of classroom management specifically warn against the use

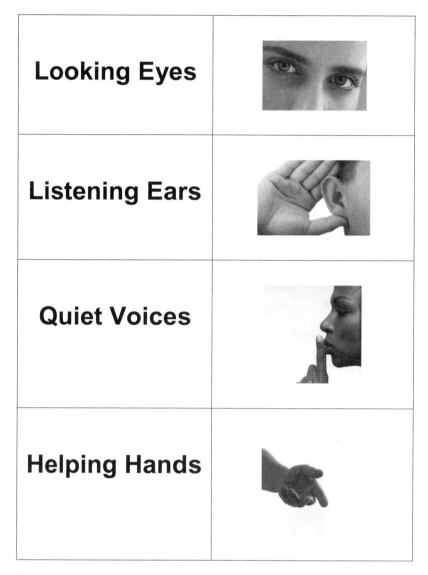

Figure 11-6. Visual rules for posting in group environments with children. Images courtesy of Microsoft Corporation © 2013.

of any of the teacher behaviors listed in Box 11–2 in response to disruptive student behavior. Instead, when student behaviors become disruptive, a Three-Step Response Plan is recommended in classroom settings (Burden, 2006; Figure 11–7). This plan employs the principles of least intervention, which states that "when dealing with routine classroom behavior, misbehavior should be corrected with the simplest, least intrusive intervention that will work" (Slavin, 2006, as cited in Burden,

> **Box 11–2. Behaviors to Avoid in Response to Disruptive Behavior** (Burden, 2006)
>
> 1. Harsh and humiliating reprimands
> 2. Threats
> 3. Nagging
> 4. Forced apologies
> 5. Sarcastic remarks
> 6. Group punishment
> 7. Assigning extra work
> 8. Reducing grades
> 9. Writing as punishment
> 10. Physical labor or exercise
> 11. Corporal punishment

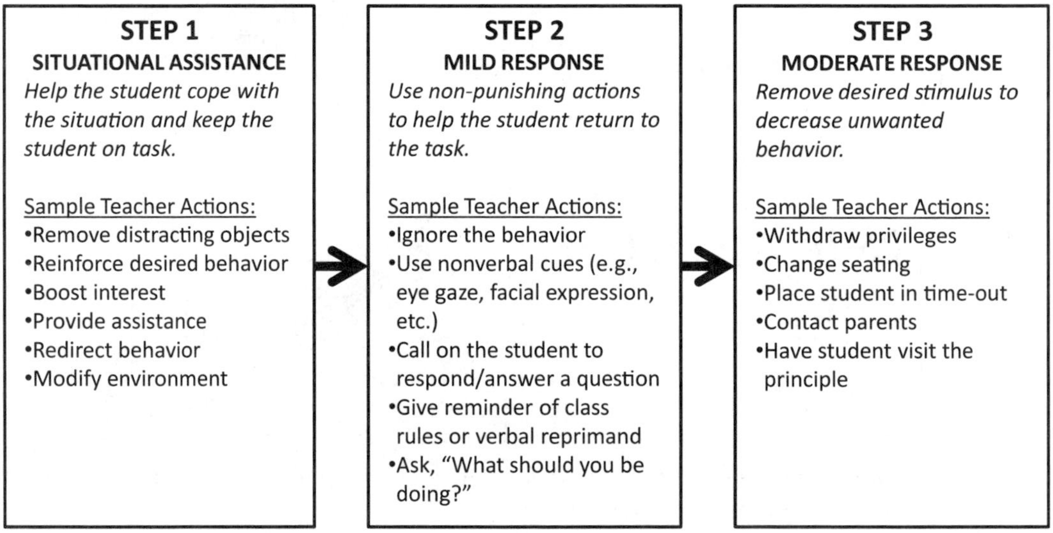

STEP 1 SITUATIONAL ASSISTANCE	STEP 2 MILD RESPONSE	STEP 3 MODERATE RESPONSE
Help the student cope with the situation and keep the student on task.	*Use non-punishing actions to help the student return to the task.*	*Remove desired stimulus to decrease unwanted behavior.*
Sample Teacher Actions: •Remove distracting objects •Reinforce desired behavior •Boost interest •Provide assistance •Redirect behavior •Modify environment	Sample Teacher Actions: •Ignore the behavior •Use nonverbal cues (e.g., eye gaze, facial expression, etc.) •Call on the student to respond/answer a question •Give reminder of class rules or verbal reprimand •Ask, "What should you be doing?"	Sample Teacher Actions: •Withdraw privileges •Change seating •Place student in time-out •Contact parents •Have student visit the principle

Figure 11–7. Illustration of Three-Step Response for addressing disruptive behavior in group settings. Adapted from Burden (2006, p. 220).

2006, p. 215). Each of these suggestions can also be used by SLPAs during group sessions to restore order when disruptive behavior is present.

4. *Matching tasks to the skills and abilities of the learners.*

In the field of education, this is known as *differentiated instruction* and is achieved when the teacher accommodates student differences in "readiness levels, interests, and learning profiles," thereby achieving an optimum learning environment for all learners (Subban, 2006, p. 940). Matching tasks to group members' skills and abilities also reduces frustration and/or boredom, which is often associated with disruptive behavior (Parsonson, 2012).

SLPs are generally very good at achieving differentiated instruction given an individual treatment session. The key is to maintain this same level of differentiation during group sessions. This requires careful planning. Just as teachers plan for their classroom activities, SLPAs must also plan carefully and work with the supervising SLP to ensure an effective lesson plan is in place for each group session. In fact, as discussed in Chapter 7, the idea of lesson planning is borrowed from the field of education and the research surrounding classroom management. Remember that one element of an effective lesson plan includes ways to modify tasks, if needed. To do this in a timely fashion requires that you carefully observe group member behavior and implement modification, as needed, *during* group sessions. Using effective data collection is also important as this information can then be used by your supervising SLP to make additional modifications prior to the next session. Chapter 10 (particularly the sections on "Things to Consider: The Client" and "Things to Consider: The Environment") offers additional suggestions in potential modifications to ensure the environment is supportive and the client is ready and able to participate fully in treatment activities.

DATA COLLECTION DURING GROUP SESSIONS

All the techniques discussed in Chapter 8 also apply to recording the performance of group members during group sessions. The importance of doing so accurately and consistently is equally important in both group and individual sessions. Collecting data during group sessions may be even more challenging, however, given the nature of the session and the need to attend to the needs of multiple members simultaneously. Appendix 11–B and the CD of this textbook contain a sample data collection sheet for use during a group session. Many of the sample data sheets provided in Chapter 8 can also be easily modified for group sessions. Box 11–3 contains some addition tips for collecting data during group treatment.

Box 11–3. Tips for Collecting Data in Group Sessions

■ Discuss with your supervising SLP employing different techniques, such as the following:
  ■ *Timed Data Collection:* Collecting data on one group member the first 5 minutes, the next group member the following 5 minutes, and so forth.
  ■ *Rotating Data Collection:* Collecting data on one goal, per client, per session and then rotating to a different goal, per client the next session, and so forth, until you have collected data on all goals for all clients, then start the rotating process all over again.
■ Make sure to prepare your data sheets in advance, completing as much as possible prior to the session, including prerecording group member names, goals, codes for scoring, and so forth.
■ Think creatively about where you will keep your data collection sheets within a group dynamic to ensure they are accessible to you but not readily in view of group members.
■ Be aware of the prompts you provide, both for data collection purposes (as recommended in Chapter 8) and also *across* group members. It may be that the prompts provided to one group member affect (either positively or negatively) the performance of another group member. For example, a student prompted using a tactile cue for the /s/ phoneme (e.g., sliding the pointer finger on the table) may influence her group mate to use the same technique for practicing her /g/ words, which would result in an error in the production of /g/. Having a way to note the relationship of all prompts is helpful if you or your supervising SLP suspect this may be the case.

REFERENCES

Adams, L. (2006). *Group treatment for Asperger syndrome: A social skills curriculum.* San Diego, CA: Plural.

American Speech-Language-Hearing Association (ASHA). (2013). *Speech-language pathology assistant scope of practice.* Retrieved from http://www.asha.org/policy

Beukelman, D. R., & Mirenda, P. (2005). *Augmentative and alternative communication: Supporting children and adults with complex communication needs.* Baltimore, MD: Paul H. Brookes.

Bradley, D. F., Pauley, J. A., & Pauley, J. F. (2006). *Effective classroom management: Six keys to success.* Lanham, MD: Rowman & Littlefield Education.

Burden, P. (2006). *Classroom management: Creating a successful K–12 learning community.* Hoboken, NY: John Wiley.

Carter, E. W., & Kennedy, C. H. (2006). Promoting access to the general curriculum using peer support strategies. *Research and Practice for Persons With Severe Disabilities, 31,* 284–292.

Cascella, R., Purdy, M. H., & Dempsey, J. J. (2007). Clinical service delivery and work settings. In R. Paul & P. Cascella (Eds.), *Introduction to clinical methods in communication disorders* (pp. 259–282). Baltimore, MD: Paul H. Brookes.

Elman, R. J. (2007). *Group treatment of neurogenic communication disorders: The expert clinician's approach* (2nd ed.). San Diego, CA: Plural.

Last, J. M. (1983). *A dictionary of epidemiology.* New York, NY: Oxford University Press.

Luterman, D. (2008). *Counseling persons with communication disorders and their families.* Austin, TX: Pro-Ed.

Mattinson, R. E. (2011). Comparison of students classified ED in self-contained classrooms and a self-contained school. *Education and Treatment of Children, 34*(1), 15–33.

McCauley, R., & Prelock, P. (Eds.). (2013). *Treatment of autism spectrum disorders: Evidence-based intervention strategies for communication and social interactions.* Baltimore, MD: Brookes.

Mire, S. (2007). Workload analysis: IEP and the group size factors in calculating workload. *School Based Issues,* 18–20.

Moon-Meyer, S. (2004). *Survival guide for the beginning speech-language clinician.* Austin, TX: Pro-Ed.

Parsonson, B. S. (2012). Evidence-based classroom behavior management strategies. *Kairanranga, 13*(1), 16–23.

Roth, F. R., & Worthington, C. K. (2001). *Treatment resource manual for speech-language pathology.* Albany, NY: Delmar.

Schubert, N. A., & Baxter, M. B. (1982). The self-contained open classroom as a viable learning environment. *Education, 102,* 411–415.

Subban, P. (2006). Differentiated instruction: A RESEARCH BASIS. *International Education Journal, 7*(7), 935–947.

Travis, L. E. (1957). *Handbook of speech pathology.* New York, NY: Appleton-Century-Crofts.

Vinson, B. P. (2009). *Workplace skills and professional issues in speech-language pathology.* San Diego, CA: Plural.

Walker, K. (2009). Self-contained classrooms: Research brief. *Education Partnerships,* 1–3.

APPENDIX 11–A

Social Skills Group Activities (Adams, 2006)

Activity	Ages	Objective	Materials	Procedure
Dice Talk	3–5 years old	Child will use eye contact in communication.	■ A small sized box ■ Plain paper to cover box ■ Marker ■ Tape	Find a small box that can be covered with paper and used as a dice for this communication game. Use a size that is easy and fun for little hands to toss. Wrap the box in plain paper. On the faces of the dice, write questions or statements to elicit answers from the children. For example, on the six faces of the dice, you could write: ■ Name an animal that lives in the zoo. ■ Tell me a food you like to eat ■ What animal lives on a farm? ■ What is something you like to drink? ■ Tell me an animal that lives on a farm. ■ Name a toy you like to play with. Explain to the children that they each will get a turn to toss the dice, and they get to answer the question that lands on top. Tell them that they will answer to you, and they must look in your eyes as they talk to you. Explain that looking at people as they talk to them is a good thing we all need to practice.
Bowling	3–5 years old	Child will learn turn-taking in a group activity.	■ Plastic bowling pins and ball ■ Masking tape	Set up the pins, placing a piece of tape on the floor to mark where the children should stand when throwing the ball. Arrange the children in a line behind the masking tape. Explain that each child will get a turn when he or she steps up to the line.

Activity	Ages	Objective	Materials	Procedure
				Show the children how to go to the back of the line after their turn. If there are so many children that the wait in line is quite long, have two bowling sets to increase the children's turn taking and lessen the demand on their patience.
Pumpkin Decorating	6–9 years old	Child will use turn-taking in group activity.	■ One large pumpkin ■ Pretty fall leaves of various shapes and colors ■ Yarn ■ Markers ■ Construction paper ■ Scissors ■ Tape ■ Slips of numbered paper and a hat to draw them out to determine turn-taking order	Tell the group they get to decorate a pumpkin, giving it a face, hair, and ears. Instruct the children that they are free to use any of the materials, but they must take turns adding decorations to the pumpkin. Allow them a brief time to discuss possible decorating ideas; if necessary, prompt their creativity with suggestions such as, "Leaves for hair? A mouth out of yarn? Draw ears with a marker?" Draw numbers out of a hat to determine the order they go in, informing them everyone may each have as many turns as necessary to fully decorate the pumpkin.
Big Muscles!	6–9 years old	Child will participate in role-play with the group.	■ Heavy objects and light objects *Heavy/Light* cans of soup/feathers detergent jug/foam cups hammer/crayon dictionary/leaf rock/cotton balls	Talk about things that are heavy and light and ask the children for the meaning of each word. Children can pretend to be weightlifters and take turns lifting the objects. Each child can win a medal for his or her big muscles.

continues

Appendix 11–A. *continued*

Activity	Ages	Objective	Materials	Procedure
I'll Be Your Server	10–12 years old	Child will use eye contact when speaking and listening.	▪ Refreshments (one item for each student to distribute to group) ▪ Server's apron (optional)	Inform students that they will each have a turn being a waiter, passing out refreshments to the rest of the group. Instruct students that good communication, including eye contact, is important to being a waiter as well as being a consumer. Have students choose the refreshment items they will distribute. Let them take turns passing out the items, using eye contact as they ask each group member, "Would you like some_____?" Remind group members also to make eye contact as they are waited on.
Student Teacher	10–12 years old	Child will use eye contact, topic maintenance, and appropriate length of communication	▪ None	Explain to the group that, for this activity, the teacher will be the student, and the students will give feedback to the teacher regarding topic maintenance. Instruct the students to think of topics for the teacher to present. Examples may include: what I did over the weekend, how to make a peanut butter and jelly sandwich, the reasons I became a teacher, my favorite foods, games I played when I was a child, and so on. Show the students a signal (such as raising a hand or pointing a finger at you) they may use if they hear the presentation go off topic. Be sure to wander off topic as you present and respond to students' signals to get back on topic.

Source: Adams (2006). Copyright. Used with permission.

Group Data Collection Sheet

Group Time: _____ Location: _____ Date: _____ (Length of Session: _____)

Members Present: _____

Group Activity: _____

Member Name: _____ NOTES FOR SESSION: _____

Objective(s)	Data Tally	Data Summary	Comments

Member Name: _____ NOTES FOR SESSION: _____

Objective(s)	Data Tally	Data Summary	Comments

Member Name: _____ NOTES FOR SESSION: _____

Objective(s)	Data Tally	Data Summary	Comments

Member Name: _____ NOTES FOR SESSION: _____

Objective(s)	Data Tally	Data Summary	Comments

CHAPTER 12

Incorporating Play and Literacy in Treatment

Sara M. Aguilar

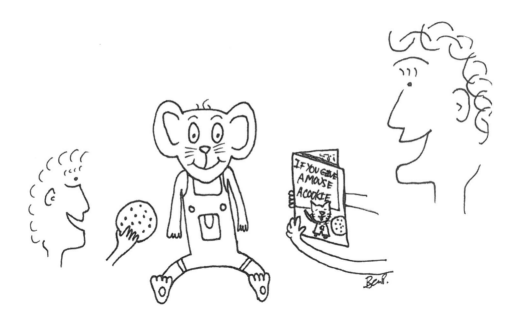

Play is a child's work.
Jean Piaget (prominent developmental psychologist)

Children learn about the world they live in through play. It provides them with a way to learn, experiment with, and use new information. Beginning in infancy with basic games, such as peek-a-boo, play goes on to assume a critical role in a child's physical, emotional, social, and cognitive-linguistic development. It is commonly believed that most of a child's linguistic knowledge develops in the context of play. The American Speech-Language-Hearing Association (ASHA) suggests that speech-language therapy within the context of play "provides both the children and their caregivers with more objects and actions to share in interactions and provides a context for enhancing the child's communication skills" (ASHA, 2008, Areas to Screen, Evaluate, and Assess, para. 2). As such, the ability to incorporate play into treatment sessions is an important skill for a speech-language pathology assistant (SLPA).

DEVELOPMENT OF PLAY

As you consider how to incorporate play into treatment, it is important to understand how play develops. A child's play begins with reflexive behaviors that initially lack inherent intentionality, such as crying, cooing, and smiling (Schwartz, 2004). When these behaviors are met with meaningful reactions from caregivers, they are treated as communicative acts. With time, these behaviors mature into

more complex cognitive processes, including representational thought, imagination, exploration, analysis, and problem solving. As such, the stages in a child's cognitive development will be reflected in that child's play. Based on Piaget's work, we know that children engage in four stages of cognitive development: sensorimotor, preoperational, concrete operations, and formal operations (Table 12–1).

The ability to engage in representational thought is a cognitive skill that typically emerges by 18 months, during the sensorimotor period of cognitive development. This period is often associated with *practice play*, Piaget's earliest classification of play (Casby, 2003). During practice play, children explore objects in an egocentric manner as they learn about the world through their physical senses (e.g., mouthing objects, banging/throwing objects). Later in this stage, children begin to engage in simple cause-effect actions, such as physically moving toward a desired

Table 12–1. Piaget's Stages of Cognitive Development

Age	Stage	Characteristics	Language Behaviors
Birth to 2 years	Sensorimotor	Begins with reflexive behaviors and motor learning. Progresses rapidly, learning object permanence, means–end behaviors, and so on.	Begins with reflexive vocal behaviors (e.g., crying/cooing) and later develops into use of true words when referents are not present (e.g., Child says "Daddy" even when he is not present).
2 to 7 years	Preoperational	Most rapid stage of language learning. Child develops representational thought and learns to solve physical problems.	Begins to engage in make believe and starts to comprehend and express temporal concepts (e.g., past, future).
7 to 11 years	Concrete Operations	Child learns to categorize and organize information; begins to be a logical thinker.	Begins to develop conversational skills; use logic to complete tasks.
11 to 15 years	Formal Operations	Learns to be an abstract thinker, tests mental hypotheses.	Uses verbal reasoning to produce "if . . . then" statements.

Source: Adapted from Casby, 2003.

object, finding a toy obscured by an object, and pulling a string to get a toy located at the end of the string (Westby, 1980).

Representational thought serves as a foundation for a child to later develop *symbolic play*. Symbolic play is associated with the preoperational period of cognitive development and includes the symbolism involved with the acquisition of true language behaviors (Westby, 1980). The presence of symbolic play indicates that a child understands that an object or entity can be used to represent something distinct from itself. For example, a child demonstrates this knowledge when using a shoebox to represent a doll's bed. This basic symbolism, used first in play, later serves as a foundation for a child's understanding of the more abstract symbols involved with language, such as the words used to represent objects, ideas, and other concepts. For instance, a pattern of sounds such as "*b-e-d*" represents *a piece of furniture used for sleeping*. Overall, symbolic play and language share the underlying ability to engage in symbolism. In fact, observation of a child's symbolic play behaviors helps determine that child's level of functioning relative to the skills required for the development of language.

The final stages of cognitive development identified by Piaget are concrete operations and formal operations. These stages are associated with more advanced types of play. During the concrete operations stage, the child learns to categorize and organize information. Later, in the formal operations stage, the child engages in abstract thought and begins to test mental hypotheses during play (Wadsworth, 2004).

One way to better understand a child's level of play and representational abilities is through careful observations, using a research-based tool, such as West-

by's (1980) Symbolic Play Scale. Westby's play scale was developed out of observational research conducted on children who are typically developing, as well as those with intellectual impairments. Interestingly, Westby found that both groups of children progressed through the same sequence of play stages. Westby's Symbolic Play Scale was originally published as an appendix in her landmark 1980 article, "Assessment of Cognitive and Language Abilities Through Play," and the scale is now easily located using an online web search. A description of the 10 stages of symbolic play, as depicted by Westby (1980), is summarized in Appendix 12–A. This summary can be used as an observational tool to determine a child's representational abilities, which can in turn guide the creation of developmentally appropriate treatment environments and materials. In addition, knowledge of the sequence of symbolic play will allow you to engage in appropriate data collection to document a child's progression through the stages of play.

PLAY IN SPEECH–LANGUAGE TREATMENT

Incorporating play in treatment can be used as a platform for intervention approaches that focus on language form (i.e., phonology, morphology, syntax), content (i.e., semantics), and use (i.e., pragmatics). Play is a natural context for all children, since it gives them an opportunity to interact and experiment with their surroundings. Children develop language during social interactions. Hence, play in treatment provides opportunities for meaningful social scenarios that encourage language. During play scenarios, a child's communication acts elicit appropriate social responses from you, the child's communication partner. Clinicians can then expand on, and enhance, a child's communication acts to support her or him in becoming a competent language user.

Intervention in the context of play requires the provision of appropriate language input and skillful selection of materials and activities, including imaginative play scenarios, toys, and books. At its core, play in treatment should be a fun, child-directed experience and involve adult guidance and scaffolding to encourage children to experiment with new language forms to understand, describe, and manipulate the world around them.

Because play involves spontaneous and fluid interaction with that child's surroundings, as intervention becomes more naturalistic and less structured, clinicians must take measures to ensure that their treatment is organized and systematic (Norris & Hoffman, 1990). Without an organized and systematic approach, play in treatment merely becomes play. The balance between the spontaneity of play and the organization and methodology of intervention is a delicate one to achieve and maintain. To achieve this balance, it is critical that you work with your supervising speech-language pathologist (SLP) to: (a) carefully determine a child's level of play, (b) create opportunities for meaningful communication, (c) provide effective scaffolding, and (d) select appropriate materials for use during play.

Determining the Level of Play

The first step in using play in treatment is to identify the child's current level of play and developmental abilities. You may identify where a child is functioning on the continuum of play by observing that child's behaviors, consulting with your supervising SLP, and using a play scale such as the one discussed above (Westby, 1980; Appendix 12–A). During observations, be aware that children typically engage in activities and interact with toys to the extent of their developmental level. In other words, an activity will be abandoned as soon as play reaches the capacity of that child's knowledge of the actions and relationships that may be performed or established with a particular toy. Consider this excellent example provided by Norris and Hoffman (1990):

The child rocks a baby doll and then abandons the activity, failing to recognize that the doll's hair can be brushed, her hat can be worn, she can be placed in a stroller and taken for a walk, etc. (p. 74)

Once a child has reached her or his level of knowledge about a given situation (i.e., relationship between objects or actions that can be performed on objects, etc.), it is your job, as the clinician, to extend that child's current knowledge to new learning opportunities. Norris and Hoffman (1990) suggest the following in relation to the scenario above:

If the child rocks the doll and begins to abandon it, the SLP might extend the child's understanding at that moment by making the child aware of some other object in relationship to the doll. The SLP can point to the doll's hair, refer to its state of messiness, and guide the child to brush the doll's hair while referring to all of the relationships between the doll and the brush

("The doll's hair is messy—it has to be brushed—You're brushing her hair—now it's looking prettier—don't brush it too hard"). (p. 74)

The actions and the accompanying language help the child to organize something about the doll in relationship to the brush that was not previously understood by the child.

Creating Communication Opportunities

Once you have extended opportunities for play, you can create the opportunity for a child to become a communicator in that environment by helping the child to: (a) understand how to control and/or manipulate activities and (b) formulate the language involved in the completion of such tasks. Norris and Hoffman (1990) point out that "the goal is not to *teach* language, but rather to provide for active experiences with the use of language so that language may *emerge*" (p. 78). One way to accomplish this is to develop a set of *communication temptations* (Wetherby & Prutting, 1984). Although originally intended to be used in the assessment of children on the autism spectrum, communication temptations can be helpful in developing play scenarios for any young child.

Communication temptations are situations devised specifically to lure the child into initiating communicative acts (Wetherby & Prutting, 1984). The procedure begins by presenting a child with a highly enticing situation that encourages communication. For instance, you may present the child with a jar of bubbles, open it and blow a few bubbles, capture one and encourage the child to pop it, then tightly close the lid on the bubble jar and hand it to the child. Next, without prompting or cueing, simply wait for the child to produce a communicative signal for help. Once the child initiates communication through vocalization, gesture, or some other means, you can respond naturally by opening the bottle and repeating the blowing/popping action with the child. After repeating this scenario a few times, you can add an additional communication temptation by bringing the bubble wand up to your lips, waiting to blow the bubble with an expectant look on your face. Once the child produces a communicative signal, you should respond naturally by blowing the bubbles. This communication temptation scenario may be applied to a number of activities, including balloons, wind-up toys, and peek-a-boo.

The key to creating this type of communication opportunity is for you to consistently view a child's behaviors as communicative (i.e., request, comment, command, question, protest, etc.) and follow through on that child's communicative act by responding in an appropriate and meaningful way. As such, play interactions should be led by the child, meaning that your goal is to focus on responding to the child's behaviors (i.e., "Oh, you want to roll the ball!") rather than requesting behaviors from the child (i.e., "What's that?" "Say *ball.*"). When you treat a child's behavior as a communicative act, it creates the opportunity to expose that child to more complex communication acts. For instance, a child's utterance of *ball* may have been merely produced as a label, but when you interpret it as a request (i.e., "You want the ball?") and provide that child with an appropriate consequence (i.e., giving the ball to the child), the child is immediately exposed to this new and more complex communication act.

Scaffolding Communication

After extending play and creating communication opportunities, you can also clarify any additional information needed by that child's communication partner (whether that may be another child, you as the clinician, an adult, a doll, etc.). This can be done by modeling the language required to express the missing information and providing support as the child attempts to engage in this more complex communication act. In this way, you are partnering with the child to assist in the communication of more complex information. This is referred to as *scaffolding* (Cazden, 1988).

Much like the scaffolding used in the construction of a building, therapeutic scaffolding temporarily provides adult support to a child who is learning how to perform more complex communication acts. Adult support ensures the opportunity to practice using language at a higher level than a child would produce independently. The amount of adult support is adjusted as the child becomes more proficient in using the targeted language forms independently. Table 12–2 outlines various approaches that may be used to support the development of complex communication acts. Furthermore, the techniques listed in Box 12–1 may be helpful during play activities.

Box 12–1

- **Self-talk:** The clinician watches the child's play and then engages in the same behavior, but while describing her or his own actions. For example, the child is playing with a tea set and the clinician begins playing with the set, stating things like, "I'm making tea. I am going to pour some tea for everyone. The tea is so yummy, but hot."
- **Parallel talk:** The clinician describes the child's behaviors during play. For example, during the above play activity with a tea set, the clinician says, "You are making tea and pouring it into each glass. Oh, the tea must be yummy, but hot."
- **Expansion:** The clinician rephrases the child's utterance but uses a grammatically correct version. For example, if the child in the above example says, "Tea hot," the clinician can expand by saying, "Yes, the tea is hot."
- **Extension or expatiation:** Similar to expansion (above), but the clinician rephrases the child's utterance, adding additional semantic information. For example, if the child said "Tea hot," the clinician could say, "Yes, we should be careful to sip the tea slowly."
- **Recast:** The clinician reformulates the child's utterance into a different form, such as a question, and so forth. For example, if the child says, "Drink tea," the clinician can say, "Are you drinking the tea?" or "Should I drink the tea?"

Adapted from Roth and Paul (2007, pp. 165–166).

Table 12–2. Scaffolding Approaches

Scaffolding Approach	Description	Example
Cloze procedures	Child and adult collaborate in creating a message. Adult omits words from phrases/sentences to allow child to provide missing information.	Adult: "Baby is tired, so she will go to _____." Child: "Bed"
Gestures and pantomime	Nonlinguistic physical cues that encourage child to produce language.	Adult: "She's tired. What should she do?" (tilting head and placing it on hands) Child: "Sleep"
Relational terms	Cues child to provide more information.	Child: "She need blanket" Adult: "So she can ... " Child: "Go bed"
Preparatory sets	Highlights important information for child, including appropriate communication acts for particular contexts.	"You can't just take the blanket, you have to *ask* baby for it."
Constituent questioning	Encourages child to produce important details about and relationships between agents, actions, objects, and locations.	Adult: "What does baby need?" Child: "Blanket" Adult: "What does she need the blanket for?" Child: "Baby go sleep"
Comprehension questions	Monitors child's level of understanding during play.	"Why did she cry?"; "Why isn't she sleeping?"; "What happens next?"
Summarization or evaluation	Encourages child to summarize or evaluate information about play activity and provides additional opportunity to practice communicating the message.	"Tell mommy what the baby did."
Binary choices	Provide child with choices for communicating a message.	"You can ask nicely—'I want blanket, please' or you can be mean—'Give me the blanket!'"
Turn-taking cues	Indirectly requests more information from child.	Child: "I want blanket." Adult: "I want the blanket ... " (with expectant pause and look) Child: "I want blanket." Adult: "Yeah?" (with rising intonation)
Phonemic cues	Provides child with beginning sound or syllable to support child's production.	Adult: "I need the bl___." Child: "-anket"

Source: Adapted from Norris & Hoffman, 1990.

Selecting Toys and Materials for Play

Another important consideration in incorporating play in treatment relates to the actual toys and materials that you employ during intervention sessions. Selection of toys should be driven by the anticipated outcome(s) targeted in your treatment session and informed by the child's interests and preferences. You must first ask yourself, "What do I want the child to do/say?" before selecting toys. Table 12–3 contains examples of possible language opportunities that may be targeted using particular toys. Be sure, however, to cautiously manage the treatment environment. It is a good idea to provide options, but be careful not to overwhelm the child with too many choices. It is also helpful to keep some toys visible but out of reach of the child to encourage the child to initiate comments and requests.

In addition, toys used in treatment must be safe for a child at a particular age (Schwartz, 2004). Clinicians should consult a toy's packaging for age recommendations; however, if packaging is not available, a good resource is the United States Consumer Product Safety Commission (2013). Be sure to take appropriate precautions when working with children with developmental delays who may continue to mouth toys past the typical age of development. Furthermore, Chapter 6 discusses additional procedures in ensuring toys and materials are properly cleaned for use in treatment.

Last, Lahey and Bloom's (1977) article is an excellent resource for determining what language input to provide to a child during play. These authors suggest that clinicians focus on using words that frequently occur in the child's environment rather than more specific and less frequently used vocabulary. For example, it is better to say *car* rather than *Toyota* or *money* instead of *quarter*. The use of more general terms is valuable because they may be used in a wider variety of situations. In addition, some words can be used to express multiple meanings and thus enable a child to use a single utterance in multiple ways. A good example of one such word is *no*, which may be used to reject, deny, or express disappearance.

SHARED READING AS PLAY

Young children with language disorders are more likely to experience academic difficulties later in life, particularly in the area of literacy, as spoken and written language have a close and interdependent relationship (Catts & Kamhi, 2005). It is common for the child with a language impairment to experience difficulties learning to read and write, just as the child who faces difficulty with reading and writing often has problems with spoken language. Furthermore, the relationship between spoken and written language is established early in a child's development and continues to grow throughout childhood and into adulthood. ASHA (2001) suggests that individuals engaging in early speech-language intervention can play a significant role in the prevention of future literacy problems. Table 12–4 lists various approaches to early literacy intervention that have been shown to be effective in preventing future literacy problems. As an SLPA, you may be asked to engage in tasks to support literacy development. To do so effectively, you will need to work with your supervising SLP to: (a) incorporate print referencing into treatment session and (b) select appropriate books for use during shared reading activities.

Table 12–3. Activities, Toys, and Language Opportunities

Activity/Toy	Language Opportunities
Peek-a-Boo	• Joint attention (fundamental skill required for language development) • Turn-taking • Cause/effect—child learns to anticipate your reappearance • Model/encourage language routines: *Where is (child's name)? Is he under the table? There you are!*
Blocks	• Cause/effect relationships: stack blocks, then knock them down • Model/encourage language routines: *Uh, oh! Fall down! Oh no!* • Color/size concepts: label and request blocks of different colors/sizes (big/small; long/short) • Prepositions: support child in understanding and/or using prepositions (e.g., *let's put it on top*)
Cars	• Cause/effect: Expand understanding of cause and effect by first stacking blocks, then using a car to knock down blocks • Model/encourage language routines: *ready, set, go!; crash!; stop/go; go fast/go slow* • Expand utterance: *yellow car; big car; fast car* • Sabotage: present car with broken wheel and see how child reacts to it. Encourage/model language: *Oh, no! What happened? It's broken! Let's fix it!*

Bubbles	• Expand utterances:
	  ○ Actions: *open/close bubbles; blow bubble; pop bubble*
	  ○ Adjectives: *big bubble; small bubble; red bubble (with colored bubbles)*
	• Request recurrence: *more bubbles*

Puzzles	• Child identifies puzzle pieces when you request them from child: *Give me the _____.* • Encourage child-initiated requests • Teach vocabulary on the puzzle pieces (e.g., farm animals, shapes, etc.) • Turn-taking

Puppets	• Feeding puppet
	  ○ Teach food vocabulary
	  ○ Identify/request foods: *Feed him the banana; What do you want to feed him?*
	  ○ Use puppet to model language: *I want more grapes! Yum, yum, yum! I like grapes!*

Balls (various sizes, textures, weights, etc.)	• Expanding utterances:
	  ○ Actions: *roll ball; bounce ball; throw ball*
	  ○ Prepositions: *ball in; ball out; ball on; ball off*
	  ○ Adjectives: *small ball; red ball; bumpy ball*

Table 12–4. Approaches to Early Literacy Intervention

Type of Approach	Description of Approach	Examples
Joint Book Reading	Shared reading between adult and child in which adult and child jointly explore content, language, and illustrations. Adult produces models by commenting on what is being read or pictured and asks questions about the book.	• Asking questions that can be answered by either looking at pictures or using information read in book (e.g., "Who is hiding under the table?" [pointing to picture of a bear under the table]) • Asking questions that require child to go beyond what is shown in pictures or given in text (e.g., "What will happen next?")
Environmental Print Awareness	Understanding the meaning of common symbols/knowledge that print communicates meaning.	• Community signs (STOP, EXIT, etc.) • Logos (restaurants, brands, etc.)
Conventions of Print	Teaching children about book handling and other common features of print and reading.	• Front-to-back direction of book reading • Left-to-right reading orientation • Meaning of punctuation (exclamations, etc.)
Phonemic Awareness/ Phonological Processing Skills	Drawing attention to sounds and encouraging sound play and sound recognition during reading.	• Alliteration in books • Nursery rhymes and other books with rhyming
Alphabetic Principle/Letter Knowledge	Recognition of letters and their corresponding sounds.	• Labeling letters • Drawing attention to words

Source: Adapted from ASHA, 2001.

Print Referencing

Print knowledge is an area of preliteracy development that involves a child's exposure to and basic understanding of written language (Storch & Whitehurst, 2002). It has received attention as a form of early literacy intervention that is associated with later success in word recognition and spelling (National Early Literacy Panel, 2004). Print referencing is an evidence-based approach for increasing print knowledge during the emergent literacy period (typically 3–5 years old) (Justice & Ezell, 2000, 2002; Justice, Kaderavek, Xitao, Sofka, & Hunt, 2009; Lovelace & Stewart, 2007). Print knowledge includes understanding the organization and functions of print in text (i.e., book title, author's name, speech bubbles, etc.), alphabet knowledge (i.e., names and features of letters), and emergent writing (i.e., expressing meaning through writing). The theory behind print referencing is that fostering a child's learning about print and literacy increases that child's awareness of, and interest in, print during shared reading activities.

Print referencing involves adult-generated cues that guide a child to notice salient features and functions of written language during shared storybook reading (Justice & Ezell, 2004). The nature of the adult-generated cues while referencing print may be either verbal or nonverbal. Verbal cues include commenting about print, asking questions about print, and making requests of the child regarding print. Nonverbal cues include drawing attention to print by pointing to text and tracking text with a finger. Table 12–5 contains examples of how to use print referencing cues in the context of shared storybook reading.

Selecting Appropriate Books for Shared Reading

Books with *print salience* lend themselves to a print referencing approach (Zucker, Ward, & Justice, 2009). Print salience refers to books that contain exciting print features, which may be used to draw a child's attention to print in books. Examples of print-salient features include: (a) bright colors, (b) interesting font changes, (c) visible speech (e.g., speech bubbles that connect illustrations and characters to text), (d) visible sounds (e.g., "meow" near a picture of a cat), and (e) environmental labels on illustrations (e.g., the word *candy* on a box). These qualities invite readers to explore, discuss, and interact with print in a meaningful way, thereby making the act of reading a rich and exciting experience rather than a passive and possibly tedious routine.

Print referencing and the use of books with print-salient material should be implemented strategically to encourage a child's understanding of the forms

Table 12–5. Print Referencing Cues

Type of Cue	Examples
Questions about print	• "Do you know what this letter is called?" • "There are words in the bear's speech bubble! What do you think he is saying?" • "Which word says *bear*?" • "What do you think this says?"
Requests of child	• "Show me where I start reading on this page." • "Look at the letters in this word. Show me one that is in your name." • "Help me read this word." • "Find the letter *C*."
Comments about print	• "This is the title of the book. It tells us what this book is called." • "This word in the title says *bear*." (points to word) • "That says *Eric Carle* (points to author's name). He's the author of this book." • "Uppercase *C* is the same shape as lower case *c*."
Nonverbal cues	• Point to words/letters • Point to the first word on page (to show where you begin reading) • Track print left to right

Source: Adapted from Zucker, Ward, & Justice, 2009.

and functions of print while introducing new vocabulary and concepts. Be mindful, though, to create a positive and fun atmosphere that encourages the child's exploration of books and fosters enjoyment in reading.

REFERENCES

American Speech-Language-Hearing Association (ASHA). (2001). *Roles and responsibilities of speech-language pathologists with respect to reading and writing in children and adolescents.* Retrieved from http://www.asha.org/policy

American Speech-Language-Hearing Association (ASHA). (2008). *Roles and responsibilities of speech-language pathologists in early intervention: Guidelines.* Retrieved from http://www.asha.org/policy

Casby, M. W. (2003). The development of play in infants, toddlers, and young children. *Communication Disorders Quarterly, 24*(4), 163–174.

Cazden, C. B. (1988). *Classroom discourse: The language of teaching and learning.* Portsmouth, NH: Heinemann.

Justice, L. M., & Ezell, H. K. (2000). Enhancing children's print and word awareness through home-based parent intervention. *American Journal of Speech-Language Pathology, 9*(3), 257–269.

Justice, L. M., & Ezell, H. K. (2002). Use of storybook reading to increase print awareness in at-risk children. *American Journal of Speech-Language Pathology, 11*(1), 17–29.

Justice, L. M., & Ezell, H. K. (2004). Print referencing: An emergent literacy enhancement strategy and its clinical applications. *Language, Speech, and Hearing Services in Schools, 35*, 185–193.

Justice, L. M., Kaderavek, J. N., Xitao, F., Sofka, A., & Hunt, A. (2009). Accelerating preschoolers' early literacy development through classroom-based teacher-child storybook reading and explicit print referencing. *Language, Speech, and Hearing Services in Schools, 40*(1), 67–85.

Lahey, M., & Bloom, L. (1977). Planning a first lexicon: Which words to teach first. *Journal of Speech & Hearing Disorders, 42*(3), 340–350.

Lovelace, S., & Stewart, S. R. (2007). Increasing print awareness in preschoolers with language impairment using non-evocative print referencing. *Language, Speech, and Hearing Services in Schools, 38*(1), 16–30.

National Early Literacy Panel. (2004, November). *The National Early Literacy Panel: A research synthesis on early literacy development.* Paper presented at the National Association of Early Childhood Specialists, Anaheim, CA.

Norris, J. A., & Hoffman, P. R. (1990). Language intervention within naturalistic environments. *Language, Speech, and Hearing Services in Schools, 21*, 72–84.

Roth, F., & Paul, R. (2007). Communication intervention. In R. Paul & P. Cascella (Eds.), *Introduction to clinical methods in communication disorders* (pp. 157–178). Baltimore, MD: Paul H. Brookes.

Schwartz, S. (2004). *The new language of toys: Teaching communication skills to children with special needs* (3rd ed.). Bethesda, MD: Woodbine House.

Storch, S. A., & Whitehurst, G. J. (2002). Oral language and code-related precursors to reading: Evidence from a longitudinal structural model. *Developmental Psychology, 38*, 934–947.

United States Consumer Product Safety Commission. (2013, June 15). *Safety education.* Retrieved from http://www.cpsc.gov/

Wadsworth, B. J. (2004). *Piaget's theory of cognitive and affective development* (5th ed.). Boston, MA: Pearson Education.

Wetherby, A. M., & Prutting, C. A. (1984). Profiles of communicative and cognitive social abilities in autistic children. *Journal of Speech and Hearing Research, 27*, 364–377.

Westby, C. (1980). Assessment of cognitive and language abilities through play. *Language, Speech, and Hearing Services in Schools, 11*, 154–168.

Zucker, T. A., Ward, A. E., & Justice, L. M. (2009). Print referencing during read-alouds: A technique for increasing emergent readers' print knowledge. *Reading Teacher, 63*(1), 62–72.

APPENDIX 12–A

Summary of Play Stages (Based on Westby, 1980)

Stage	Typical Age of Acquisition	Description	Examples
I	9–12 months	■ Development of object permanence ■ Means-ends behaviors ■ Uses some toys appropriately/ceases to mouth/bang all toys ■ Vocalizations begin to function as requests or commands	■ Child finds toy covered by scarf ■ Moves to desired object/pulls string to attain toy at end of string ■ Rolls car on table (rather than putting it in his or her mouth)
II	13–17 months	■ Explores toys ■ Understands that adults are entities who can act upon objects ■ Single words emerge but are context dependent ■ Communication becomes increasingly intentional (gestures/vocalizes to request, command, gain attention, initiate interactions with others, protest, and label)	■ Identifies part of toy responsible for operation and attempts to physically activate it (push, pull, turn, pound, or shake) ■ Seeks help from adult when child is unable to operate it independently
III	17–19 months	■ Representational abilities begin to emerge (pretend play) ■ Autosymbolic play emerges ■ Begins to exhibit tool use ■ True verbal language emerges ■ Marked growth in vocabulary/a variety of words used for various functions/semantic roles	■ Child pretends to sleep, eat, etc. ■ Finds toy hidden out of view ■ Obtains toy with use of a stick
IV	19–22 months	■ Symbolic play extends beyond himself or herself ■ Word combinations used to express semantic relations (possessive relation is most common) ■ Child has combined sensorimotor concepts and has acquired internalized action schemas and is now able to refer to objects/individuals who are not physically present in play scenario	■ Child pretends doll is sleeping or pretends to feed communication/play partner ■ Child says, "my baby," "my car," etc.

continues

Appendix 12–A. *continued*

Stage	Typical Age of Acquisition	Description	Examples
V	24 months	■ Child engages in pretend play scenarios about other individuals ■ Simple sequences emerge (not able to perform more complex realistic sequences) ■ Emergence of present progressive *-ing*, plural and possessive *-s* ■ Begins to use short sentences to describe what is presently occurring ■ Communicative acts begin to include simple interrogatives, often lacking proper syntactic form	■ Child plays house and pretends to be mommy ■ Child puts food in bowl, then uses a spoon to feed doll/stacks blocks, then knocks them down ■ With rising intonation, child says, "The doggy sleepy" in order to ask "Is the doggy sleepy?"
VI	2½ years	■ Child begins to depict less common events ■ Child's role in play changes quickly ■ Associative play begins to emerge (though parallel play remains most common) ■ Uses language to analyze experiences ■ Begins to provide syntactically and semantically appropriate answers to "who, whose, what, where, and what . . . do" questions ■ Begins to ask "why" questions, especially in response to negative statements, but may not understand adult's answer to "why" question	■ Child engages in pretend play involving doctor/sick child, or teacher/student ■ Child switches from being teacher to child often with little indication/warning ■ Child asks, "Where the doggy is?" ■ Child participates in the same activity as another individual but plays independently (without working together cooperatively)
VII	3 years	■ Begins to link several play schemas in a sequence ■ With the use of sequences, the child begins to talk about past and future events using past and future verb tenses ■ Play becomes increasingly associative	■ Child pretends to make a pizza, bake it, cut it, serve it, and wash the dishes ■ Child says, "He ate pizza." and "He will eat pizza."

Stage	Typical Age of Acquisition	Description	Examples
VIII	3–3½ years	<ul><li>Plays with less realistic toys, which involves abstraction in order to identify similarities and differences between real and pretend objects</li><li>Descriptive vocabulary increases</li><li>Begins to take another's perspective and develops the metalinguistic ability to think about and talk about language</li><li>Dolls are given personalities and begin to participate in play scenarios</li></ul>	<ul><li>Child plays with doll house, barn</li><li>Child uses blocks to construct enclosures (house, fence, etc.)</li><li>Child pretends a row of chairs is a bus</li><li>Child provides dialogue during play</li></ul>
IX	4 years	<ul><li>Child begins to consider future events and solve problems for novel events</li><li>Child begins to use modal verbs*: *can, may, might, could, would, will* (*these will not be mastered until 10–12 years)</li><li>Child begins to use conjunctions, including *and, but, if, so, because*</li></ul>	<ul><li>Child begins to consider and verbalize, "What would happen if . . . ?" or "If I do this, then . . . "</li><li>Child builds increasingly elaborate structures with blocks and other 3D objects</li><li>Uses dolls to test out hypotheses ("What would happen if . . . ")</li></ul>
X	5 years	<ul><li>Child begins to plan out sequences and play scenarios in advance</li><li>Identifies what will be required to carry out planned play scenarios</li><li>Play becomes more imaginative and the child is able to manage more than one event at a time</li><li>Child begins to use relative and subordinate clauses in order to link two or more prepositions</li><li>Child begins to use relational terms,* including *then, when, first, while, next, before, after* (*these will not be mastered until 12 years)</li></ul>	<ul><li>Child states that she will be the mother and while she is feeding the baby, her other children clean their room and daddy works in the yard</li><li>Child produces phrases such as, "I'm the princess who lives in the castle."</li></ul>

CHAPTER 13

Speech Sound Remediation

Lei Sun

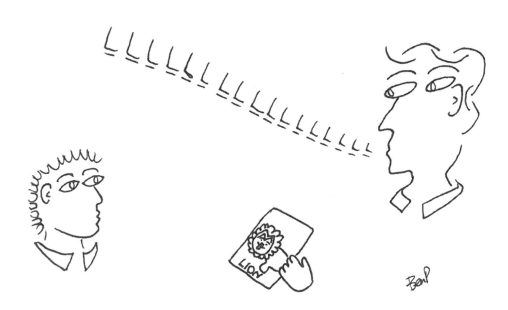

Words mean more than what is set down on paper. It takes the human voice to infuse them with deeper meaning.

Maya Angelou (American author, poet, and recipient of the National Medal of the Arts and the President's Medal of Freedom)

The caseload of speech-language pathologists (SLPs) commonly includes individuals with speech sound disorders (SSD), especially for SLPs working in school settings, with preschoolers and young school-age children (ages 3–9 years). According to the American Speech-Language-Hearing Association's (ASHA's) 2012 schools survey, students with articulation and phonological disorders were the most commonly reported individuals on the caseload of school-based SLPs (ASHA, 2012). As such, speech-language pathology assistants (SLPAs) working in school settings must be knowledgeable about this topic. This chapter provides an overview of SSD, including speech sound development and classification, as well as general and specific guidelines in the treatment of SSD. This chapter is not meant to be a substitute for more in-depth reading and resources in this area; rather, it can serve as a complement to your introductory coursework on the topic.

Before we discuss sound remediation, it is important to review some key concepts in this area. A *phoneme* is a family of very similar sounds. For example, we produce the /t/ in *tea, tool,* and *take* slightly different, but we all perceive the first sound as /t/. A phoneme is the smallest linguistic unit of sound that can signal a difference in meaning. As an example, if we change the first sound of *tea* to /k/, then it will be a different word, *key,* which has a totally different meaning from *tea.* The concept of signaling a difference in meaning, through a change of sound, is very important for speech intervention. Usually, we use *virgules* such as /t/ for the ideal transcription of the sound (e.g., the way the sound should be produced) and *brackets* [t] for the actual sound produced by an individual. The International Phonetic Alphabet (IPA) is commonly used to represent the sounds of oral language. Appendix 4–B in Chapter 4 contains a list of core IPA symbols.

Speech intelligibility relates to how much a listener can understand a child's speech. It can be treated directly or indirectly, depending on the goals/objectives set by an SLP. Children in speech and language therapy have different priorities. In some instances, speech sounds are not necessarily targeted if the child has limited verbal output or if language intervention is the priority. Speech intelligibility is often addressed in younger children because of the significant negative impact it can have on social interaction and future academic performance (e.g., literacy). Usually, a child can be easily understood by age 5 years, except for some later developing sounds, such as /s,

z, ʃ, θ, ð/ (misarticulations of these sounds are appropriate for a 5-year-old) (Peña-Brooks & Hegde, 2007). Children who are diagnosed with intellectual disabilities, early speech/language delay, autism, and other speech/language-related impairments may require a longer time to develop speech sounds (Bernthal, Bankson, & Flipsen, 2013). In some instances, inconsistent speech sound production and persistent use of age-inappropriate phonological processes (e.g., error patterns such as liquid gliding—use /w/ to replace /r/, final consonant deletion—deleting sounds in the final position) may be observed beyond age 9 years. For children with speech and/or language disorders, speech can be targeted directly or indirectly, depending on the overall speech intelligibility and how much speech errors negatively affect the child's daily life, social interaction, and academic performance.

To consider individual differences in acquiring speech sounds, it is important to become familiar with speech acquisition norms and realize that there is no cutoff age for the development of a single sound. For example, /s/ starts to emerge around age 3 years and may not be mastered until the age 8 years. It usually takes longer to develop later developing sounds compared with early developing sounds, such as /h, m, w, p/. As a foundation for a discussion of speech sound remediation, the following section provides an overview about speech sound classification, speech sound acquisition, and common phonological processes.

SPEECH SOUND CLASSIFICATION

Classifications of sounds, using their place (where along the vocal tract the consonant is formed), voicing (whether the vocal folds are vibrating during the production), and manner (how the sound is formed) (Peña-Brooks & Hegde, 2007, p. 71), is an important foundation in understanding how to elicit target sounds. Figure 13–1 contains a place-voice-manner (PVM) chart, denoting place of articulation, whether the consonant shown is voiced or voiceless, and manner of articulation. This chart is provided by Bowen (2011) and is available on Dr. Bowen's website (http://speech-language-therapy.com/images/pvmchart.png).

Being familiar with this classification is helpful in understanding the similarity and differences across sounds. For example, if the child's target sound is /s/ and the child is able to produce /t/ consistently, clinicians can take advantage of place similarity to use /t/ to elicit /s/. Similarly, clinicians can use voice on and off to train the voiced sounds by helping the child to feel the vibration of the voice box by, for example, placing the child's hand on her or his neck when producing voiced sounds. A vowel chart is also provided for review, as vowels can be used to elicit some consonant production (Figure 13–2).

SPEECH SOUND DEVELOPMENT

Consonants

Several speech sound developmental norms/sequences are frequently used by SLPs to determine the eligibility for treatment of SSD, such as Sander (1972), Templin (1957), and Smit, Hand, Freilinger, and Bird (1990) (Gordon-Brannan & Weiss, 2007, p. 63). Due to different methodologies and criteria used when researchers develop speech norms, different sequences of speech sound acquisition have been reported. Despite these minor differences, the order of acquisition of

			PLACE						
MANNER		VOICING	Bilabial	Labiodental	Interdental	Alveolar	Palatal	Velar	Glottal
OBSTRUENTS	Stop	Voiceless	p			t		k	ʔ
		Voiced	b			d		g	
	Fricative	Voiceless		f		s	ʃ		h
		Voiced		v	ð	z	ʒ		
	Affricate	Voiceless					tʃ		
		Voiced					dʒ		
SONORANTS	Nasal	Voiced	m			n			
	LIQUID Lateral	Voiced				l			
	LIQUID Rhotic	Voiced						r	
	Glide	Voiced	w				j	w	

Figure 13–1. Place-Voice-Manner (PVM) Chart (Bowen, 2011). Used with permission.

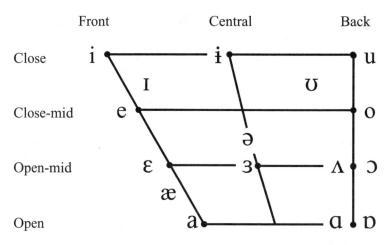

Figure 13–2. English vowels, classified based on position of the tongue. Image courtesy of Wikimedia Commons.

sounds and sound classes is very similar. For example, in general, stops, nasals, and glides develop early, and liquids, fricatives, and affricates develop later. Clinicians must keep in mind, though, that the position of the sound (e.g., whether the sound appears in the initial, medial, or final position of a word) will further affect how long it may take the child to acquire the sound. As an example, /t/ in initial position (*tea, toy, tale*) may be mastered around age 3 years, but /t/ in final position (*cat, feet*) may not be mastered until around age 4 years. Generally speaking, if the sound emerges in one position, sound production in other positions should be expected soon. Medial sounds usually (but not always) take slightly longer to acquire compared with sounds in initial and final positions.

A helpful classification of sound development was that developed by Shriberg (1993), which divides the 24 English speech sounds into three categories: early eight, middle eight, and late eight. Lof (2004) used this classification to compare common speech acquisition norms and found that children master the early eight sounds around age 3 years, the middle eight sounds between ages 3 and 7 years (with /t, k, g, ŋ, f/ often acquired by age 4 and / v, tʃ, dʒ / developing between ages 5 and 7), and the late eight sounds usually between 6 and 8 years of age (Table 13–1).

Consonant Clusters/Blends

Consonant clusters or blends (e.g., combination of consonants) usually develop after the child's oral motor control and coordination is more mature. Box 13–1 contains a list of common consonant clusters.

Consonant clusters can be in the initial position and final position (-pt, -ks,

Table 13–1. Shriberg's Three Categories of Speech Sound Developmental Sequence

Early eight	/m, b, j, n, w, d, p, h/
Middle eight	/t, k, g, ŋ, f, v, tʃ, dʒ/
Late eight	/ s, z, l, r, ʃ, ʒ, θ, ð/

Source: Shriberg, 1993, as cited in Lof, 2004.

Box 13–1.
Common Consonant Clusters

- L blends: pl-, kl-, fl-
- S blends: sp-, sm-, sn-, st-, sk-
- R blends: gr-, br-, dr-, kr-

-ft, -sk, etc.) and can be the combination of two consonants and three consonants (spr-, spl-, thr-, -kst). Like consonant acquisition, consonant clusters follow a general acquisition sequence, which varies based on the position of the cluster. Usually, consonant clusters begin to develop around age 4 years, when the child has developed a good amount of consonants and is ready to combine them. Therefore, it is unrealistic to work on consonant clusters when the child has only a limited number of consonants in her or his phonetic inventory (e.g., sounds that the child is able to produce consistently), has not yet developed the sounds included in the clusters, or when the child is too young. It is always good to practice single consonants (e.g., /s/) until the sound production is stabilized and then introduce associated consonant clusters (e.g., sm-, sn-, sp-, st-, etc.).

Keep in mind that consonant clusters take longer to develop, and some may be mastered after age 8 years for some children (e.g., thr-, skw-, str-, spr-, etc.) (Peña-Brooks & Hegde, 2007). In addition, clinicians generally consider consonant acquisition when working on clusters. As an example, it is appropriate for a 5-year-old to say *fwog* instead of *frog*, as /r/ is still developing. In general, it is more important to help the child be aware of a cluster that has two or three sounds in it, rather than the perfect production of each individual phoneme in the cluster.

For example, it is more critical t[...] /f/ and /r/ in *frog* even though it[...] like *fwog* than only producing one s[...] in the cluster as in *fog,* because *fog* is a d[...] ferent word and carries a very different meaning from *frog*. In contrast, *fwog* still carries the meaning of *frog* even though it does not sound the way it should be produced.

Vowels

Most children have no difficulty acquiring vowels. Vowels usually develop early, except /ɚ, ɝ/, which are usually mastered before age 5 years because tongue retraction is required to produce these two r-colored vowels. If a child has trouble producing vowels, minimal contrasts/pairs (which will be reviewed under the phonemic/linguistically-based/phonology treatment approach) are often used in treatment to target perception and production training.

COMMON PHONOLOGICAL PROCESSES

While children learn to talk like adults, they simplify adults' speech by using predictable "error" patterns called *phonological processes*. The use of phonological processes is related to speech sound acquisition. For example, a child uses /t/ to replace /k/ (velar fronting) when the child is still in the process of developing the /k/ sound. Some phonological processes may be eliminated early, such as initial/final consonant deletion and velar fronting, but some phonological processes may take longer to be suppressed, such as liquid gliding and stopping of voiced/

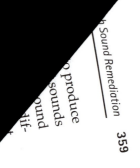

ch, sometimes ific patterns/ stead of par- will improve ing final con- it is impor- ...ept of some com- ...nological processes (Table 13–2).

GENERAL TREATMENT PRINCIPLES

In general, treatment may be viewed as "a continuum of activities comprising three stages: establishment, facilitation of generalization and maintenance" (Bernthal et al., 2013, p. 270). Figure 13–3 represents this continuum. Treatment starts with eliciting the target sound, gradually moves to stabilizing the speech sound production in all positions and increasing linguistic levels (from words to conversation), and then maintaining consistent speech sound production in different settings, contexts, and with different communication partners through self-monitoring.

The first step in the treatment process is to establish appropriate treatment goals and objectives. This is the job of your supervising SLP (ASHA, 2013). As an SLPA, it is critical that you are able to accurately identify target sounds, production level (syllable, word, phrase/sentence, spontaneous speech), accuracy level (e.g., 70% accuracy, 7 of 10 trials), prompt level (e.g., minimal, maximal prompting), and setting (usually in speech therapy) from each treatment objective. Chapter 7 offers general suggestions in this area. Remember that a goal may be written in various ways, but it should always contain these elements. An example of a common speech sound remediation goal is, "L.B. will produce /s/ and /s/ blends at word level with 80% accuracy with minimal

Table 13–2. Common Phonological Processes

Phonological Process	Description	Examples
Final consonant deletion	A final consonant is omitted/deleted from a word	ca for cat, cu for cup
Initial consonant deletion	An initial consonant is omitted/deleted from a word	at for fat, ake for lake
Syllable deletion	A syllable (especially weak/unstressed syllable) is omitted/deleted from a word	puter for computer, nana for banana
Cluster reduction	One phoneme of the cluster is deleted from the cluster	fag for flag, fog for frog
Stopping of fricatives	Uses stops to replace fricatives and affricates	top for sop, poo for zoo
Velar fronting	Uses alveolar stops (/t, d/) to replace velar sounds (/k, g, ŋ/)	tea for key, do for go
Liquid gliding	Uses a glide (/w, j/) to replace a liquid (/l, r/)	wake for lake, yeg for leg
Devoicing	Uses a voiceless consonant to replace a voiced consonant	nos for nose, pik for pig
Assimilation	One sound changes to another sound more like its neighboring sound. It could be due to place or manner.	lellow for yellow, take for cake

Source: Peña-Brooks & Hegde, 2007.

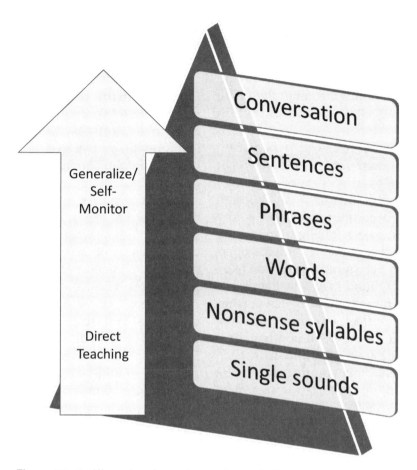

Figure 13–3. Hierarchy of speech sound remediation.

promoting in three consecutive speech therapy sessions." Using this goal as an example, can you identify the elements listed above?

Intervention targeting remediating SSD is generally divided into two major treatment approaches: phonetic/motor-based/articulation treatment approaches and phonemic/linguistically-based/phonologic treatment approaches. Although different treatment approaches stem from distinctive theories and clinical observation, it is impossible to separate the function (linguistic/phonemic) from the form (motor-based/phonetic), as they are two sides of the same coin. As you implement treatment, it is important to keep this in mind. Phonology is one aspect of language, and intervention to remediate SSDs should always be considered in the larger scope of language and its purpose. The ultimate goal is to improve a child's overall speech intelligibility, in order to convey meaning efficiently and effectively, and to assist the child function better in her or his daily life. The World Health Organization's *International Classification of Functioning, Disability and Health* (World Health Organization, 2001) highlights this relationship and should be the cornerstone of speech sound remediation (Figure 13–4). Effective and functional intervention targets both form (body structures and functions) and function (use of speech sounds meaningfully, along with language rules, to function well in daily activities).

A traditional view of remediating speech errors used discrete skills (e.g., not viewing phonology as part of language) and a "drill-and-kill" method. Although maximizing accurate production is key to improving speech intelligibility, it may be that with this method, students overgeneralize speech sound production (e.g., use the target sound in words that do not contain the target sound). This further compromises effective communication. Students may also respond poorly to drill activities. The gold standard in speech sound remediation should always be effective, efficient, and *functional* treatment activities. Box 13–2 depicts an example of this approach within a treatment session.

PRIMARY TREATMENT APPROACHES

Although we divide treatment approaches into two main categories, phonetic/motor-based/articulation and phonemic/linguistically-based/phonologic, it is impossible to work on form and function separately. The difference across different treatment approaches is how each approach organizes and sequences treatment targets, according to the child's severity of SSD, rather than using specific techniques to elicit speech sounds. For example, clinicians use phonetic treatment approaches, such as using a variety of cues (e.g., visual, tactile, verbal) or external tools (e.g., tongue depressor), to elicit a target sound. Once the sound is stimulable, phonemic treatment approaches should be used to facilitate target discrimination and sound production. Therefore, a combination of the phonetic and phonemic approaches is recommend-

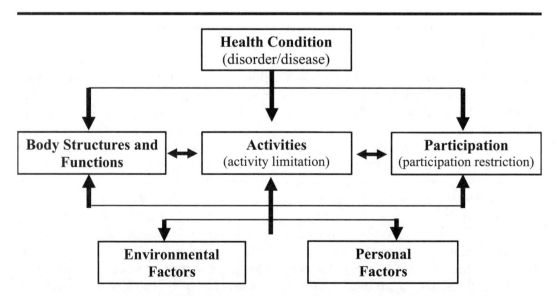

Figure 13–4. Model of the *International Classification of Functioning, Disability, and Health.* Copyright World Health Organization (WHO). Used with permission.

Box 13–2. Sample Speech Sound Remediation Session

1. Start the treatment session by having the child practice target sounds at the appropriate linguistic level (e.g., word/phrase/sentence, etc.) for a short amount of time.
2. Have the child use target words in naturalistic activities. For younger children, play-based activities are an excellent option. Language-based activities, such as shared book reading, are especially good for children with language impairments (LI) and SSD. Literacy-based treatment activities, incorporating phonological awareness activities for preschoolers and conventional reading and writing for older children, are also highly valuable. Chapter 12 offers additional suggestions in these areas.
3. End the session with reviewing target sounds and speech homework.

ed, depending on the child's needs and strengths. Table 13–3 briefly summarizes the general differences between the phonetic and phonemic treatment approaches.

Phonetic/Motor–Based/Articulation Treatment Approach

A traditional approach to phonetic training has been commonly used since the 1970s (Van Riper & Erickson, 1996). Using this approach, the child gradually moves along the continuum of treatment from perceptual/ear training, sound establishment, sound stabilization, transfer/carryover, and then maintenance. Some elements of the traditional approach can be separately incorporated into treatment as needed.

Perceptual Training/Ear Training

Perceptual training is used at the beginning of a traditional approach if the child has difficulty discriminating between

Table 13–3. Core Differences: Phonetic Versus Phonemic Approaches

Phonetic Approach	Phonemic Approach
Focus on teaching correct production of an individual sound	Focus on learning correct production through contrasting sounds
Use of nonsense/made up syllables/words is allowed	Only use meaningful real words
Appropriate for limited speech errors	Appropriate for identified erred patterns
Good for nonstimulable sounds	Good for stimulable sounds
Start with phonemes or nonsense syllables	Start with words

Sources: Bernthal, Bankson, & Flipsen, 2013; Peña-Brooks & Hegde, 2007.

the desired sound (e.g., the target speech sound) and the undesired sound (e.g., the sound that the child produces instead). If the child does not have auditory discrimination problems, treatment moves forward to the sound establishment phase. As perceptual training requires a certain level of metalinguistic skills, the child's age is usually taken into consideration and different perceptual training activities recommended, based on the child's age and how the child responds to the training activity. It is important to keep in mind that working on perceptual training does not automatically lead to correct sound production and improved speech intelligibility. However, perceptual training may be used to increase awareness of the target phoneme and may be added before production training or incorporated into production training. The use of perceptual training may or may not be evident in a child's treatment objectives. An example of an objective including perceptual training may be, "XX will independently distinguish ___ sound (desired sound) from ___ sound (undesired sound) when presented with picture cards, with 80% accuracy in two consecutive sessions." Table 13–4 summarizes different methods for ear training.

Sound Establishment/Sound Elicitation

Sound elicitation often starts with a phoneme (e.g., fricatives), syllable (i.e., target

Table 13–4. Perceptual Ear Training Methods

Traditional Approach	Identification	Clinician directs the child's attention to how the speech sound feels in the mouth. Clinician uses objects to describe the characteristics of the speech sound (e.g., /t/ is a ticking sound, /f/ is an angry cat sound). A common task may be for the child to ring a bell or raise his or her hand when hearing a target sound.
	Isolation	Child is asked to identify the target sound in increasing linguistic levels (syllables, words, phrases, sentences).
	Stimulation	Similar to auditory bombardment, child is provided with maximal auditory stimuli of the target sound, through varying loudness, stress (e.g., add stress to syllable containing the target sound), and duration of the sound (prolong the target sound).
	Discrimination	Child is asked to make judgments of correct and incorrect productions made by the clinician.
Auditory Bombardment		Tasks blend the target sound into all activities and emphasize the target sound through shared book reading, language/literacy games, play, conversation, and so forth. For example, if the target sound is /s/, the clinician may read a book about superheros (Superman, Spiderman, Sandman, etc.), highlighting /s/ while reading the book. Similarly, the clinician may emphasize /s/ in conversation (it'S Super Silly, iSn't it? That'S hiS not yourS).
Minimal Pair		Clinician uses pairs of words containing undesirable sound (e.g., use [t] to replace /s/, [t] is the undesirable sound) and desirable sound (/s/ is the desirable sound) along with written words and corresponding pictures. As an example, the child is asked to hand pictures named to the clinician (sea-tea, sue-two).

Source: Bernthal, Bankson, & Flipsen, 2013.

phoneme + schwa, especially stops—/pə/ and liquids /lə/), or word (i.e., meaningful and functional CVC words). Your supervising SLP will determine which level facilitates production more easily for each child and the child's ultimate goal in communication. A common treatment objective at this level of training may be, "XX will produce ___ sound in ___ position (initial or final) at word (or syllable-CV, VC) level with minimal prompting with 70% accuracy in two consecutive sessions." Table 13–5 summarizes several techniques used to elicit target sounds. Keep in mind, though, that more than one technique may be needed. The combination of techniques depends on the child's

needs and how the child responds to each technique. All the techniques listed are used to elicit speech sounds in isolation. Conversational speech is dynamic and variable, considering the influence from neighboring sounds (e.g., the consonant or vowel that comes before and after the sound) and suprasegmental features (e.g., stress, intonation, etc.), rather than the combination of isolated speech sounds. Therefore, additional attention is generally given to transferring learned, isolated speech sounds to more connected running speech, and then to generalization to different settings and with varied communication partners. As an additional reference, readers are referred to *Articulatory*

Table 13–5. Common Techniques for Eliciting Speech Sounds

Sound-Evoking Techniques	Procedures
Imitation	Ask the child to watch, listen, and repeat the target sound. A mirror can be used (e.g., watch me, listen, and make the sound just like I do-/s/).
Phonetic Placement	Clinician describes where to place the articulators in order to produce the target sound, along with visual and tactile cues. A mouth puppet and mirror can be used with younger children. Oral structure graphs can be used with older children (first grade and up). External tools such as a tongue depressor should be used as the last resort.
Contextual Cues/ Co-articulation	Clinician identifies key words (words in which the child can produce the target sound correctly) and word contexts (the neighboring sounds that can facilitate the correct production of the target sound, without additional training). Clinician uses this advantage to help the child feel and hear the target sound and attempt to transfer the correct target production to other words. Usually the information can be gathered from contextual testing done by the SLP. For example, /s/ may be produced easily in clusters/blends (st, sp, sn, etc) rather than singletons (sun, sit, etc) (Williams, 1991). /s/ may be produced easily after /t/ due to similar placement (bright-sun, hot-soup, etc.). Velar sounds may be easily produced after high-back vowels (/u, ʊ/).
Sound Modification/ Shaping	Clinician uses the sound that is already in the child's phonetic inventory (the child can produce the sound correctly and independently) and shapes it to the target sound.
	For example, if the child can produce /l/, /l/ is shaped into /r/ by asking the child to slide the tongue tip slowly back along the roof of the mouth.
Tactile-Kinesthetic	Clinician manipulates the child's articulators externally on the face and neck to guide the speech sound production.

Sources: Bernthal, Bankson, & Flipsen, 2013; Bauman-Waengler, 2012; Gordon-Brannan & Weiss, 2007).

366 *Speech-Language Pathology Assistants: A Resource Manual*

and *Phonological Impairments: A Clinical Focus* by Jacqueline Bauman-Waengler (2012) and *Eliciting Sounds: Techniques and Strategies for Clinicians* by Secord, Boyce, Donohue, Fox, and Shine (2007).

Sound Stabilization

Once the target sound is successfully elicited, phonetic treatment then focuses on stabilizing sound production in all positions of words and at varied levels of complexity. Generally, objectives start with the lowest level (i.e., when the child requires great assistance from the clinician) and then progresses to higher levels (i.e., when the clinician starts to fade prompting, in order to achieve correct *independent* speech sound production). For example, if the child successfully produces /s/ in final position (*kiss, face*), treatment then moves forward to initial (*sun, see*) and then medial position (*seesaw, castle*) which automatically incorporates two-syllable words. Once the child finishes the sound production in one position or one level (syllable, word), a review is incorporated to ensure sound stabilization while moving forward to the next level. An example of a common treatment objective at this level would be, "XX will produce ___ sound in ___ position (initial, medial or final) at word level with minimal prompting with 70% accuracy in two consecutive sessions" or "XX will produce ___ sound in all positions at sentence level with minimal prompting with 70% accuracy in two consecutive sessions." Table 13–6 provides treatment suggestions in this area.

Speech Homework

To improve speech intelligibility, clients must practice correct speech sound production. Because 30 minutes or an hour a week of treatment does not provide sufficient practice, speech homework is necessary. Creating a speech file for the child and sending home a list of practice words after each session is recommended. As an SLPA, you may be asked to assist your supervising SLP in creating these materials (ASHA, 2013). The practice words should be the words that have been practiced in treatment sessions and for which correct sound production has been established. Usually 10 to 15 minutes a day is sufficient to maintain and stabilize correct sound production. A note for the parent or caregiver regarding how to use the speech homework and a signature and/or initial line for the parent or caregiver to confirm the completion of the speech homework is recommended. Appendix 13–A contains a sample speech homework sheet.

Phonemic/Linguistically–Based/ Phonologic Treatment Approach

The focus of phonemic/linguistically based/phonology treatment is used to replace erred patterns and to establish sound contrasts (Bernthal et al., 2013). These treatment approaches are more appropriate for children whose speech errors can be identified by patterns/phonological processes, such as final consonant deletion, velar fronting, liquid gliding, cluster reduction, and so forth. Because the child uses patterns, his or her speech intelligibility is usually much lower than the child who has articulation disorders with fewer speech errors. Children with phonological disorders usually have difficulty distinguishing the target sound from the error sound. For example, a child who uses liquid gliding may have difficulty distinguishing the difference between

Table 13–6. Sound Stabilization Sample Activities

Level	Treatment Suggestions
Word	*Target sound can first be elicited in final or initial position and then gradually moved to medial position. The purpose of treatment is to stabilize the sound production in all word positions.* *Potential Activities:* 1. Incorporate target words into board games or any type of game. For example, use target words to play Go Fish (e.g., the child must produce the word correctly to receive the correct card). 2. Use games as reinforcement to elicit maximal correct sound production. For example, the child must produce the word correctly for three times before moving the pawn. *Suggested games:* Go Fish, fishing game, memory game, bowling, safari, Hangman (good for children with a large vocabulary size), etc.
Phrase/sentence	*Incorporate phrases that contain the target sound. Carrier phrases start with the same phrase and only fill in different words that contain the target sound to complete the sentence.* *Potential Activities:* 1. Set a scene that facilitates the use of carrier phrases. e.g., I see a _____ (target sound /l/: lake, lamp, line, etc). 2. To increase the difficulty, two target words can be included in one phrase. e.g., I "like" the _____ (target sound /l/: lake, lamp, line, etc).
Sentence	*Start with simple and short sentences containing one target word and then gradually increase the complexity of the sentence and the number of target words.* *Potential Activities:* 1. Use ready-made materials and ask the child to read the sentences if the child is able to read. 2. If the child has higher language abilities, ask the child to make up a sentence using the practiced target word. For example, I like to go to beach and pick up "seashells" out of the "sand."
Conversation	*The purpose of conversation level is to help the child be more aware of his or her own speech errors and develop effective self-monitoring strategies. It requires a certain level of metalinguistic skills and may be more appropriate for older children and children with good language skills.* *Potential Activities:* 1. Use audio recording: record part of the session, play it back to the child, identify and discuss the speech errors. We must be cautious about the child's emotional and psychological changes when using this method. Do not make the child feel that he or she is the center of the attention (put the child on the spot). 2. Ask the child to fill out the speech rating chart to evaluate his or her own speech for each session using letter grade (A, B, C). A speech diary can be created to use at home to continue the self-monitoring process. 3. Discuss with the child to develop effective strategies tailored specifically for him or her. For example, use of the secret visual code shared between the classroom teacher, the child, and the clinician as a reminder when needed.

Source: Bernthal, Bankson, & Flipsen, 2013.

lake and *wake* that results in incorrect production. In contrast, a child with an articulation disorder may be able to differentiate the difference between /w/ and /r/ but struggles to produce /r/. Therefore, which treatment approach (phonetic or phonemic) is most effective and beneficial depends on the child's ability to contrast the sounds and the ability to produce the target sound with minimal assistance (i.e., the sound is stimulable). If a child understands the difference between the sounds, the sound-evoking techniques reviewed earlier to facilitate sound production are used. If the child struggles with differentiating the error sound and the target sound, training on perception of contrasts and then production of contrasts will be the focus. Your supervising SLP will determine the most appropriate approach for each client (ASHA, 2013).

Providing the treatment that meets the child's needs to improve the child's overall speech intelligibility is the ultimate goal. An indication of using phonologically based treatment activities may not always be evident in an objective. An objective using this approach may look like the examples presented in the sound stabilization section, such as "XX will produce ___ sound in ___ position (initial, medial, or final) at word level with minimal prompting with 80% accuracy in two consecutive sessions." The use of treatment approaches depends on the child's deficits and severity of SSD. An overview of three evidence-based phonologically based treatment approaches is reviewed in the sections that follow.

Minimal Oppositions/Minimal Pairs

Word pairs are used in a minimal opposition/minimal pair contrast approach.

A phoneme that is already in the child's inventory is used to contrast with the target sound/desired sound (Barlow & Gierut, 2002). For example, if the child uses /w/ to replace /r/, it shows that the child is able to produce /w/ (in the child's inventory) but may not understand the contrast between /w/ and /r/. Treatment then focuses on the use of /w/ in the child's inventory to contrast the target sound /r/. The goal of this treatment is to help the child understand that different sounds represent different words and meanings and correct sound production is important for successful communication. Therefore, a change of one sound will change the word and intended meaning, which may cause communication breakdowns. As an example, if the child asks for a picture of *tea* instead of *key* when she really wants *key*, receiving the wrong picture card of *tea* will be the consequence of incorrect sound production. The procedure of minimal pair training is presented in Figure 13–5.

Maximal Oppositions Contrast

Maximal oppositions contrast uses the same procedure as minimal oppositions contrast (above). The only difference is in the selection of word pairs (Gierut, 1989). The word pair *tea-key* is different only on one feature: that of place. If "k-m" pairs are used, greater phonological change in the phonology system can be made, because /k/ and /m/ differ on place, manner, and nasality of production. Therefore, in maximal opposition training, /m/ would be used, if it was already in the child's inventory, to contrast with /k/ (the target sound). The purpose of this approach is to promote better generalization to other sounds through maxi-

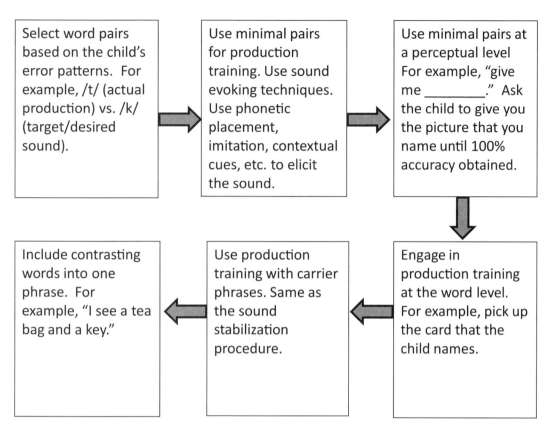

Figure 13–5. Minimal opposition/minimal pairs approach flowchart, based on Bernthal, Bankson, and Flipsen (2013).

mal contrast to promote greater overall change of the child's phonological system. The same flowchart for minimal oppositions contrast (see Figure 13–5) can be used for maximal oppositions contrast as well, with the only difference being the selection of a sound already in the child's repertoire that maximally contrasts with the target sound.

Multiple Oppositions Therapy

The multiple oppositions approach is based on minimal oppositions (as above). The aim of this approach is to reorganize the child's phonological system in a systematic way. Instead of targeting one contrast each time, this approach targets several contrasts simultaneously (Williams, 1993, 2003). This approach is good for children who have multiple sound errors and tend to use one sound to replace several sounds. For example, if the child uses /t/ to replace /s, f, k/, it is most efficient and effective to target all three substitutions at once. In this instance, three different pairs of contrasts are used, including t-s (*cheat-cheese*), t-f (*cheat-chief*), and t-k (*cheat-cheek*), with 10 words in each pair. The therapy procedure is similar to minimal oppositions (see Figure 13–5). First, the child would sort the words that the clinician names into different piles (three target sounds: /s, f, k/) for perception training. Once the child is able to successfully differentiate these sound contrasts, treatment would work on production training. Clinicians can also ask the child to sort the words that she or he names into different piles to work on perception and production simultaneously.

ADDITIONAL TREATMENT CONSIDERATIONS

Working With Children With Limited Language Ability

Tying speech therapy to daily life and functional communication is the goal when working with children who have limited language ability. Being able to communicate needs and wants is a priority. Therefore, targeting functional words/ phrases and high-frequency words is highly recommended. Treatment begins with CVC words that are highly functional and frequently used in daily life such as *hi, bye, no, help, want, go, me, mom, dad*, and so forth. How intelligible the word and phrase should be depends on the child's current function in speech and language and other related health issues. Sometimes, approximation (i.e., close production of the target word) is acceptable if the child is not able to produce clear speech sound but approximation of the sound/ word serves the communication purpose.

Working With School-Age Children With SSD

Children who start to develop phonics and phonological awareness may benefit from using phonological awareness activities to improve speech sound production. Phonological awareness is the individual's awareness of the sound structure of spoken words (Justice, Gillon, McNeill, & Schuele, 2013). Development of phonological awareness is important for learning to read. Working on phonological awareness may facilitate speech sound production. As phonological awareness brings the child's attention to the sound and syllable (e.g., alliteration of the sound at the beginning/at the end, syllable segmenting/blending, etc.), it is beneficial to incorporate these tasks into treatment to facilitate speech sound production and phonological awareness simultaneously. If the child uses syllable deletion, writing down the words and clapping out the syllables may increase the child's awareness of the syllable boundary and syllable structure. An example of this would be for the word *computer*. This is a three-syllable word. If the child tends to say *puter*, clinicians can show the child a picture along with the written word and then clap out or highlight the syllables. Some children can quickly "fix" their speech errors through auditory and visual prompting. For alliteration, clinicians can ask the child to sort the cards into different piles based on the position of the sound and then use these target words to practice sound production. If the child starts and enjoys spelling, spelling can also be used as a building block to facilitate awareness of speech sounds and speech errors.

Targeting Grammatical Morphemes

Final consonant deletion (FCD) is a one of the common phonological processes that may persist beyond appropriate age. What makes FCD important as a treatment target is its negative impact on grammatical morphemes. Grammatical morphemes carry additional meaning like plurals (indicates number) and tense markers (indicates time). If a child tends to delete all final sounds, it will not only significantly affect the child's speech intelligibility but also prevent the child from delivering meaningful messages. For example, when the child is explaining what happened last night to her friend, deletion of final consonants has a negative impact, as in "I play Candyla__ wi__ my mo__ an__ da__ la__ ni__" versus "I played Candyland with my mom and dad last night. Without the final consonants, the intended message is confusing. Another example is the deletion of plurals. If the child says, "my dog like to fight with each other" for "my dogs like to fight with each other," without the producing /s/ at the end, the listener may be puzzled with how many dogs the child has. Therefore, /t, d, ŋ s, z/ in the final position are very important because they carry additional grammatical meaning for present progressive tense (wash<u>ing</u>), regular past tense (walk<u>ed</u>) and plurals (dog<u>s</u>). According to Tyler, Lewis, Haskill, and Tolbert (2002), working on morphosyntax (morphology and syntax) can lead to cross-domain change in phonology. Therefore, instead of working on final consonant deletion *in general*, clinicians can target those specific final sounds that carry additional grammatical meanings to also facilitate positive changes in phonology and other language components (morphosyntax and pragmatics).

The Use of Nonspeech Oral Motor Exercises/Activities (NSOME)

Nonspeech oral motor exercises (NSOME) are activities, such as blowing bubbles,

sucking straws, chewing tube, tongue wagging, and kissing, used to improve speech intelligibility. NSOME are frequently questioned by researchers regarding the direct relationship between NSOME and improving speech intelligibility (Forrest, 2002; Lof, 2003). The rationales behind not using NSOME with children with SSD are as follows (Forrest, 2002, cited in Bernthal et al., 2013):

1. Speech needs more than the strength of articulators. One purpose of NSOME is to strengthen oral muscles to improve speech intelligibility.
2. Breaking speech production down into individual and isolated motor components is not sufficient to learn the overall skill. Speech production requires very sophisticated fine motor control and coordination in a timely fashion. Therefore, exercising each articulator does not improve overall skills required for speech.
3. Even though the structures used in speech and nonspeech activities may be the same, the structures are used differently in these two types of activities.

The best way to improve speech intelligibility is to actually work on speech sounds and practice the sounds in a meaningful context (e.g., words, phrases) daily, because speech movement is different from other gross motor and fine motor movements. Effective ways of treating speech errors include the following:

1. Providing ear training, if necessary
2. Working on speech sound production intensively using meaningful words at different levels (i.e., word, phrase, sentence, conversation)

3. Incorporating curriculum-based and literacy-related activities to work on generalization of correct sound production
4. Providing speech homework for daily practice under the parent's or caregiver's supervision
5. Helping the child develop and implement self-monitoring strategies to self-correct error sounds in daily life

Selecting Treatment Materials

A wide selection of articulation cards is available. However, as an SLPA, you will be required to select *appropriate* training words for the child, either in support of your supervising SLP's session or before you implement treatment with a client (ASHA, 2013). Box 13–3 contains a list of important elements to consider in selecting these materials.

When selecting stimuli, the target word should be easily identified. Real objects or pictures of real objects/actions that contain the target sound may be more effective and functional for younger children. Line drawing pictures, word lists, or reading passages may be more suitable for older children who are reading or are beginning to read. Ready-made articula-

---

Box 13–3. Things to Consider When Selecting Treatment Materials

- **Syllable shape:** Syllable shape is the number of syllables in the word. Fewer syllables will make it easier for the child to produce the target sound.
- **Neighboring sounds:** Neighboring sounds are the sounds that come before and after the target sound. These may influence the target sound. For example, /uk/ will be easier than /ek/ when eliciting /k/ in VC syllable production because the tongue position of /u/ is closer to the tongue position of /k/ (high-back vowel /u/ vs. mid-front vowel /e/).
- **Stress:** Stress can be used to highlight the target sound. If the target sound is stressed, it may be easier for the child to pick up the sound.
- **Cluster or singleton:** The use of singletons or blends depends on the easiness of facilitating the production of the target sound. For example, /s/ may be produced more easily in consonant clusters (st-, sn-) than singleton (Williams, 1991).
- **Frequency:** High-frequency words are more functional and commonly used in daily life. However, error production from old habits may be more difficult to correct. In that case, staying away from the high-frequency words that are consistently produced incorrectly should be considered, until the target sound can be produced consistently.

tion cards are convenient and can save time on preparation. However, it is important to keep in mind that selection of these materials must be done *before* each session to maximize learning outcomes. Appropriate training words should be selected to best facilitate target sound production. Functional target sounds used frequently in the child's daily life and words, selected from the child's curriculum should be used to facilitate generalization and maximize treatment gains.

Individualized training materials are highly recommended. Training materials should always be meaningful to the child. Therefore, selection of words based on the child's language level is important in facilitating both speech and language development. Using pictures with written words printed on the top or bottom may increase print awareness and sight word learning while working on the target sound. Choosing target words meaningful for the child or appropriate for the child's language level will facilitate generalization of the sound production and increase the child's vocabulary repertoire. Starting with early developing words, such as concrete objects and visible action words, especially for younger children, may be helpful. If the child does not know the target word (e.g., *seesaw*), clinicians can talk about the word (e.g., "you can find it in the playground, one end goes up and on end goes down," etc.) and link it to the child's personal experience. Speech therapy should never be only drill and sound practice. When a child makes the link between the word, the letter, the sound, and the concept, the word will be stored in long-term memory more easily and become part of the child's vocabulary repertoire.

As most children who have SSD may have comorbid language delays/disorders, addressing distorted speech sound(s) through language/literacy-based treatment activities may be more effective. Even for children who have only SSD, without other developmental or language learning issues, language/literacy-based treatment can also facilitate and support the child's language development and learning. The focus of the language/literacy-based treatment goes beyond correct speech production. For example, through shared book reading, the target sound(s) can be highlighted and related word and content knowledge can be emphasized and elaborated. These types of activities can be blended into the treatment session to facilitate speech and language development simultaneously. Box 13–4 contains suggestions for creating language/literacy-based treatment activities. Chapter 12 (particularly the sections in this chapter on books as play) also provides additional suggestions in this area.

Making Speech Sessions Fun and Motivating

Treatment sessions should never be "drill-and-kill," but to stabilize the target sound production, maximal training opportunities and practice must be provided. As maximum repetition is inevitable, clinicians must keep the speech session interesting and motivational. If the child is also working on language, then fun activities can be blended into the session to make the session not that "work-like." As stated earlier, language/literacy-based activities should always be part of the treatment to facilitate both speech and language production. How to divide the session and how much time to spend on speech sound production and language learning depends on the child's therapy priority

Box 13–4. Suggestions of Language/Literacy-Based Treatment Activities

1. *Select a book that is appropriate for the child's language and reading level.* The book can be chosen from the pool of reading materials used in the classroom or home. That way, the teacher or parent can carry over the learning into different settings to promote generalization. Collaboration with other professionals and the parent to select appropriate and motivating treatment materials is crucial.
2. *Preread the book and highlight the words containing the target sound.*
3. *While you read the book with the child, emphasize the target sound and talk about the target words* (e.g., definition, synonym, antonym, homonym).
4. *After reading the book, help the child to retell the story, using target words and pictures from the book.*
5. *Incorporate arts and crafts after the reading activities to make retelling the story fun and easy.*

and how the child responds to the treatment. You can work with your supervising SLP in discussing a good balance for each child. No matter the type of activities, keeping them fun and motivational is critical. Short games and language/literacy-based activities can be used creatively to keep the speech session fun and provide maximal opportunity for practice. Table 13–7 provides sample activities that can be easily modified and expanded. The purpose of these activities is to use simple and easy games/activities that do not create additional cognitive and linguistic demands and focus on maximizing opportunity for target sound production.

Keep in mind that treatment is a dynamic process. As such, clinicians need to have an open mind regarding the "trial-and-error" process. Keeping the speech session fun and effective is the goal; thus, finding an effective approach to facilitate a target sound production through a short

and quick "experimental trial" may be required. It is also critical to keep in mind that every child needs be treated individually, even though she or he may have the same goal or work on the same sound(s). It is very common to see that children respond to the same treatment approach or treatment activity differently. Therefore, creating individualized treatment activities is necessary.

Remember, too, that in a school setting, treatment in a group session may be used instead of individual sessions. Many of the activities discussed in Table 13–7 can also be adopted for groups of children. Chapter 11 also offers suggestions in this area. How to group children to address each child's speech/language goal(s) can be very challenging, but effective group sessions have the advantage of facilitating speech or language development through peer modeling. Using peers to model correct production and transfer practice into

Table 13–7. Sample Games and Treatment Activities

Sample Activity	Materials	General Procedure
Finishing	Fish-shape magnets Fishing poles Training words	Attach target words on the back of fish-shape magnets. Child uses fish pole to catch the fish and says the target words.
Bowling	Bowling ball and pins Training words	Attach target words on the bowling pins. Child knocks down bowling pins and says the word on the pin.
Safari	Flashlight(s) Training words	Place target words around the room. Give the child a flashlight. Turn off the light. Ask the child to find all target words using the flashlight.
Art & Craft	Scissors, glue, materials vary, Training words	Procedure varies depends on the art project. Use target words as part of the materials to complete the project.
Board game	Candyland, Chutes & Ladders, Bingo, etc.	Procedure varies depends on the board game. Child has to produce the target word(s) before moving the pawn.
Card game	Memory Games, Go Fish, etc.	Procedure varies depends on the card game. Use target words as game cards to compete with each other. Minimal pairs can be used as cards for Go Fish game.
Toys/Games	Train Set, Genga, etc.	Procedure varies depends on the game. Various toys and games can be used. Child has to produce the target words before receiving or moving a game piece.

fun and competitive games may make training more fun and motivational.

Last, iPad or other high-technology devices can be attractive and fun for children. Several apps designed for speech sound remediation can be used along with ready-made articulation cards. However, some children may be distracted by these devices, which may result in difficulty managing the session. Therefore, how to best use these devices without creating a negative impact on speech/language learning must be considered.

Monitoring Progress/ Tracking Clinical Data

To ensure the effectiveness of the intervention, clinicians must consistently track the frequency of the correct production of the target sound in relation to the child's progress toward speech goal(s). Creating a general clinical data sheet that can be quickly modified for each child is highly recommended. Clinical data must be collected in each session. Audio recording each session to ensure the accuracy of the data is also necessary. Appendix 13–B contains a sample data sheet. Any data sheet should include quantitative data (e.g., numbers, such as percentages, number of prompts, etc.) and qualitative data (e.g., clinical observations that cannot be quantified easily in numbers). Chapter 8 offers additional suggestions in this area. The appendices of Chapter 8 also contain generic data sheets that can be modified for SSD treatment. Data sheets with the following components are very helpful:

1. Target sound: the sound(s) the child was working on in the session
2. Position: initial (I), medial (M), or final (F) position
3. Accuracy of production
4. Type of prompt provided
5. Qualitative clinical observation. Clinical observation should be brief but informative. Information should include the client's level of participation (e.g., attention, behavior), the training materials used and any noted client strengths and/or weaknesses evident while implementing treatment.

If language is also addressed in the session, progress regarding language learning should be documented separately. A separate data sheet for each goal addressed in the child's treatment plan can be used. As stated earlier, the purpose of data collection is to ensure the effectiveness of the intervention. Therefore, if a child does not progress at a desired and reasonable pace, treatment activities will need to be modified by your supervising SLP. Last, these data will need to be effectively conveyed to your supervising SLP. Chapter 9 contains additional suggestions on how to summarize this information in a modified SOAP note format.

REFERENCES

American Speech-Language-Hearing Association (ASHA). (2012). *2012 Schools survey report: SLP caseload characteristics*. Retrieved from http://www.asha.org/research/mem berdata/schoolssurvey/

American Speech-Language-Hearing Association (ASHA). (2013). *Speech-language pathology assistant scope of practice*. Retrieved from http://www.asha.org/policy

Barlow, J., & Gierut, J. (2002). Minimal pair approaches to phonological remediation. *Seminars in Speech and Language, 23*(1), 57–67.

Bauman-Waengler, J. (2012). *Articulatory and phonological impairments: A clinical focus* (4th ed.). Boston, MA: Pearson.

Bernthal, J., Bankson, N., & Flipsen, P. (2013). *Articulation and phonological disorders: Speech sound disorders in children* (7th ed.). Upper Saddle River, NJ: Pearson.

Bowen, C. (2011). *Communication disorders glossary*. Retrieved August 10, 2013, from http://www.speech-language-therapy.com/index.php?option=com_content&view=article&id=14&Itemid=123

Forrest, K. (2002). Are oral-motor exercises useful in the treatment of phonological/articulatory disorders? *Seminars in Speech and Language, 23,* 15–25.

Gierut, J. (1989). Maximal oppositions approach to phonological treatment. *Journal of Speech and Hearing Research, 54,* 9–19.

Gordon-Brannan, M. E., & Weiss, C. E. (2007). *Clinical management of articulation and phonologic disorders* (3rd ed.). Baltimore, MD: Lippincott, Williams & Wilkins.

Justice, L., Gillon, G., McNeill, B., & Schuele, C. M. (2013). Phonological awareness: Description, assessment, and intervention. In J. E. Bernthal, N. W. Bankson, & P. Flipsen (Eds.), *Articulation and phonological disorders: Speech sound disorders in children* (7th ed., pp. 355–382). Upper Saddle River, NJ: Pearson.

Lof, G. (2003). Oral motor exercises and treatment outcomes. *Perspectives on Language, Learning, and Education, 10*(1), 7–12.

Lof, G. (2004). *Confusion about speech sound norms and their use* [PowerPoint slides]. Retrieved from http://poti.wikispaces.com/file/view/confusion+about+speech+sound+norms+and+their+use.pdf

Peña-Brooks, A., & Hegde, M. N. (2007). *Assessment and treatment of articulation and phonological disorders in children: A dual-level text* (2nd ed.). Austin, TX: Pro-Ed.

Sander, E. (1972). Do we know when speech sounds are learned? *Journal of Speech and Hearing Disorders, 37,* 55–63.

Secord, W. A., Boyce, S. E., Donohue, J. S., Fox, R. A., & Shine, R. E. (2007). *Eliciting sounds: Techniques and strategies for clinicians* (2nd ed.). Clifton Park, NY: Delmar Cengage Learning.

Shriberg, L. (1993). Four new speech and prosody-voice measures for genetics research and other studies in developmental phonological disorders. *Journal of Speech and Hearing Research, 36,* 105–140.

Smit, A., Hand, L., Freilinger, J., Bernthal, J., & Bird, A. (1990). The Iowa articulation norms project and its Nebraska replication. *Journal of Speech and Hearing Disorders, 55,* 779–798.

Templin, M. (1957). *Certain language skills in children.* Minneapolis: University of Minnesota Press.

Tyler, A., Lewis, K., Haskill, A., & Tolbert, L. (2002). Efficacy and cross-domain effects of a morphosyntax and a phonology intervention. *Language, Speech and Hearing Services in School, 33,* 52–66.

Van Riper, C., & Erickson, R. (1996). *Speech correction: An introduction to speech pathology and audiology* (7th ed.). Englewood Cliffs, NJ: Prentice-Hall.

Williams, A. (1991). Generalization patterns associated with training least phonological knowledge. *Journal of Speech and Hearing Research, 34,* 722–733.

Williams, A. L. (1993). Phonological reorganization: A qualitative measure of phonological improvement. *American Journal of Speech-Language Pathology, 2,* 44–51.

Williams, A. L. (2000). Multiple oppositions: Case studies of variables in phonological intervention. *American Journal of Speech-Language Pathology, 9,* 289–299.

World Health Organization. (2001). *International Classification of Functioning, Disability and Health (ICF).* Geneva, Switzerland: Author.

APPENDIX 13–A

Sample SSD Homework Sheet

Please give this speech homework to your parent. Say each word correctly **10 times** a day with your parent. Pay attention to the sound you make. Remember to show your parent what you have learned in your speech session. Please ask your parent to put **a checkmark for each word** after you say the word correctly 10 times. After you finish saying all the words correctly, please ask your parent to **initial on the bottom for each day you practice**. Please remember to bring your speech folder with you next time when you come to speech room.

Keep up the good work!! _____/Speech teacher

Target words—/s/ in initial position	Day 1	Day 2	Day 3	Day 4	Day 5	Day 6	Day 7
Sun							
Sea							
Say							
Saw							
Parent's Initials							

APPENDIX 13–B

Sample SSD Treatment Data Collection Form

Target Sound	Position (I/M/F)	Speech sound production (+ correct production, – incorrect production) Prompt system 1. Physical (placement) 2. Visual 3. Verbal 4. No prompt/ independent
/k/	I (initial)	–/3 (explanation: incorrect with physical prompt provided), –/2, –/2+3 (incorrect with visual and verbal combined), +/3 (correct with physical prompt provided), +/3, +/3 . . . _____ *correct production* / _____ *total number of production in one session (correct + incorrect)* = _____*% accuracy*

Clinical Observation (qualitative)

Fully participated. Word level: one- and two-syllable words used. Responds best to physical prompt (articulation placement with tongue depressor). Starting to positively react to visual prompt. Mirror used throughout.

CHAPTER 14

Augmentative and Alternative Communication

Margaret Vento-Wilson

Just as a dance couldn't be possibly be a dance unless people moved to it, so language doesn't become communication until people grow to express it back. It has to be a two-way exchange.
Blackstone, 2000, p. 3, as cited in Beukelman & Mirenda, 2005

The position statement of the American Speech-Language-Hearing Association (ASHA) asserts that "communication is the essence of human life and that all people have the right to communicate to the fullest extent possible" (ASHA, 2001, Position Statement, para. 2). For people with significant congenital or acquired communication impairments, this directive presents greater challenges and increased complexity than for those for whom communication occurs through typical development and normal channels. Approximately 0.3% to 1.3% of the U.S. population experiences communication impairments that impede their ability to produce and/or comprehend spoken, written, or signed language (ASHA, 2004; Beukelman & Mirenda, 2005). These percentages translate into an estimated two million individuals who are unable to use speech or handwriting as a means to communicate about their daily needs (ASHA, 2004). Through the effective intervention of trained professionals, including speech-language pathology assistants (SLPAs), at least some of these communication barriers may be overcome through the use of assistive technology (AT) or augmentative and alternative communication (AAC) (ASHA, 2004; Glennen & DeCoste, 1997).

Based on research conducted by ASHA (2004), 45% of speech-language pathologists (SLPs) surveyed reported that they provide services to individuals with AAC needs, with the occurrence being slightly higher in hospitals than in school settings (ASHA, 2004). In health care settings, SLPs surveyed reported that 66% of referrals received were for patients who were likely AAC candidates, with the majority of these referrals being from pediatric hospitals (ASHA, 2002). In the school setting, approximately 0.3% to 1% of school-aged children are identified as unable to speak (Matas, Mathy-Laiddo, Beukelman, & Legresley, 1985, as cited in Glennen & DeCoste, 1997). Given the high level of need these figures represent, it is very likely that as an SLPA, you will encounter individuals with AAC needs in your employment and training settings.

As an SLPA, you will be expected to be knowledgeable and competent in AAC concepts and implementation practices. As discussed in Chapter 2, in the area of service delivery, ASHA specifically states that, provided training, supervision, and planning are appropriate, one of the tasks that may be delegated to an SLPA is to "program and provide instruction in the use of augmentative and alternative communication devices" (ASHA, 2013b, Responsibilities Within the Scope of SLPAs, para. 1). In addition, the following list provides a general description of the potential roles of an SLPA in AAC intervention (ASHA, 2013a; Beukelman, Ball, & Fager, 2008):

- Support of multimodality intervention
- Preparation of low-tech materials
- Integration of low- and high-tech materials into developmental/restorative/compensatory intervention
- Instruction to communication partners in AAC use
- Maintenance of AAC technology
- Serving as a liaison between AAC commercial companies and related AAC personnel.

This chapter provides an overview of AAC concepts and practices. While this topic may initially seem daunting, as you read this chapter and become more familiar with AAC, you may find that this challenging topic offers an opportunity for you to grow as an SLPA. AAC intervention can and often does have a profound effect on the lives of your clients. The journey you are undertaking by reading this chapter is very similar to the journey your clients undertake, whether they come to you as a toddler with complex communication needs, or as an adult who has experienced an abrupt or gradual, but nonetheless devastating, loss of speech and language. With the appropriate guidance and support, they too will evolve from a novice AAC user into an experienced AAC user, with the ability to maintain and develop relationships and remain relevant and involved with their world (Beukelman & Mirenda, 2005). AAC offers them the opportunity to experience language, the quintessential tool of mankind, "which is so tightly woven into human experience that it is scarcely possible to imagine life without it" (Pinker, 1994, p. 17).

ASSISTIVE TECHNOLOGY

Assistive technology (AT) can be defined broadly as an item, piece of equipment, or system that can be used as a means to preserve, enhance, or improve the functional capabilities of an individual (Bugaj & Norton-Darr, 2010). Examples of AT include the use of eyeglasses, hearing aids, enlarged handles on kitchen utensils, walkers, wheelchairs, and Braille codes on elevator buttons (Glennen & DeCoste, 1997). Specific to communication, AT includes the use of a broad range of AAC devices or systems (Glennen & DeCoste, 1997; Parette & Sherer, 2004).

AUGMENTATIVE AND ALTERNATIVE COMMUNICATION

The term *AAC* is defined as a system that can be used to temporarily or permanently compensate for the impairments, activity and participation limitations, and restrictions of individuals with severe expressive or receptive impairments in speech, language, or communication (ASHA, 2004). AAC is also defined as a dynamic, multimodal communication continuum that evolves based on a user's growth and development, the situation, and the communication partner. Its ultimate purpose is to minimize barriers to successful communication (Glennen & DeCoste, 1997). Before delving further into a discussion of AAC, it is essential to have an understanding of the distinctions among the terms *speech, language,* and *communication.*

Speech is the individual sounds and sound patterns of any given language. It is a vocal production and it is comprehended auditorily. *Language* is symbolic and is used to convey messages through a rule-governed system, which involves syntax, semantics, phonology, morphology, and pragmatics. Language can occur

independent of speech, as evidenced when individuals use American Sign Language (ASL) (Figure 14–1) to communicate, either in addition to or instead of spoken language. *Communication* is the act of conveying a message that establishes a shared understanding between the message sender and the message receiver. Communication can occur without speech or language, such as when two people who speak different languages use gestures or pictures to ask or answer a question. For people with deficits in the production or comprehension of speech, language, or communication, AAC offers users the opportunity to create intelligible and comprehensible messages through a combination of symbols and then to use those symbols with their communication partners in multiple settings and circumstances (ASHA, 2004).

AAC Users

AAC users encompass a wide range of heterogeneous individuals, whose only shared links are the presence of severe communication impairments (ASHA, 2004) and "an inability to communicate vocally" (Glennen & DeCoste, 1997, p. IX). Additional factors that contribute to the need for AAC include challenging communicative behavior that is unacceptable in society, involves the use of unusual or reflexive movement, fatigues the user, is so unconventional or idiosyncratic that only familiar communicators can interpret it, is inefficient, or is potentially harmful to the user (ASHA, 2004). Severe communication impairments requiring the use of AAC can be congenital or acquired. Common congenital and acquired impairments that can cause severe communication impairments, necessitating the

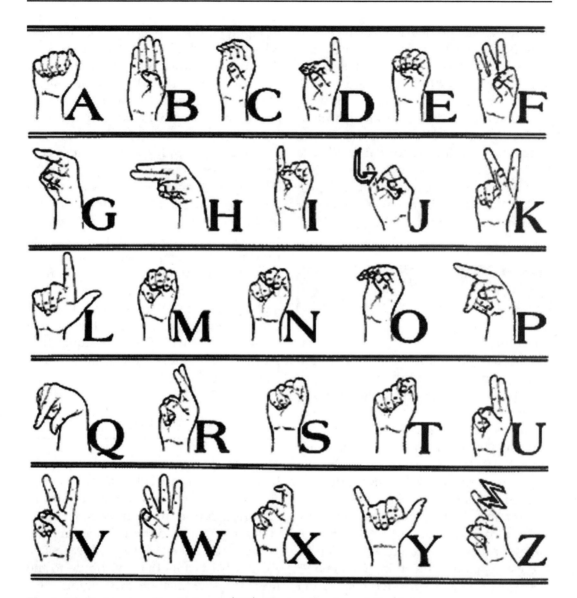

Figure 14–1. American Sign Language (ASL) alphabet. Courtesy of Bing Images.

needed for AAC, are listed in Table 14–1. When working with individuals with severe communication impairments, it is vital to keep in mind that these impairments do not always suggest a concomitant cognitive impairment (Fried-Oken, Beukelman, & Hux, 2012). As Chapter 5 recommends, you must view all individuals as unique in their needs, preferences, *and abilities.*

Purpose of AAC Intervention

When working with individuals with severe communication impairments, it is

Table 14–1. Common Congenital and Acquired Impairments That May Benefit From Augmentative and Alternative Communication

Congenital Impairments	Acquired Impairments
• Cerebral palsy (CP) • Autism spectrum disorder (ASD) • Intellectual disability (ID) • Childhood developmental apraxia of speech (CAS) (ASHA, 2004; Beukleman & Mirenda, 2005)	• Cancer • Acquired apraxia of speech (AOS) • Amyotrophic lateral sclerosis (ALS) • Multiple sclerosis (MS) • Traumatic brain injury (TBI) • Cerebral vascular accident (CVA) • Primary progressive aphasia (PPA) • Dysarthria • Spinal cord injury • Locked-in syndrome (Beukelman & Mirenda, 2005; Hux, Weissling, & Wallace, 2008)

important to be mindful of the primary purpose of AAC intervention, which extends significantly beyond the directive to find a technical solution to communication problems (Beukelman & Mirenda, 2005). While AAC intervention involves language organization, strategies, and techniques, it also involves the emotional and social issues that surround receptive and expressive language impairments (Cress, 2004). The broadly stated and humanistic purpose of AAC intervention is to enable people to engage efficiently and effectively with others in a variety of situations and contexts of their choice. It allows the user to participate in conversations at home and in their communities, learn their native language, and initiate and maintain relationships (Beukelman & Mirenda, 2005). To fully accomplish these goals, AAC intervention needs to incorporate not just the AAC user but must take into consideration and integrate family members and other communicative partners—AAC cannot be taught or used in isolation (Cress, 2004).

Myths About AAC Use

One of the basic theoretical constructs of AAC is that all individuals have the right to communicate, regardless of the method and regardless of a perceived ability to communicate. Although the effectiveness of AAC has been demonstrated through an extensive body of literature (ASHA, 2004; Beukelman & Mirenda, 2005; Glennen & DeCoste, 1997), there is a high level of misunderstanding about its assessment and intervention among related professionals, family members, and even users themselves. Table 14–2 identifies some of the more commonly encountered myths and provides research-based data that dispel these myths and offer support for the use of appropriate AAC assessment and intervention. While this table highlights many of the myths regarding AAC use, various researchers have indicated that a minimal level of speech comprehension and the ability to use distal gestures, such as pointing, may be suggestive of greater success in AAC use (ASHA,

Table 14–2. Common Myths and Truths About Augmentative and Alternative Communication (AAC)

Myth	Truth
There are prerequisite skills, cognition levels, and communicative abilities required for AAC assessment and intervention.	Although language and cognition are interrelated, it remains unclear which force drives the other, and without a method of communication, cognition cannot be demonstrated.
	AAC access has been demonstrated to support the early cognitive and linguistic skills necessary for the development of language.
There is a minimum age for AAC assessment and intervention.	The earliest AAC intervention can apply to a child's behaviors, gestures, cooperative actions, and sounds.
	AAC use benefits infants and toddlers, based on evidence suggesting that a child's early learning experiences in the first 3 years of life are foundational to subsequent brain development.
Language acquisition follows a symbolic representational hierarchy that flows from objects to written words.	During the early phases of language development, symbol type (i.e., iconic or abstract) may not be a significant factor in intervention since, ultimately, all symbols function the same.
AAC use will interfere with a child's speech or vocal development.	AAC use does not impede vocalizations or oral language. AAC has been shown to encourage vocalizations and oral language by increasing communication opportunities.
	Children typically use the most efficient method of communicating, and with the inherent advantages that speech offers over AAC, children will move to speech when possible.
AAC implementation should be delayed until a consistent verbal communication delay is confirmed over time.	Communication across all modes in the early childhood years should be made available to the child.
	Delaying AAC implementation, when behaviors and physical limitations suggest a risk for impaired speech, can have a negative effect on the long-term development of speech and language.
The introduction of AAC decreases the users' need to work on speech.	Natural speech improvements often correlate with the introduction of AAC.
	AAC users typically use multiple communication modes, including technology, gestures, and natural speech.
Speech, regardless of how limited it is, should be the primary mode of communication.	Children and adults who are left without a reliable means to communicate even their basic wants and needs have the potential to demonstrate behavior problems, social failure, academic challenges, and learned helplessness.
The use of AAC makes individuals look "different" from their peers.	Rather than inhibiting language production, the implementation of AAC has the potential to inhibit challenging communicative behavior and build more socially acceptable behaviors.
	Ultimately, individuals look more atypical when they are unable to express themselves.
AAC use represents the last resort in speech-language intervention.	Early introduction of AAC fosters communication and language skills, as well as diminishes communication failure for both beginning communicators and those with acquired disabilities.
	AAC intervention is holistic in that it addresses improving communication skills across all modes, including verbal skills.

Table 14–2. *continued*

Myth	Truth
AAC, if unsuccessful, can be considered a failure after the implementation of only a limited set of AAC strategies or techniques.	Because AAC is a continuum that may involve a variety of strategies and support levels, multiple attempts may be necessary to find the right combination of strategies, aids, support, and techniques.

Sources: ASHA, 2004; Beukleman and Ball, 2002; Beukelman, Fager, Ball, and Dietz, 2007; Branson and Demack, 2009; Cress and Marvin, 2003; Light and Drager, 2007; National Scientific Council on the Developing Child, 2007; Romski and Sevcik, 2005; YAACK, 2013.

2004). For individuals with congenitally based communication disabilities, it is never too early to introduce AAC into comprehensive communication and language intervention (Cress & Marvin, 2003; Romski & Sevcik, 2005). For individuals with acquired communication disabilities, early introduction of compensatory AAC strategies can also support remaining verbal comprehension and expression abilities (Hux, Weissling, & Wallace, 2008).

AAC Components

AAC should be thought of as a system composed of the following primary components or modes: symbols, aids, strategies, and techniques, rather than a single device (ASHA, 2004; Beukelman & Mirenda, 2005).

Symbols

Symbols can be graphic, auditory, gestural, or textured/tactile and can be unaided, such as facial gestures, or aided, such as pictures (ASHA, 2004). Examples include printed or spoken words, photographs, gestures, and objects. The concept of symbols is multifaceted and can be described given their visual relationship to the actual concept (also known as iconicity); their level of stability or transience; and their acquisition hierarchy (ASHA, 2004; Beukelman & Mirenda, 2005; Glennen & DeCoste, 1997).

Iconicity can be thought of as how "guessable" the symbol is, without assistance (ASHA, 2004). Symbol iconicity ranges from transparent, where the symbol demonstrates a clear relationship to the concept (e.g., a drawing of a house that represents *home*) (Figure 14–2A), to opaque, where the symbol does not demonstrate a clear relationship to the concept without an established meaning (e.g., the American Sign Language sign for *home*) (Figure 14–2B) (Beukelman & Mirenda, 2005; Glennen & DeCoste, 1997).

Symbol stability refers to how dynamic or static a symbol is. Spoken symbols (i.e., words) and manual signs are very dynamic and transient, whereas graphic symbols are considered static or permanent (Glennen & DeCoste, 1997). Symbols that are more static and permanent place lower cognitive demands on both the sender and the receiver than do dynamic or transient symbols. Dynamic symbols require sustained attention, memory, and sequencing abilities, which can exceed developing or preserved skills (Fager, Hux, Beukelman, & Karantounis, 2006).

As to acquisition hierarchy, symbols can be arranged in order, given their visual relationship to the actual concept, progressing from real objects (i.e., realia) to a signed representation of a concept (e.g., Amerind, ASL) (ASHA, 2004). Symbols that are more concrete, such as a juice box that represents "juice," are easier to comprehend than more abstract signs, such as a Blissymbol for "elephant" (Figure 14–3) or the signed Amerind symbol for "more" (Figure 14–4). Abstract symbols typically require training to use and understand. Box 14–1 contains a generally accepted symbol hierarchy with respect to ease of acquisition, starting with symbols

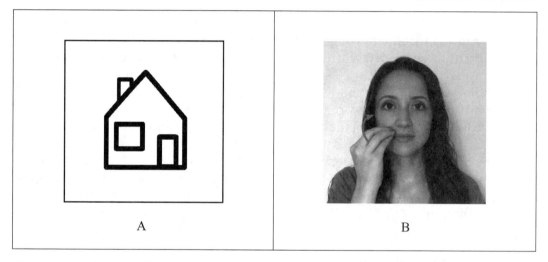

Figure 14–2. Example of transparent versus opaque symbol iconicity. **A.** Black and white icon of "home." The Picture Communication Symbols ©1981–2010 by Mayer-Johnson LLC. All rights reserved worldwide. Used with permission. Boardmaker is a trademark of Mayer-Johnson LLC. **B.** American Sign Language (ASL) sign for "home."

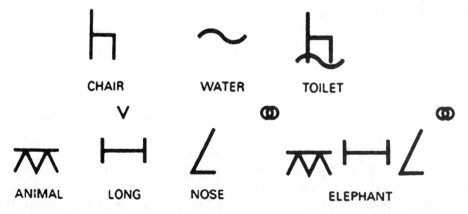

Figure 14–3. Examples of Blissymbols. Blissymbols included with the permission of Blissymbolics Communication International (BCI), http://www.blissymbolics.org

that are more easily acquired (i.e., objects) and progressing to symbols requiring more effort to acquire (i.e., traditional orthography). Research conducted about symbol use for people with acquired communication impairments also suggests that the inclusion of contextually rich photographs (Figure 14–5) may lead to more successful expressive and receptive symbol use (Fried-Oken et al., 2012).

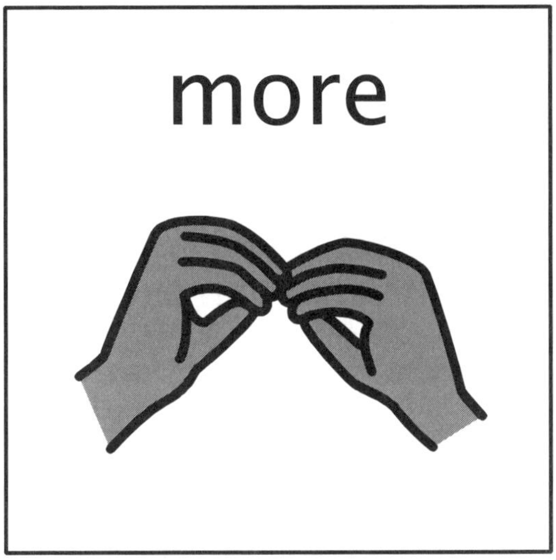

Aids

Aids, or devices, are used to convey or receive the actual message, such as switch-activated devices or a series of symbols that convey meaning (ASHA, 2004). AAC aids can be categorized as aided and unaided, although most people who are nonverbal use multiple communication modalities that incorporate both aided and unaided systems (Glennen & DeCoste, 1997).

Unaided Communication. Unaided communication methods involve solely the individual's body (Glennen & DeCoste, 1997). Box 14–2 contains examples of unaided communication. Unaided communication methods offer an efficient communication method without the need for external devices. Successful unaided communication requires a shared understanding between communication partners of the meaning or situational context represented by the nod, gesture, vocalization, or symbol. This requirement makes

Figure 14–4. Amerind symbol for "more." The Picture Communication Symbols ©1981–2010 by Mayer-Johnson LLC. All rights reserved worldwide. Used with permission. Boardmaker is a trademark of Mayer-Johnson LLC.

Box 14–1. Symbol Acquisition Hierarchy

1. Objects
2. Color photographs
3. Black and white photographs
4. Miniature objects
5. Black and white line drawings
6. Blissymbols
7. Traditional orthography

Sources: Beukelman and Mirenda (1997); Glennen and DeCoste (1997).

Box 14–2. Examples of Unaided Communication

- Speech
- Eye movements
- Head nods
- Gestures
- Vocalizations
- Sign language
- Facial expressions

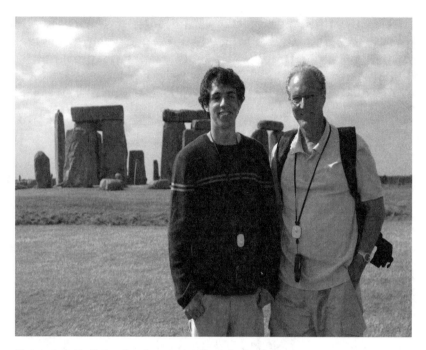

Figure 14–5. Example of contextually rich photograph.

communication with an unfamiliar partner more difficult, unless the communicative act is transparent or "guessable" enough to establish a clear meaning.

Unaided communication strategies require at least a minimal level of motoric ability. Typical users may include people with dysarthria or people who have experienced a stroke or a traumatic brain injury who are able to at least partially use their preserved cognitive, linguistic, visual, and motoric abilities to convey their messages (Beukelman & Mirenda, 2005; Glennen & DeCoste, 1997).

Aided Communication. Aided communication methods involve the use of tools, equipment, or devices in addition to an individual's body (Glennen & DeCoste, 1997). Aided AAC systems offer increased message length, complexity, speed, and comprehensibility to the communication partner. Aided communication strategies also require at least a minimal level of motoric ability and cognition, but it is important to remember that as the complexity of the device increases, cognitive demand increases as well. Typical users may include people with a variety of disorders (e.g., childhood apraxia of speech, apraxia of speech, amyotrophic lateral sclerosis, etc.) who are able to use preserved cognitive, linguistic, visual, and/or motoric abilities to communicate with this strategy (Beukelman & Mirenda, 2005; Glennen & DeCoste, 1997).

The category of aided systems can be further broken down into the categories of low tech and high tech (Glennen & DeCoste, 1997). *Low-tech* AAC systems are typically handmade and not computer based. Box 14–3 lists examples of low-tech, aided communication. The appendices of this chapter contain samples.

Box 14–3. Examples of Low-Tech Aided Communication

■ Paper and pencil (e.g., for use in writing and drawing)
■ Communication books (Appendix 14–A)
■ Eye-gaze boards (Appendix 14–B)
■ Alphabet boards (Appendix 14–C)
■ Choice boards (Appendix 14–D)
■ Real objects
■ Remnant books (e.g., movie tickets, concert programs, menus, and so forth from recent life events)

An additional set of aided low-tech communication devices are those that use an electronic component but are limited in their output (Glennen & DeCoste, 1997). Examples of these include the following:

■ Clock communicator (Appendix 14–E)
■ Switch and button communicators (Appendix 14–F)

High-tech AAC systems typically contain microcomputer chips, can be dedicated solely to AAC use, or can be a program or app on a nondedicated mobile device or a computer (Glennen & DeCoste, 1997). High-tech devices typically offer message retrieval and storage, stored or synthetic speech, prediction features, and complex vocabulary (Beukelman & Mirenda, 2005). A significant benefit of AAC systems with speech-generating devices or voice output is their ability to enhance communicative interaction between people (Cress & Marvin, 2003). Voice output can be accomplished through stored speech, also called digitized speech, which is similar to a tape recording, and synthesized speech, which is generated by a computer. The quality of synthesized speech will vary based on the system used. Typically, AAC systems offer several prestored voices, which can be customized by altering loudness, rate, and/or pitch. Some synthesized voices are very intelligible to the listener, while others can be robot-like, requiring careful listening. An example of digitized speech is when a classmate or peer prerecords a short phrase (e.g., I want milk) within an AAC device, which can then be selected and played by the AAC user in a communicative context. Recent advances in technology also allow AAC users, such as individuals who are diagnosed with a progressive disease (e.g., amyotrophic lateral sclerosis, multiple sclerosis, etc.), to preserve samples of their speech within a computer system, to be retrieved at a later date, when they are no longer able to communicate vocally. It can be very comforting for AAC users and their communication partners to hear the voice they have become familiar with over the years.

Box 14–4 lists examples of high-tech aided communication. The appendices of this chapter contain samples. These are but a few examples of the many high-tech communication devices available to AAC users. As you grow in your skills and experience with AAC, you will no doubt learn about many more options in this area.

Box 14–4. High-Tech Aided Communication Examples

- Speech-generating devices (SGDs) and voice output communication aids (VOCAs) (Appendix 14–G)
- Text-to-speech devices (Appendix 14–H)
- Computers, iPads, and tablets, adapted with software or apps for communication purposes (Appendices 14–I and 14–J)

Strategies

Because AAC users typically communicate at a fraction of the rate of natural speakers (2–15 words per minute vs. 200 words per minute), *strategies,* which are used to improve and refine messages and increase the rate of communication, are of high value to AAC users and their communication partners (ASHA, 2004; Beukelman & Mirenda, 2005). Furthermore, strategies can be used across aided and unaided communication and low- and high-tech devices and may decrease the cognitive and motoric demands on the AAC user. Although a complete review of all available strategies is beyond the scope of this chapter, Table 14–3 contains a few examples. Additional methods of refining and improving messages and enhancing the rate of communication are topic identification and the use of partner-focused questions (Beukelman & Mirenda, 2005).

Techniques

Techniques are used to transmit the message itself (ASHA, 2004). AAC users can make their communication choices through access methods called direct or indirect selection.

Direct selection involves an interaction between the motoric abilities of the AAC user and the manual, mechanical, or technological options offered by the communication device. Direct selection can be high tech or low tech and allows the user to make a direct communication choice via a body part, such as a hand or the head, or some form of technical aid, such as a light pointer, adapted mouse, or a switch. Examples of direct selection techniques are highlighted in Box 14–5.

Recent advances in computer technology also allow for an additional avenue of direct selection using the eyes, referred to as eye tracking. Using eye tracking, high-tech devices track the movements of the eye and register a location on the screen where an AAC user gazes. If the user holds her or his gaze in that position or blinks, the system registers that as a selection (e.g., activation of a symbol on the screen) (Fager, Bardach, Russell, & Higginbotham, 2012). Examples of this technology can be found in Appendices 14–K and 14–L.

For those individuals who do not possess sufficient motoric abilities to allow them to make a direct selection, *indirect selection* offers options that compensate for these limitations. Indirect selection, also called scanning, entails making a communication choice through intermediary steps by the communication partner or with the device (Beukelman & Mirenda, 2005). When using indirect selection, symbols are presented and

Table 14–3. Examples of Augmentative and Alternative Communication (AAC) Strategies

Strategy	Definition	Example
Encoding	The use of a prestored, shortened code to represent a longer, stored message.	The use of the letters *GG* to represent the phrase, "Please get my glasses."
		The use of the alphanumeric symbol *B2* to represent, "I need to take a shower."
Prediction	A dynamic interaction between the AAC user and the AAC device or communication partner that allows for prediction of the balance of a partially formulated message at the letter, word, or phrase level.	Letter: Based on rules of spelling and letter patterns.
		Word: Based on context and rules of grammar.
		Phrase: Based on context and topic and sophisticated computer algorithms that incorporate natural language constructs.
Sequencing	When using symbols to communicate and moving beyond the single-symbol level, symbols can be combined to create novel phrases.	An example of a sequenced phrase can be seen in Figure 14–6.

Sources: Beukelman & Mirenda, 2005; Glennen & DeCoste, 1997.

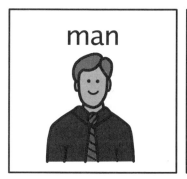 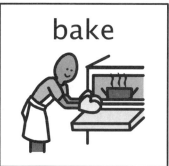 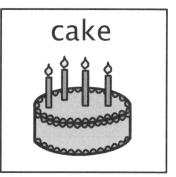

Figure 14–6. Example of symbol sequencing. The Picture Communication Symbols ©1981–2010 by Mayer-Johnson LLC. All rights reserved worldwide. Used with permission. Boardmaker is a trademark of Mayer-Johnson LLC.

Box 14–5. Examples of Direct Selection Methods

- Eye gaze
- Physical contact
  - Manual touch or pressure on keyboard or switch
- Pointing (no contact)
- Voice recognition

Source: Glennen and DeCoste (1997).

the AAC user makes a selection from the options presented. Symbols can be presented auditorily, as when a communication partner calls out the individual letters of the alphabet and waits for confirmation/rejection of a specific letter choice. Symbols can also be presented visually, as when a communication partner points to the symbols on a communication board or when a high-tech system highlights a symbol by changing its background color, placing a dark outline around the symbol, and so forth. The AAC user selects a desired symbol using some form of physical confirmation to the listener, such as a head nod or eye blink, or with some form of minimal motor movement (e.g., tap with the finger, wrist, head, etc.) on a "switch" (Appendix 14–F), which then activates a switch-enabled AAC device. The speed and timing of the auditory or visual scanning can be individualized to reflect the cognitive, linguistic, visual, auditory, and motoric abilities of the user.

AAC Intervention Guidelines

AAC intervention occurs within the context of a team of professionals that include the AAC users and their families (ASHA, 2004). In addition to you and your supervising SLP, this team of related professionals can also include general and special education teachers, physical therapists, occupational therapists, and rehabilitation engineers (Beukelman & Mirenda, 2005). As with all other speech-language intervention, AAC intervention revolves around the individualized goal written by the SLP. For your reference, Chapter 8 contains sample AAC objectives. AAC intervention looks much like other speech-language intervention with the

exception that the input and/or output can be mediated through alternate means, such as vocalizations, signs, objects, or a low- or high-tech device. One of the basic premises of AAC intervention, which mirrors a basic premise of all speech-language intervention, is that the intervention should be functional, take place in naturalistic contexts and situations (Beck, Stoner, & Dennis, 2009), and be led by the AAC user's interests, innate curiosities, actions, and behaviors (Cress & Marvin, 2003; Hourcade, Everhart, Pilotte, West, & Parette, 2004; Romski & Sevcik, 2005).

Best practices suggest that the clinician overlay targeted language or provide a verbal model in parallel with symbol manipulation or referencing (Beck et al., 2009; Beukelman & Mirenda, 2005; Dada & Alant, 2009). This method of evidence-based intervention, called augmented input strategies, has the potential to enhance both expressive and receptive language skills. Modeling language allows the user to learn, restore, and/or use language. An example of this method can be seen where the clinician points to the icon for baby and crib and comments to the child, "Oh look, the baby is sleeping," or, when working with adults, asking the individual, "What did you think of that song?" while pointing to icons representing "good" and "bad" (Figure 14–7) (Beck et al., 2009). When implementing AAC intervention with adults who have cognitive/communication impairments and may have difficulty with symbolic representation (e.g., aphasia), augmented input strategies increase the likelihood of symbol comprehension and communication.

An additional factor to consider for AAC intervention is the dynamic aspect of AAC in that users may need to use multiple AAC systems, based on their

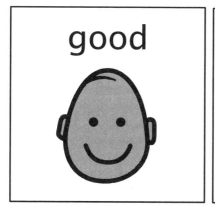 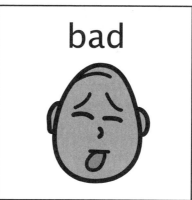

Figure 14–7. Boardmaker choice icons. The Picture Communication Symbols ©1981–2010 by Mayer-Johnson LLC. All rights reserved worldwide. Used with permission. Boardmaker is a trademark of Mayer-Johnson LLC.

audience and their communication partners. For example, individuals may use vocalizations and signs with familiar communication partners (i.e., home), yet may use a picture-based system with unfamiliar communication partners (i.e., community members) (ASHA, 2013a). Similarly, because AAC is dynamic and multimodal, it is likely that over the course of intervention, modifications to the AAC system may need to be made. These modifications can involve all components of the AAC system, such as the symbols used and the strategies and techniques employed. For children developing their speech, language, and communication abilities, the AAC components may increase in complexity and the messages increase in length. For adults with acquired communication impairments, AAC modifications may need to be made due to speech, language, and communication improvements or due to diminishing capabilities that may accompany degenerative conditions (Beukelman & Ball, 2002).

As discussed in greater detail in Chapter 6, an individual's cultural experiences and background will also influence intervention. While much of the research on AAC use has focused on the Anglo-European culture, ideals and values, SLPAs must be aware of the values, ideals, and considerations of other cultures, ethnicities, and languages (Beukelman & Mirenda, 2005; Glennen & DeCoste, 1997) since cultural norms have a significant effect on the implicit and explicit rules of communication and language (Hetzroni & Harris, 1996). The concepts of collectivism, cooperation, interdependency, family hierarchies, respect/politeness, and levels of directness within the communication cycle vary across cultures, social communities, customs, and languages and must be considered by the SLPA involved in the implementation of AAC systems. Best practices in AAC implementation allow users to code-switch, or to adjust the content and complexity of their communication based on their communication partner/partners, whether they be peers, family members, or health care or educational professionals (ASHA, 2004). Additional factors to consider include user and family attitudes toward technology and the possible stigmatization of disabilities, rehabilitation services, and education (ASHA, 2004; Beukelman & Mirenda, 2005; Glennen & DeCoste, 1997; Parette & Scherer, 2004). These factors should be carefully considered, especially given the fact that stigmatization is closely associated with abandonment of assistive technology (Parette & Scherer, 2004).

Last, vocabulary selection and organization also play a key role in AAC intervention. It is generally accepted that both adults and children with complex communication needs benefit from AAC intervention when a meaningful, functional, individualized, and motivating vocabulary is made available to them. Vocabulary selection, which is an ongoing process, is typically accomplished with the participation of the AAC user and people significant to the user, including their family, friends, and related professionals, including SLPAs. Assessing vocabulary needs can involve ecological inventories or questionnaires (Fallon, Light, & Paige, 2001), communication diaries, and standardized vocabulary lists (Glennen & DeCoste, 1997). Factors to consider in making vocabulary selections may include where the vocabulary is being used (e.g., home vs. school), age, gender, and literacy level (Beukelman & Mirenda, 2005).

Once established, the vocabulary should be broken down into the categories of core and fringe vocabulary for purposes of organization within the AAC device. *Core vocabulary* refers to words or messages that are highly functional, occur frequently across individuals,

and relate to basic functional needs and social exchanges. *Fringe vocabulary* refers to words or messages that are specific to an individual or context (Beukelman & Mirenda 2005; Glennen & DeCoste, 1997). Table 14–4 contains examples of core vocabulary for toddlers and adults.

Once the vocabulary has been defined, it must be organized physically and linguistically to promote efficient and effective communication. Whether creating a communication book or installing software or an application, the vocabulary must be organized based on the cognitive/communicative and motoric abilities of the user, the knowledge and experience level of the communication partners, the communicative context, and frequency of use (Beukelman & Mirenda, 2005; Glennen & DeCoste, 1997). Vocabulary can be organized by semantics and syntax (e.g., parts of speech), categories (e.g., people, locations, actions), or activities (e.g., holidays, vacations). Box 14–6 contains some basic tenets for vocabulary organization.

Table 14–4. Examples of Core Vocabulary (Toddlers and Adults)

Toddler	Adult
• All done	• Go
• Different	• Eat
• Help	• Yes
• Mine	• No
• More	• Stop
• Not/don't	• Home
• Stop	• Restroom
• That	(Glennen & DeCoste, 1997)
• Want	
• What	
(Van Tatenhove, 2007)	

Box 14–6. Vocabulary Organization

- Core vocabulary with broad language functions should be placed in prominent positions that can be accessed quickly and easily, and extended vocabulary can be placed in secondary positions that may be accessed through multiple steps or on subsequent pages.
- Words or phrases that regulate activities or behaviors (e.g., *more, again, help, all gone, all done*) should hold prominent positions.
- Words used to comment and relate to others (e.g., *fun, good, bad, like*) can hold secondary positions.
- The words *yes* and *no* do not need to be in prominent positions if the user has an alternate and reliable method to communicate these words.

Source: Van Tatenhove (2007).

Helpful Tips

Chapter 5 includes tips for communicating with individuals with disabilities. These recommendations are applicable to AAC users as well. In addition, when communicating with an AAC user, it is important to keep in mind that they expend a considerable amount of energy and cognitive resources on communication, and they must adapt their communicative choices based on these decreased resources (Fried-Oken et al., 2012). Best practices suggest the following (Accessible Technology Coalition, 2011):

- Face the person.
- Treat AAC users with the same manners and level of respect you use with others.
- Speak directly to the AAC user; never talk about them with someone else when they are present.
- Communication with the use of AAC takes additional time and energy—allow the AAC user time to compose and communicate his or her message.
- Do not limit your questions to a simple "yes/no" format.
- Do not be afraid to ask for clarification.
- Always ask permission to provide assistance or touch their AAC device.
- Be patient when experiencing technological glitches.
- Do not be condescending to AAC users.
- Remember at all times that a person's silence does not necessarily reflect his or her desire to communicate.

REFERENCES

Accessible Technology Coalition. (2011). *Etiquette in communicating with AAC users.* Retrieved from http://atcoalition.org/article/etiquette-communicating-aac-users

American Speech-Language-Hearing Association (ASHA). (2001). *Scope of practice in speech-language pathology.* Rockville, MD: Author.

American Speech-Language-Hearing Association (ASHA). (2002). *2002 Omnibus survey caseload report: SLP.* Rockville, MD: Author.

American Speech-Language-Hearing Association (ASHA). (2004). Roles and responsibilities of speech-language pathologists with respect to augmentative and alternative communication: Technical report. *ASIIA Supplement, 24,* 1–17.

American Speech-Language-Hearing Association (ASHA). (2013a). *Communication services and supports for individuals with severe disabilities: FAQs.* Retrieved from http://www.asha.org/NJC/faqs-aac-basics.htm

American Speech-Language-Hearing Association (ASHA). (2013b). *Speech-language pathology assistant scope of practice.* Retrieved from http://www.asha.org/policy

Beck, A. R., Stoner, J. B., & Dennis, M. L. (2009). An investigation of aided language stimulation: Does it increase AAC use with adults with developmental disabilities and complex? *Augmentative and Alternative Communication, 25*(1), 42–54.

Beukelman, D. R., & Ball, L. J. (2002). Improving AAC use for persons with acquired neurogenic disorders: Understanding human and engineering factors. *Assistive Technology, 14,* 33–44.

Beukelman, D. R., Ball, L. J., & Fager, S. (2008). An AAC personnel framework: Adults with acquired complex communication needs. *Augmentative and Alternative Communications, 24*(3), 255–267.

Beukelman, D. R., Fager, S., Ball, L., & Dietz, A. (2007). AAC for adults with acquired neurological conditions: A review. *Augmentative and Alternative Communications, 23*(3), 230–242.

Beukelman, D. R., & Mirenda, P. (2005). *Augmentative and alternative communication: Supporting children and adults with complex communication needs.* Baltimore, MD: Paul H. Brookes.

Blackstone, S. (Ed.). (2000). *Beneath the surface: Creative expression of augmented communicators.* Toronto, Canada: ISAAC.

Branson, D., & Demchak, M. (2009). The use of augmentative and alternative communication methods with infants and toddlers with disabilities: A research review. *Augmentative and Alternative Communications, 25*(4), 274–286.

Bugaj, C. R., & Norton-Darr, S. (2010). *The practical and fun guide to assistive technology in public schools: Building or improving your district's AT team.* Washington, DC: International Society for Technology in Education.

Cress, C. J. (2004). Augmentative and alternative communication and language: Understanding and responding to parent's perspectives. *Topics in Language Disorders, 24*(1), 51–61.

Cress, C. J., & Marvin, C. (2003). Common questions about AAC services in early intervention. *Augmentative and Alternative Communication, 19*(4), 254–272.

Dada, S., & Alant, E. (2009). The effect of aided language stimulation on vocabulary acquisition in children with little or not functional speech. *American Journal of Speech-Language Pathology, 18,* 50–64.

Fager, S., Bardach, L., Russell, S., & Higginbotham, J. (2012). Access to augmentative and alternative communication: New technologies and clinical decision-making. *Journal of Pediatric Rehabilitation Medicine: An Interdisciplinary Approach, 5,* 53–61.

Fager, S., Hux, K., Beukelman, D. R., & Karantounis, R. (2006). Augmentative and alternative communication use and acceptance by adults with traumatic brain injury. *Augmentative and Alternative Communications, 22*(1), 37–47.

Fallon, K. A., Light, J. C., & Paige, T. K. (2001). Enhancing vocabulary selection for preschoolers who require augmentative and alternative communication (AAC). *American Journal of Speech-Language Pathology, 10*(1), 81–94.

Fried-Oken, M., Beukelman, D. R., & Hux, K. (2012). Current and future AAC research considerations for adults with acquired cognitive and communication impairments. *Assistive Technology, 25,* 56–66.

Glennen, S. L., & DeCoste, D. C. (1997). *Handbook of augmentative and alternative communication.* New York, NY: Del Mar Cengage Learning.

Hetzroni, O. E., & Harris, O. L. (1996). Cultural aspects in the development of AAC users.

Augmentative and Alternative Communication, 12(1), 52–58.

Hourcade, J., Everhart Pilotte, T., West, E., & Parette, P. (2004). A history of augmentative and alternative communication for individuals with severe and profound disabilities. *Focus on Autism and Other Developmental Disabilities, 19*(4), 235–244.

Hux, K., Weissling, K., & Wallace, S. (2008). Communication-based interventions: Augmentative and alternative communication for people with aphasia. In R. Chapey (Ed.), *Language intervention strategies in aphasia and related neurogenic communication disorders* (pp. 813–836). Baltimore, MD: Lippincott Williams & Wilkins.

Light, J. C., & Drager, K. (2007). AAC technologies for young children with complex communication needs: State of the science and future research directions. *Augmentative and Alternative Communication, 23*(3), 204–216.

National Scientific Council on the Developing Child. (2007). *The timing and quality of early experiences combine to shape brain architecture* (Working Paper No. 5). Retrieved June 21, 2013, from http://developingchild.harvard.edu

Parette, P., & Sherer, M. (2004). Assistive technology use and stigma. *Education and Training in Developmental Disabilities, 39*(3), 271–226.

Pinker, S. (1994). *The language instinct.* New York, NY: William Morris.

Romski, M., & Sevcik, R.A. (2005). Augmentative communication and early intervention: Myths and realities. *Infants and Young Children, 18*(3), 174–185.

Van Tatenhove, G. M. (2007). *Normal language development, generative language & AAC.* Retrieved from http://vantatenhove.com/files/NLDAAC.pdf

Wu, Y., & Voda, J. A. (1985). User friendly communication board for nonverbal, severely physically disabled individuals. *Archives of Physical Medicine and Rehabilitation, 66*, 827–828.

YAACK. (2013). *Does AAC impede natural speech? —and other fears.* Retrieved from http://aac.unl.edu/yaack/b2.html

APPENDIX 14–A
Example of Communication Book

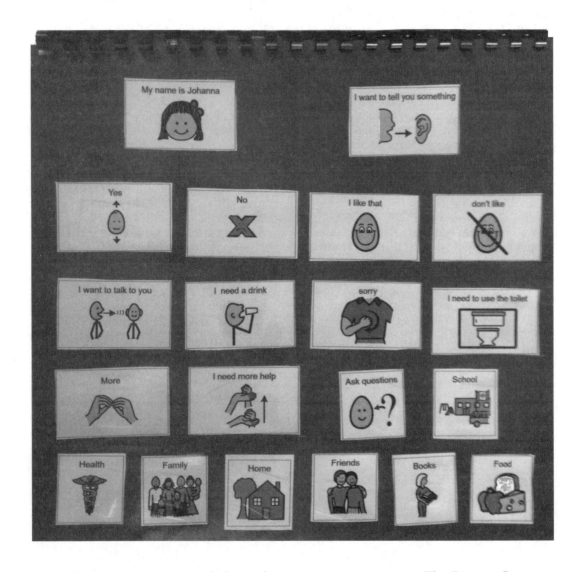

Note: The user points to symbols on the page to communicate. The Picture Communication Symbols ©1981–2010 by Mayer-Johnson LLC. All rights reserved worldwide. Used with permission. Boardmaker is a trademark of Mayer-Johnson LLC. Image courtesy of Bing Images.

APPENDIX 14–B
Eye-Gaze Board: SpeakBook

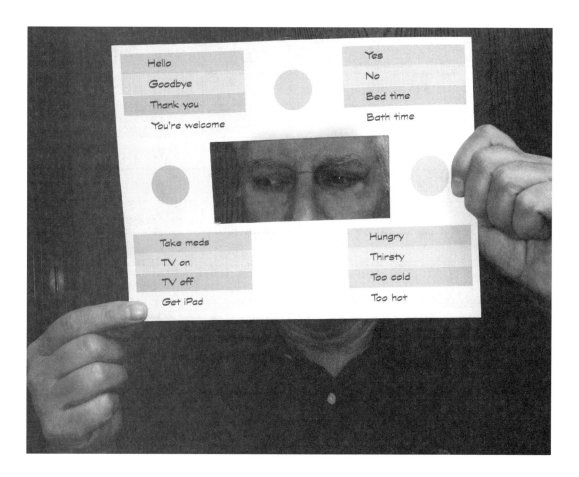

Note: The eye-gaze board is held up between the augmentative and alternative communication (AAC) user and the communication partner. The communication partner places her or his face within the boundaries of the hole in the center of the board and locks gaze with the AAC user before posing a question. The AAC user indicates his or her communication choice by gazing at the desired box and the communication partner confirms the choice verbally. Used with express permission: Patrick Joyce, Speakbook; Nonprofit Communication Tools (http://www.speakbook.org).

APPENDIX 14–C

Example of Alphabet Boards

Traditional Alphabet Board

A	B	C	D	E	F
G	H	I	J	K	L
M	N	O	P	Q	R
S	T	U	V	W	X
Y	Z				
0	1	2	3	4	5
6	7	8	9		

Vowel-based Alphabet Board (Wu & Voda, 1985)

A	B	C	D		
E	F	G	H		
I	J	K	L	M	N
O	P	Q	R	S	T
U	V	W	X	Y	Z

Note: Alphabet boards can be used to communicate messages by either having the augmentative and alternative communication (AAC) user point to each letter to form words and phrases or by having the letters presented auditorily and having the AAC user indicate his or her choice with an agreed-upon method (e.g., blinking, finger raising, nodding, etc.).

APPENDIX 14-D

Example of Choice Board

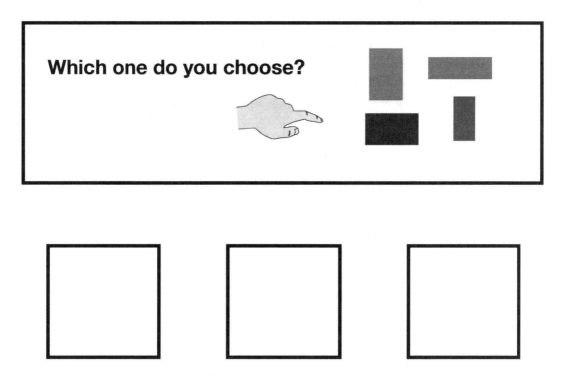

Note: The blank boxes could contain words or visual icons of desired items or activities that the user points to in order to indicate a specific choice.

APPENDIX 14–E
Example of Clock Communicator

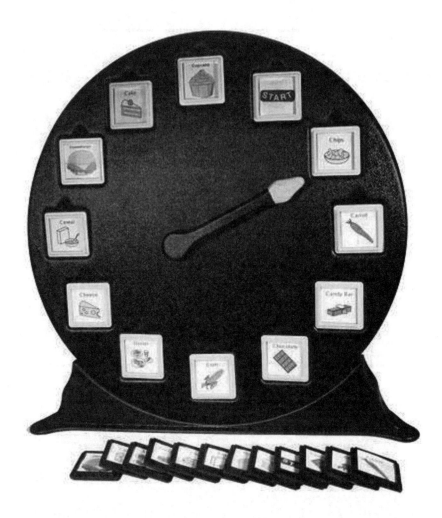

Note: The user selects the position for a desired icon and a corresponding (digitized) message plays. This device can also be accessed using a switch. When using a switch, the hand moves slowing around the dial of choices. The user selects the icon (thereby playing the corresponding message) by depressing a switch when the hand reaches the desired symbol. Used with express permission: manufactured by Enabling Devices, 50 Broadway, Hawthorne, NY. 800-832-8697 (http://www.enablingdevices.com).

APPENDIX 14–F
Example of Switch Communicator

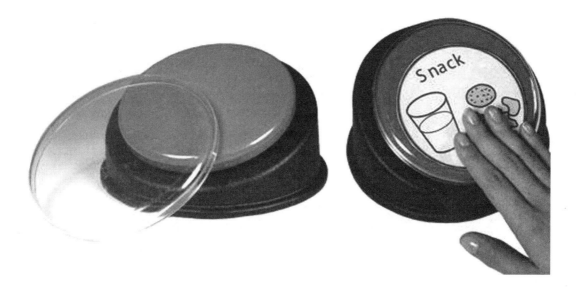

Note: The message is recorded using digitized speech. The augmentative and alternative communication (AAC) user presses a button to play a message in a communicative context. Can also be used as a switch, when attached with a wire to a switch-enabled device. Switch-enabled devices systematically present options to the AAC user. When the desired item is highlighted, pressing this switch activates a corresponding symbol on the switch-enabled system. This process is also known as scanning. Used with express permission: manufactured by Enabling Devices, 50 Broadway, Hawthorne, NY. 800-832-8697 (http://www.enablingdevices.com).

APPENDIX 14-G
Speech-Generating Device: GoTalk Express 32

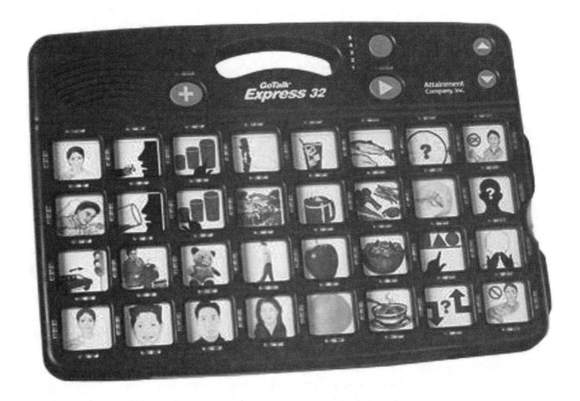

Note: The user selects the desired icon and the system speaks out a prerecorded message (also known as "digitized speech"). Used with express permission by Attainment Company (http://www.attainmentcompany.com/gotalk-express-32).

APPENDIX 14–H
Text-to-Speech Device: LightwriterSL40

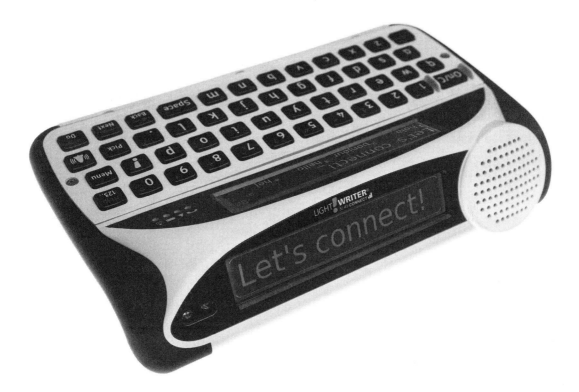

Note: The user types words and the device converts written text into voice output. LightwriterSL40-Connect. Copyright. Used with permission of Toby Churchill House, Ltd., Cambridge, England.

APPENDIX 14–I

Visual Scene Display: Speaking Dynamically Pro

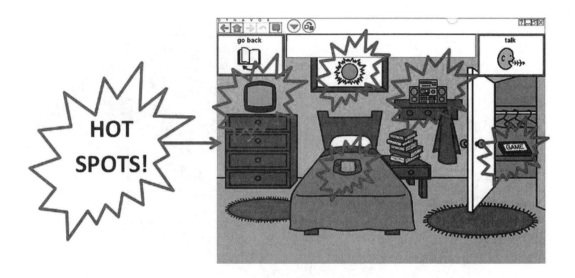

Note: The user selects a "hot spot," and the software is programmed to speak out an associated phrase, such as "TV" or "I want to play a game," using either digitized or synthesized speech. Copyright. The Picture Communication Symbols ©1981–2010 by Mayer-Johnson LLC. All rights reserved worldwide. Used with permission. Boardmaker is a trademark of Mayer-Johnson LLC.

APPENDIX 14–J
iPad Tablet With the Proloquo Application

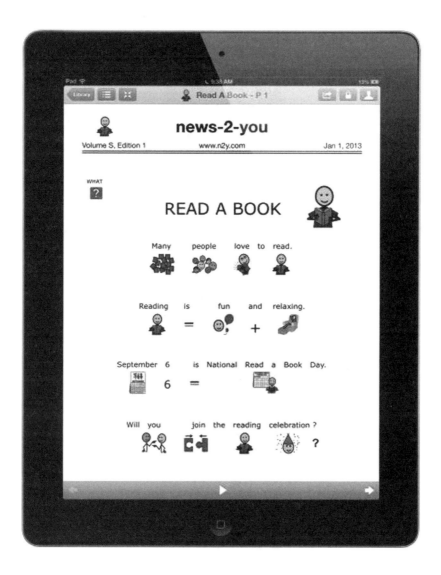

Note: The user generates voice output by selecting the desired icon(s). Proloquo2Go is an AssistiveWare product. Copyright. Used with permission.

APPENDIX 14–K
Eye Tracking Device (Mouse Control): Enable Eyes Control Bar

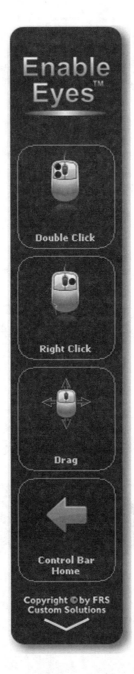

Note: These tools allow the user to perform all of the common types of mouse clicks, using his or her eyes rather than hands/fingers. Enable Eyes Control Bar. Copyright. Used with express permission: manufactured by FRS Custom Solutions, 49 S. Illinois Ave., Mansfield, OH 44905; 888-884-2190. http://www.frs-solutions.com. Enable Eyes is a trademark of Forbes Rehab Services, Inc.

APPENDIX 14–L

Eye Tracking Device (Keypad Access): Enable Eyes Control Bar

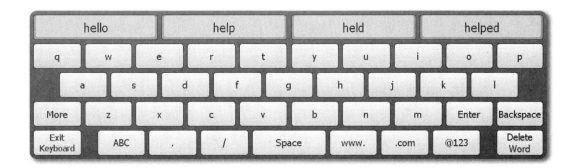

Note: The system allows the user to enter text into any Windows application, using eye tracking software that registers the user's eye gaze and snaps to the nearest key, eliminating unwanted selections between keys. Enable Eyes Control Bar. Copyright. Used with express permission: manufactured by FRS Custom Solutions, 49 S. Illinois Ave., Mansfield, OH 44905; 888-884-2190. http://www.frs-solutions.com. Enable Eyes is a trademark of Forbes Rehab Services, Inc.

CHAPTER 15

Autism Spectrum Disorder (ASD)

Jodi Robledo

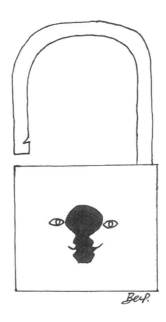

Autism isn't something a person has, or a "shell" that a person is trapped inside. There's no normal child hidden behind autism. Autism is a way of being. It is pervasive: It colors every experience, every sensation, perception, thought, emotion, and encounter, every aspect of existence. It is not possible to separate the autism from the person—and if it were possible, the person you'd have left would not be the same person you started with.

Sinclair, 1993, p. 1, as cited in Kluth, 2010, p. 3

As a speech-language pathology assistant (SLPA), you will have the opportunity to work with individuals with autism spectrum disorder (ASD). According to the Centers for Disease Control and Prevention (CDC), one of every 88 children in the United States has been identified as on the autism spectrum, a 10-fold increase in prevalence in 40 years (CDC, 2012). It is four to five times more common in boys than in girls and can be found in all cultures across the world. Researchers believe that the cause or causes of ASD involve both genetic and environmental factors. The focus of current research continues to search for both the cause and cure of ASD, as well as evidence-based practices in supporting individuals with ASD across the life span.

The purpose of this chapter is to give you a general overview of the definitions and common characteristics of ASD, as well as foundational supports that will benefit individuals with ASD. The goal of this chapter is *not* to simply present a list of deficits that distinguish individuals with ASD from those without ASD. Rather, the goal of this chapter is to present you with information that will guide your learning regarding the *individuals* with ASD that you will support. Remember this famous saying about ASD—if you know one individual with autism, then you know *one* individual with autism. As professionals, we must continue to learn and grow in relationship with and understanding of the individuals we support. As the disability rights movement reminds us, it is imperative that we work *with* individuals, rather than working *on* them.

DEFINITIONS OF AUTISM SPECTRUM DISORDER

Clinical Definitions

Within a medical (or clinical) model, autism is described as a "spectrum" disorder, implying that individuals will range in intensity of characteristics. According to the fifth edition of the *Diagnostic and Statistical Manual of Mental Disorders* (*DSM-5*; American Psychiatric Association [APA], 2013), individuals with ASD will display persistent deficits in social communication and social interaction across multiple contexts as well as restricted, repetitive patterns of behavior, interests, and activities. Severity is described in three levels: Level 1 requiring support, Level 2 requiring substantial support, and Level 3 requiring very substantial support. In addition, the *DSM-5* outlines that symptoms must be present in the early developmental period; cause clinically significant impairment in social, occupational, or other important areas of current functioning; and are not better explained by intellectual disability or global developmental delay.

Challenges within the category of social communication and social interaction may include challenges with reciprocity; reduced sharing of interests, emotions, or affect; challenges with initiation or response to social interactions; challenges with nonverbal communication, eye contact, and understanding and using gesture and facial expressions; and deficits in developing, maintaining, and understanding relationships.

Challenges within the category of restrictive, repetitive patterns of behavior, interests, and activities may include stereotyped or repetitive motor movements, use of objects, or speech; insistence on sameness, inflexible adherence to routines, or ritualized patterns of verbal or nonverbal behavior; highly restricted, fixated interests that are abnormal in intensity or focus; and hyper- or hyporeactivity to sensory input or unusual interests in sensory aspects of the environment.

Educational Definition

The category of autism was added to the Individuals With Disabilities Education Act (IDEA) in 1990 under PL 101-476 (Hall,

2009; Knoblauch & Sorenson, 1998). To receive supports and services from special education, individuals must meet the following three criteria: Individuals must be eligible in a disability category as defined in IDEA, there must be an adverse impact on educational performance, and there must be an actual need for special education and related services to achieve a free and appropriate public education. Autism is specifically defined in IDEA as a developmental disability significantly affecting verbal and nonverbal communication and social interaction, repetitive activities, stereotyped movements, resistance to environmental change or change in daily routines, and unusual responses to sensory experiences. Generally, autism is evident before age 3 years and adversely affects an individual's educational performance (Hall, 2009).

An Insider's Perspective

I think that much of the characteristics of autism is a result of not being able to cope with the neurological impairment which autistic people seem to have. I expect that withdrawal of an autistic person into his own world is a result of the impairment. I also believe that an autistic person's inability to cope makes them less able to concentrate and therefore to learn. I hope this evaluation by an autistic individual will help other people to understand that we are intelligent even though we may not always appear to be. (Hale & Hale, 1999, p. 60)

I believe that autism results when some sort of mechanism that controls emotion does not function properly, leaving an otherwise relatively normal body and mind unable to express themselves with the *depth that they would otherwise be capable of.* (Williams, 1992, p. 203)

I believe Autism is a marvelous occurrence of nature, not a tragic example of the human mind gone wrong. In many cases, Autism can also be kind of genius undiscovered. (O'Neil, 1999, p. 14)

Although clinical and educational definitions are most commonly associated with the "definition of ASD," these definitions leave out one of the most important aspects of truly understanding what ASD is—the perspective and experiences of individuals with ASD—the true experts. One important aspect of including the insider's perspective in the definition of ASD is that we can better understand how ASD affects individuals in different ways—that no two people with ASD experience it the same way. As we move on to explore the common characteristics of ASD, we must remember that individuals will vary greatly in the intensity or type of characteristic and that if we are truly hoping to understand the individuals we support, we must understand *their* strengths and challenges.

COMMON CHARACTERISTICS

As noted earlier, no two individuals experience ASD in the same way. Nonetheless, there are common characteristics that many individuals with ASD share. These include social differences, communication differences, sensory differences, movement differences, learning differences, and passions, interests, and rituals. Common characteristics presented in this chapter include both the clinical description and an insider's perspective.

Social Differences

I can't speak for other kids, but I'd like to be very clear about my own feelings. I did not ever want to be alone. And all of those child psychologists who said, "John prefers to play by himself" were dead wrong. I played by myself because I was a failure at playing with others. (Robison, 2007, p. 211)

Some people have said that autistic people don't care about friendships. That wasn't true at all for me. I tried to make as many friends as possible . . . I just want to say that people mean more than anything to me. I always try to be as friendly as I can to people I meet. However, I still need to work more on my social skills. They are not as good as a lot of people's. (McDonnell, 1993, p. 363)

Challenges with social relationships and interactions have been paramount to the definition of ASD since it was first described. In 1943, Leo Kanner suggested that the social impairment in autism was the defining component of the disorder (Heflin & Alaimo, 2007; Kanner, 1943; Waterhouse, Fein, & Modahl, 1996). Social challenges associated with ASD are well documented within the literature (Attwood, 1998; Baron-Cohen, 1989; Bellini, 2008; Brown & Whiten, 2000; Dawson & Fernald, 1987; Rogers, 2000; Travis, Sigman, & Ruskin, 2001; Wing & Gould, 1979).

The major social challenges of ASD are those in nonverbal communication, social initiating, social reciprocity, social cognition, behavior associated with perspective taking and self-awareness, and social anxiety and withdrawal (Bellini, 2006, 2008).

Nonverbal Communication

Individuals with ASD often have difficulty reading body language and non-verbal cues from others. Many individuals with ASD also report that they can attend better to the speaker when they are looking away from the person's face (Robledo, Strandt-Conroy, & Donnellan, 2012). However, in avoiding direct eye contact, individuals may miss nonverbal communication. Individuals with ASD may struggle to read and understand subtle social signals or to decode what they experience as social secrets (Kluth, 2009, 2010). Other individuals with ASD report that they also have trouble using nonverbal communication such as gestures, body language, and facial expressions (Kluth, 2009, 2010).

Social Initiation

There are two common categories of social initiation challenges for individuals with ASD: those who rarely initiate interactions with others and those who initiate frequently but inappropriately (Bellini, 2006, 2008). Individuals in the first category often demonstrate fear, anxiety, or apathy regarding social interactions. Within the second category, individuals may initiate often but might do so by interrupting, repeating phrases or questions, or violating other social rules or norms when initiating. In addition, some individuals with ASD may attempt to initiate, but others might not recognize their attempts to be social or interact.

Social Reciprocity

Challenges associated with social reciprocity involve the give-and-take, turn-taking, mutuality, and back-and-forth exchanges of social interactions. Many individuals with ASD engage in one-sided conversations, forgetting to ask the perspective of their social partner

(Bellini, 2008). Individuals with ASD may fail to jointly attend, meaning they are not always able to jointly attend in unison to an object, event, or person with their social partner. Many individuals with ASD report that they have difficulty keeping up with the rhythm or pace of the conversation and struggle to know when it is appropriate to jump into a conversation. Others report challenges with knowing when to terminate an interaction, often reporting difficulty determining the social cues that signal the end of the conversation. Knowing how to appropriately terminate an interaction can also be challenging. An individual with ASD may walk away, change topics, or hang up the phone before the social partner believes the conversation is near a close.

Social Cognition

Researchers have suggested that many social challenges displayed by individuals with ASD are due to challenges with social cognition (Baron-Cohen, 1989; Bellini, 2006, 2008). Social cognition refers to understanding the thoughts, intentions, motives, and behaviors of ourselves and others (Flavell, Miller, & Miller, 1993), as well as the social norms, customs, and values of our culture (Resnick, Levine, & Teasley, 1991). Challenges related to difficulty with social cognition could include difficulty with analyzing social situations, understanding the jokes or humor of others, or correctly interpreting the intentions of others (Bellini, 2008).

Perspective Taking and Self-Awareness

Individuals with ASD often make socially inappropriate comments, have challenges expressing sympathy for others, have difficulty maintaining personal hygiene or personal space, or may fail to talk about or acknowledge the interests of others (Bellini, 2008). Difficulty with taking the perspective of another has been described as lacking a theory of mind (Baron-Cohen, 1989). However, we must consider that some of these problems might simply be problems of *showing* concern and care and might not reflect a lack of perspective taking or self-awareness. Many individuals with ASD have reported being so attuned to the feelings of others that they themselves can feel emotional distress just by being around others who feel this way (Kluth, 2009).

Social Anxiety and Performance Fears

Individuals with ASD may experience social anxiety, or intense fears of social situations (Bellini, 2008). Due to intense fears, they might avoid interacting with peers and might engage in solitary activities instead. It is important to remember that many of these individuals do want to engage in social interactions, but a lack of social skills or intense fears might be holding them back.

Communication Challenges

My speech really just bulges out of my mouth like a balloon, and the real thoughts in my head just keep on a direct line. The direct line and the balloon are related, but they do not correspond, and the more the balloon bulges, the less sense it makes, until it bursts, leaving nearly all my thoughts scattered, and me wild with anger and shame. (Blackman, 1999, p. 135)

There are, on occasion, still times when I want to talk, but I can't. I can try and try and try, but I can't talk. There is a fear holding me back. I do not know what it is I am afraid of, I only know that it is a feeling of fear unlike any other feeling of fear I have ever known. It is not that I do not want to talk, it is that I am unable to at that moment. (McKean, 1994, p. 39)

I am very fortunate that my friends and family are people who know me very intimately. Many times I feel as if oral communication is over rated. Much of how I express myself is through my eyes. Those close to me are easily able to tell if I am sick, tired, or happy, by just looking at my face. My expressions are not always appropriate yet my eyes are the windows to my soul. (Rubin, in Biklen, 2005, p. 89)

For most individuals with ASD, there are no problems with the physical form or function of the mouth, vocal cords, or other parts of the anatomy involved in speech and communication. Nonetheless, challenges with both nonverbal and verbal communication are a defining characteristic of ASD. Approximately 33% to 50% of individuals with ASD do not develop functional speech (Noens & van Berckelaer-Onnes, 2005). If an individual with ASD does use speech, there may be impairments in the ability to initiate or sustain conversations (Paul & Sutherland, 2005).

The quality or tone of voice of an individual with ASD may be monotone, singsong, flat, husky, or unusual sounding. Fay (1980) described that the prosody, pitch, or volume in speech may be unusual. Intonation may be mechanical, wooden, or arrhythmic. This can be problematic, as others may believe that the individual is cold, aloof, or odd.

Individuals with ASD may also use immediate or delayed echolalia (Fay,

1980; Prizant & Rydell, 1993). Immediate echolalia refers to repeating sounds or speech that the individual has just heard. Delayed echolalia refers to repeating sounds or speech that the individual has heard in the past. There is great debate as to the purpose of echolalia. Some researchers believe that echolalia serves different functions for individuals with ASD (Prizant & Rydell, 1993). Some have described it as attempts to communicate with those around them or as self-stimulatory or calming, whereas others have called echolalia "words of annoyance" that are not volitional and have little meaning.

Individuals with ASD have also reported difficulty with processing speech (Kluth, 2009, 2010). They have reported challenges with hearing and processing all aspects of speech. Many report that they hear bits and pieces of a conversation and have trouble processing and understanding the general message of the speaker. Understanding different types of language can also be challenging. In addition, individuals with ASD often have trouble with figurative language, idioms, metaphors, jokes, slang, and sarcasm (Kluth, 2009).

A review by Hall (2009) summarized common communication challenges associated with ASD. For example, challenge in the use of pronouns has been reported, with the individual with ASD often using the third person when talking about himself or herself (Scheuermann & Webber, 2002). Gender is also commonly confused in the speech of individuals with ASD, with words such as *he, she,* or *it* being used incorrectly. Difficulty with word boundaries and a tendency to comprehend phrases as single chunks of speech are also common in individuals with ASD (Fay, 1980). Using bound morphemes can also be challenging. Answering *Wh-*questions can also present challenges for individuals with ASD (Koegel & Koegel, 1995). It has also been reported that individuals with ASD have a greater capacity for learning nouns over verbs.

Sensory Differences

The unmodulated sensory input often overwhelmed me, causing me mental torture, and I would begin feeling mentally confused and sluggish. My head would feel fogged so that I could not think. My vision would blur, and the speech of those around me would become gibberish. My whole body buzzed. The slight tremor that always plagued me would worsen. My hands would feel detached from my body, as if they were foreign objects. I would be paralyzed, unable to comprehend my own movements unless I could see them. I could not tell where my hand started and the table ended, or what shape the table was, or even if it was rough or smooth. I felt like I was in a cartoon world. (Hawthorne, as cited in Gillingham, 2000, pp. 21–22)

Individuals with ASD have reported a variety of sensory differences. Most often, individuals report hypo- or hyper-responses to stimuli affecting their sense of smell, touch, vision, taste, temperature, and hearing (Gillingham, 2000). In addition, individuals with ASD have reported differences with their vestibular system and proprioception (Gillingham, 2000). The impact of sensory differences in the everyday life of an individual with ASD should not be underestimated and is an area in need of support. The description of each area of sensory differences will focus heavily on the experience of individuals with ASD to give you a rich understanding of how these differences affect them.

Tactile Sensitivity

Individuals with ASD can experience the sensation of touch in different ways (Robledo et al., 2012). Some may crave and seek out touch, whereas others may avoid touch in any way. On the same hand, individuals with ASD may seek out deep-pressure touch, like a firm hug or handshake, while at the same time pull away from light or soft touch. Unexpected touch can startle many individuals with ASD and should be avoided. Many individuals report avoiding activities or situations where touch may become unbearable. Sean Barron and Temple Grandin described their experiences with tactile sensitivity:

I felt acutely uncomfortable sitting upright in the bathtub, so I didn't enjoy taking a bath in the least. I absolutely hated the way my bottom felt against the tub, and I couldn't make myself think about something else so I wouldn't feel it. When I tried to sit normally it felt "squishy" and I was extremely sensitive to this feeling. I couldn't shake it off. It was the same feeling I used to have when I couldn't stand to touch our rug with my bare feet. To make it more bearable, I shifted most of my weight onto one side so that only a part of me came into contact with the bathtub. When they insisted I "sit right," it only compounded the problem. (Barron & Barron, 1992, p. 96)

"I'll miss you, Temple." She walked quickly to my side and kissed my cheek. I ached to be enfolded in her arms, but how could she know? I stood rigid as a pole trapped

by the approach avoidance syndrome of autism. I drew back from her kiss, not able to endure tactile stimulation—not even loving, tactile stimulation. (Grandin & Scariano, 1986, p. 65)

Individuals with tactile sensitivities also describe challenges with personal hygiene such as brushing teeth and hair. Others have also reported avoiding certain fabrics and/or preferring to wear similar clothing again and again. Tactile sensitivities have also been reported in eating. Many individuals with ASD seek or avoid particular food textures. This sensitivity may limit their diet.

Auditory Sensitivities

Auditory input such as noises and sounds typically causes anxiety for individuals with ASD. Donna Williams (1992, 1994) and Temple Grandin (1995) explained that hearing certain sounds created painful experiences. Williams (1992) expressed that the tone of someone's voice can disturb her. Grandin (1992) described her hearing as feeling "like having a hearing aid with the volume control stuck on super loud" (p. 107) and expressed that "sudden loud noises hurt my ears like a dentist's drill hitting a nerve" (p. 107). She further described her dislike for environments that had many different noises, "such as shopping centers and sports arenas. High pitched continuous noise, such as bathroom vent fans or hair dryers, are annoying" (p. 2).

Lucy Blackman (1999) described her auditory differences:

Because other people's sound processing was alien to me, I had no idea that sound should not be like a pressure-cooker lid.

I put my hands to my ears for loud sudden noises, but the continuous clamour of everyday life was only relieved by movement. Even in the classroom there was visual stimulation and noise, which combined with my own breathing and a buzzing effect that I think was my own inner ear. (p. 51)

Matt Ward explained that sudden loud noises were very stressful:

Especially things like gunshots, loud motors, and brass bands. My mom took me through a drive-thru car wash once when I was in grade school and I was terrified. The brushes sounded to me like the sound of intense machine gun fire, but I could not communicate well enough to explain why I got so upset. (Robledo et al., 2012, p. 4)

Other individuals with ASD noted that at times, their ability to process auditory input was inconsistent. Darren White explained a "trick which my ears played was to change the volume of sounds around me. Sometimes when other kids spoke to me I could scarcely hear them and sometimes they sounded like bullets" (White & White, 1987, p. 225). Donna Williams (1992) also expressed difficulties in understanding people. She sometimes needed people to repeat a particular sentence several times because she heard the message in bits. She stated that her mind segments sentences into words. This leaves her with a strange and sometimes unintelligible message. She described it as a "bit like when someone plays around with the volume switch on a TV." (p. 69). In fact, she described that she would sometimes turn the sound up and down on the television, breaking up people's voices while keeping the picture intact. This seemed to imitate the difficulty she sometimes had hearing people consistently.

Visual Sensitivities

Individuals with ASD have described several different types of visual differences, including unique interactions with colors, stimulation or pain caused by visual stimuli, different responses to lighting, and challenges with eye contact.

Sean Barron described his intrigue with colors and the positive emotions he felt when comparing colors for hours at a time (Barron & Barron, 1992). Donna Williams (1992) also discussed her unusual interaction with colors. Her early memories included spending hours looking at bright spots of color that made her laugh. Years later she learned that the spots of color were air particles of reflected light, which she was able to see due to her hypersensitivity to color and light.

Other individuals with ASD experienced colors quite differently. Darren White described a situation where he received a bike as a Christmas present. He explained that he could not look at the yellow color on his bike because it was too painful. Extra red was added to make the color look orange and that color "blurred upwards making it look like it was on fire" (White & White, 1987, p. 226). Other colors were also problematic for him; he could not see blue clearly because it "looked too light and it looked like ice" (p. 227).

Many individuals report sensitivity to lights, particularly fluorescent light. A participant in Robledo et al. (2012) pointed out, "There are certain types of light I cannot tolerate—they make me nervous . . . If I am in a hall and it is too bright, I can't handle it, I have to put a sun hat on. Fluorescent light absolutely turns my stomach into knots. It does a trip on my nervous system" (p. 5). A variety of colors and patterns have also been reported as problematic.

A common visual characteristic in ASD is a lack of eye contact (Kluth, 2009; Robledo et al., 2012). The following individuals with ASD shared their perspective on lack of eye contact related to visual sensitivity:

When I concentrated on the sound, I felt my eyes and nose shutting off. I could never do everything together at the same time. That is, I could not see you and at the same time hear you. My sense of hearing was always sharper than my sight. This is the reason I never used my eyes to interact with anybody. Psychologists call it "lack of eye contact." The result was the knowledge of a fragmented world perceived through isolated sense organs. (Mukhopadhyay 2000, p. 74)

Sometimes, eye contact literally is painful for me to achieve. This has become easier for me to achieve however with those in my life with whom I am extremely comfortable. There are certain days, though, where eye contact is not something I am able to achieve, regardless of who the person is. (Rubin, in Biklen, 2005, p. 89)

Olfactory Sensitivities

Individuals with ASD have also reported sensitivities to smell. Some smells may be unbearable, whereas others are pleasing. Intense smells such as perfume or air fresheners may be highly distracting for individuals with ASD. It is important to note that many of these smells do not bother individuals without ASD. Therefore, it is critical to examine the environment for potential sensory triggers.

Other Areas of Sensitivity

Additional areas of sensitivity that individuals with ASD have report include sensitivities to taste, temperate, pain, vestibular system, and proprioception (Gillingham, 2000). It is critical to become aware of the particular sensitivities an individual with ASD may experience. As well, variables such as emotion, fatigue, and hunger can greatly affect a person's ability to regulate their sensory system.

Movement Differences

I often can't control my body and make jerky weird movements. I believe the problem is with purposeful movement. Sadly we cannot even move from one place to another when we want to. We compensate by going where a movement takes us and actually use our weird movements to get where we want to go. For example, when I want to move from one area on the keyboard to another I will jerk and have my hand land where I want it to. Movements appear as mental retardation when we can't get our bodies to follow directions. Movement disorders make it appear that we don't understand what is being asked or we are being non-compliant. (Rubin et al., 2001, p. 426)

I cannot seem to tell my right from my left although I know my right from my left. I cannot seem to find my mouth upon command. I have trouble finding where my nose is when I am asked. I find that my breath will not come when I am asked to blow or when I am asked to take a deep breath. I am unable to draw through a straw. I have trouble sticking out my tongue. I cannot seem to spit the water out when brushing my teeth. I cannot

purse my lips when I want to drink out of a bottle. I don't seem to get the message to wave or to smile when I should be responding to someone or something. My autism seems to be apparent in my random use of my hands and feet. My habit of biting is a symptom of my being nonverbal and is mostly due to frustration. (Hale & Hale, 1999, p. 60)

They asked him to point at his body parts, but the boy could not do it. Not that he was ignorant of the parts of the human body, but he was unable to point and identify them in his own self. Pointing at objects was difficult too, as he pointed only at the letters on the board and could not generalize it with the other things. Then the doctors asked the other way around. They touched his legs and hands and so on. They asked him to point on the board. This he did with ease. (Mukhopadhyay, 2000, p. 26)

At times, individuals with ASD may move their bodies in ways that seem atypical to individuals without ASD. They might rock, or flap, or jump, or repeatedly touch an object. We might assume that these behaviors are communicative attempts to interact or volitional behaviors that demonstrate a diminished cognitive ability. Movement differences are the least understood characteristic of ASD. However, many researchers (Leary & Donnellan, 2012; Torres et al., 2013) have indicated that our understanding of these movement differences will not only help us better support individuals with ASD but will also play a significant role in objectively measuring and standardizing ASD—its treatment and the tracking of an individual's changes over time.

Donnellan, Leary, and Robledo (2006) have defined a movement difference as a difference, interference, or shift in the efficient, effective utilization and integration of movement—a disruption in the organization and regulation of perception, action, posture, language, speech, thought, emotion, and/or memory. Movement differences are manifested in a wide range of behaviors, including the more easily identifiable activities such as unusual gait and posture, constant physical movement, or repetitive rocking. Other movement differences tend to become evident at transition points. Among these are the following:

- Starting—difficulty initiating
- Executing—difficulty with the rate, rhythm, target, and so on of movement
- Continuing—difficulty "staying on track," not taking alternative paths, and so forth
- Stopping—difficulty terminating a movement; the tendency to "perseverate"; getting "stuck" in one sensory mode like staring into space
- Combining—difficulty adding a sensory mode or a movement (e.g., listening to someone speak while watching his or her gestures and facial expression, doing two things at once, etc.)
- Switching—difficulty "letting go" of one perception or movement and initiating a new one.

Many individuals without ASD also experience movement differences from time to time. However, the intensity, duration, rhythm, rate, frequency, and/ or timing of these movement differences are exacerbated in individuals with ASD, affecting their ability to communicate, relate, and function in their communities.

Learning Differences

I think in pictures. Words are like a second language to me. I translate both spoken and written words into full-color movies, complete with sounds, which run like a VCR tape in my head. When somebody speaks to me, his words are instantly translated into pictures. (Grandin, 1995, p. 19)

All of the previous described characteristics of ASD can affect an individual's ability to learn. Many individuals with ASD have reported experiencing learning challenges similar to those with learning disabilities. Difficulty with input, organization, memory, and output can occur (Kluth, 2009). Difficulties with generalization have often been reported (Kluth, 2009). Many individuals have learning strengths in concrete thinking and have more difficulty with abstract thinking, awareness, and judgment. It is critical to remember that lack of cognitive ability might not be the area of challenge. Rather, an individual may not be performing academically due to other challenges of ASD, such a sensory sensitivities, movement differences, or communication skills.

Individuals with ASD also have learning strengths, including highly developed text reading, word recognition, and precocious reading development. In addition, many display advanced skills with memorizing chunks or language, including songs. Many have excellent mathematical skills or can write beautiful poetry.

Passions, Interests, and Rituals

People with autism like routines, and if those routines are broken it does not mean that we don't understand what is happening it just means that it is harder for us than most to stop our brains from spinning off into their regular patterns. (Rubin, in Biklen, 2005, p. 88)

Many individuals with ASD have intense passions, fascination, and interests (Kluth, 2009). Some may have only a few interests over their life, while others vary. The most common fascinations across individuals with ASD are trains, vehicles, transportation systems, machines, weather, natural disasters, geography, animals, drawings, music, pop stars, and television shows (Hippler & Klicpera, 2004; Mercier, Mottron, & Belleville, 2000).

Individuals with ASD often follow specific rituals in their lives. These might involve how objects, space, and time are organized or may involve repetitive types of behavior. Passions, interests, and rituals clearly serve a specific purpose to the individual with ASD. As such, it is critical to understand the role these are playing within their lives.

FOUNDATIONAL SUPPORTS

Individuals with ASD can be successful in any and every environment. The following section will highlight some foundational strategies and supports that will enable you to support individuals with ASD. Although there are numerous methodologies and packaged programs available to support individuals with ASD, this section focuses on foundational supports that should be involved in every interaction and intervention.

Inclusion and Collaborative Teaming

Inclusion supports and benefits all learners. It stresses interdependence and inde-

pendence, views all students as capable and complex, values a sense of community, and promotes civil rights and equity (Doyle, 2008; Falvey, Givner, & Kimm, 1995; Kluth, 2010; Sapon-Shevin, 2007; Udvari-Solner, 1997; Villa & Thousand, 1995). For individuals with ASD, access to the least restrictive environments will help them learn and grow. Opportunities to practice and learn from typically developing peers are invaluable for individuals with ASD. Supporting individuals with ASD requires a collaborative team approach. Professionals, parents, peers, and the individuals themselves should all be on the same page when designing supports across the life span.

Relationships and Belonging

Developing, maintaining, and facilitating relationships and belonging are critical for building community for individuals with ASD. Relationships with parents, therapists, teachers, peers, and others should guide all supports for individuals with ASD. When an individual with ASD feels he or she is in a safe, supportive, and trusting relationship, learning and growth will occur. Collaboration and connection with families and individuals with ASD is key—they are the true experts in ASD.

Social Communication Supports

As many individuals with ASD struggle to communicate and interact socially, communication and social support must be at the forefront of any intervention. It is critical to take the perspective of the individual with ASD and focus on what communication and social skills are important and meaningful to his or her life. Fitting students with ASD into packaged communication or social skills programs does not take into account the individual variability that all individuals with ASD present. Our challenge is to determine what supports and strategies work best for *this* individual with ASD. It is a difficult yet fruitful task.

Sensory and Movement Supports

Understanding each individual's unique sensory system and patterns of movement is critical for truly offering personalized supports and accommodations. This will require that you get to know the individual you work with by listening and observing. As you become more familiar with the individual and build a relationship with that individual, you will be able to partner as a team to discover the best accommodations, modification, and adaptations to fit the individual needs of the person you support.

Positive Behavior Supports

It is important to remember that individuals with ASD are trying their best to behave appropriately. Often what looks on the surface like a problem behavior is actually a manifestation of a sensory or movement problem, physical discomfort, and/or an inability to communicate effectively or to understand or perform what is being asked (Kluth, 2010). Be sure you spend ample time *teaching* and *reinforcing* desired behaviors. When trouble does arise, employ strategies that are respectful and promote learning and growth. Behavioral support should not be about control; rather, it should be about collaboratively teaming to support dreams.

Learning and Environmental Supports

By understanding the many characteristics of ASD, you can help create environments and supports that will enable individuals with ASD to function effectively. Think about the sensory systems of the individuals with ASD who you support—what types of sensory sensitivities do they have and in what ways can they be accommodated in the environment? Individuals with ASD have typically reported that they learn best when materials are presented clearly and visually. Active learning that provides visuals, examples, manipulatives, and interaction will be most successful. Do not forget to use your most valuable resource—the individuals with ASD. Elicit their perspective on ways they might be better supported. Be creative and flexible in all supports.

CONCLUDING THOUGHTS

This chapter presented a general overview of ASD, including definitions, characteristics, and foundational supports. Effective support requires true understanding of each and every individual that you work with. As SLPAs, your growth in understanding will come from working with, listening to, and knowing individuals with ASD in your daily practice.

REFERENCES

American Psychiatric Association. (2013). *Diagnostic and statistical manual of mental disorders* (5th ed.). Washington, DC: Author.

Attwood, T. (1998). *Asperger's syndrome: A guide for parents and professionals*. Philadelphia, PA: Kingsley.

Baron-Cohen, S. (1989). The autistic child's theory of mind: A case of specific developmental delay. *Journal of Child Psychology and Psychiatry, 30*, 285–297.

Barron, J., & Barron, S. (1992). *There's a boy in here.* New York. NY: Simon & Schuster.

Bellini, S. (2006). Social challenges of children and youth with autism spectrum disorders. In E. Boutot & B. Myles (Eds.), *Autism spectrum disorders: Foundations, characteristics, and effective strategies* (pp. 201–222) Upper Saddle River, NJ: Pearson.

Bellini, S. (2008). *Buildings social relationships: A systematic approach to teaching social interaction skills to children and adolescents with autism spectrum disorders and other social difficulties.* Shawnee Mission, KS: Autism Asperger Publishing.

Biklen, D. (2005). *Autism and the myth of the person alone.* New York, NY: New York University Press.

Blackman, L. (1999). *Lucy's story: Autism and other adventures.* Brisbane, Australia: Book in Hand.

Brown, J., & Whiten, A. (2000). Imitation, theory of mind and related activities in autism: An observational study of spontaneous behavior in everyday contexts. *Autism: The International Journal of Research and Practice, 4*, 185–205.

Centers for Disease Control and Prevention. (2012). *Prevalence of autism spectrum disorders—Autism and Developmental Disabilities Monitoring Network, 14 sites, United States, 2008.* Retrieved from http://www.cdc.gov/ncbddd/autism/data.html

Dawson, G., & Fernald, M. (1987). Perspective taking ability and its relationship to the social behavior of autistic children. *Journal of Autism and Developmental Disorders, 17*, 487–489.

Donnellan, A., Leary, M., & Robledo, J. (2006). I can't get started: Stress and the role of movement differences for individuals with the autism label. In G. Baron, J. Groden, G. Groden, & L. Lipsitt (Eds.), *Stress and coping in autism* (pp. 205–245). Oxford, UK: Oxford University Press.

Doyle, M. (2008). *The paraprofessional's guide to the inclusive classroom: Working as a team* (3rd ed.). Baltimore, MD: Brookes.

Falvey, M., Givner, C., & Kimm, C. (1995). What is an inclusive school? In R. Villa & J. Thousand (Eds.), *Creating an inclusive school* (pp. 1–12). Alexandria, VA: ASCD.

Fay, W. (1980). Aspects of language. In W. Fay & A. Schuler (Eds.), *Emerging language in autistic children* (pp. 51–85). Baltimore, MD: University Park Press.

Flavell, J., Miller, P., & Miller, S. (1993). *Cognitive development* (3rd ed.). Upper Saddle River, NJ: Prentice-Hall.

Gillingham, G. (2000). *Autism: A new understanding!* Edmonton, Canada: Tacit.

Grandin, T. (1992). An inside view of autism. In E. Schopler & G. B. Mesibov (Eds.), *High-functioning individuals with autism* (pp. 105–126). New York, NY: Plenum.

Grandin, T. (1995). *Thinking in pictures: And other reports from my life with autism.* New York, NY: Doubleday.

Grandin, T., & Scariano, M. (1986). *Emergence: Labeled autistic.* Novato, CA: Arena.

Hale, M., & Hale, C. (1999). *I had no means to shout!* Bloomington, IN: 1st Books.

Hall, L. (2009). *Autism spectrum disorders: From theory to practice.* Upper Saddle River, NJ: Pearson.

Heflin, L., & Alaimo, D. (2007). *Students with autism spectrum disorder: Effective instructional practices.* Upper Saddle River, NJ: Pearson.

Hippler, K., & Klicpera, C. (2004). A retrospective analysis of the clinical case records of "autistic psychopaths" diagnosed by Hans Asperger and his team at the University Children's Hospital, Vienna. In U. Frith & E. Hill (Eds.), *Autism: Mind and brain* (pp. 21–42). Oxford, UK: Oxford University Press.

Kanner, L. (1943). Autistic disturbances of affective contact. *Nervous Child, 2*, 217–230.

Kluth, P. (2009). *The Autism Checklist: A practical reference for parents and teachers.* San Francisco, CA: Jossey-Bass.

Kluth, P. (2010). *'You're going to love this kid!' Teaching students with autism in the inclusive classroom* (2nd ed.). Baltimore, MD: Paul H. Brookes.

Knoblauch, B., & Sorenson, B. (1998). IDEA's definition of disabilities. *ERIC Digest.* Reston, VA: ERIC Clearinghouse on Disabilities and Gifted Education.

Koegel, R., & Koegel, L. (1995). *Teaching children with autism: Strategies for initiating positive interactions and improving learning opportunities.* Baltimore, MD: Brookes.

Leary, M. R., & Donnellan, A. M. (2012). *Autism: Sensory-movement differences and diversity.* Cambridge, WI: Cambridge Book Review Press.

McDonnell, J. (1993). *News from the border.* New York, NY: Ticknor & Fields.

McKean, T. (1994). *Soon will come the light.* Arlington, TX: Future Horizons.

Mercier, C., Mottron, L., & Belleville, S. (2000). Psychosocial study on restricted interest in high-functioning persons with pervasive developmental disorders. *Autism, 4,* 406–425.

Mukhopadhyay, T. R. (2000). *Beyond the silence.* London, UK: National Autistic Society.

Noens, I., & van Berckelaer-Onnes, I. (2005). Captured by details: Sense-making, language and communication in autism. *Journal of Communication Disorders, 38,* 123–141.

O'Neil, J. (1999). *Through the eyes of aliens: A book about autistic people.* Philadelphia, PA: Jessica Kingsley.

Paul, R., & Sutherland, D. (2005). Enhancing early language in children with autism spectrum disorder. In F. Volkmar, R. Paul, A. Klin, & D. Cohen (Eds.), *Handbook of autism and pervasive developmental disorders* (3rd ed., pp. 925–945). New York, NY: John Wiley.

Prizant, B., & Rydell, P. (1993). Assessment and intervention strategies for unconventional verbal behavior. In J. Reichle & D. Wacker (Vol. Eds.), *Communication approaches to challenging behavior: Integrating functional assessment and intervention strategies* (pp. 263–297). Baltimore, MD: Brookes.

Resnick, L., Levine, J., & Teasley, S. (1991). *Perspectives on socially shared cognition.* Washington, DC: American Psychological Association.

Robinson, J. (2007). *Look me in the eye: My life with Asperger's.* New York, NY: Crown.

Robledo, J., Strandt-Conroy, K., & Donnellan, A. (2012). An exploration of sensory and movement differences from the perspective of individuals with autism. *Frontiers in Integrative Neuroscience, 6,* 1–13.

Rogers, S. (2000). Interventions that facilitate socialization in children in autism. *Journal of Autism and Developmental Disabilities, 30,* 399–409.

Rubin, S., Biklen, D., Kasa-Hendrickson, K., Kluth, P., Cardinal, D., & Broderick, A. (2001). Independence, participation, and the meaning of intellectual ability. *Disability and Society, 16,* 425–429.

Sapon-Shevin, M. (2007). *Widening the circle: The power of inclusive classrooms.* Boston, MA: Beacon.

Scheuermann, B., & Webber, J. (2002). *Autism: Teaching does make a difference.* Belmont, CA: Wadsworth/Thomson Learning.

Sinclair, J. (1993). Don't mourn for us. *Our Voice, 1*(3). Retrieved September 8, 2013, from http://ani.autistics.org/don't_mourn.html

Torres, E., Brincker, M., Isenhower, R., Yanovich, P., Stigler, K., Numbereger, J., . . . Jose, J. (2013). Autism: The micro-movement perspective. *Frontiers in Integrative Neuroscience, 7,* 1–26.

Travis, L., Sigman, M., & Ruskin, E. (2001). Links between social understanding and social behavior in verbally able children with autism. *Journal of Autism and Developmental Disorders, 31,* 119–130.

Udvari-Solner, A. (1997). Inclusive education. In C. Grant & G. Ladson-Billings (Eds.), *Dictionary of multicultural education* (pp. 141–144). Phoenix, AZ: Oryx.

Villa, R., & Thousand, J. (1995). *Creating an inclusive school* (pp. 1–12). Alexandria, VA: ASCD.

Waterhouse, L., Fein, D., & Modahl, C. (1996). Neurofunctional mechanisms in autism. *Psychological Review, 103,* 457–489.

White, G. B., & White, M. S. (1987). Autism from the inside. *Medical Hypothesis, 24,* 223–229.

Williams, D. (1992). *Nobody nowhere.* New York, NY: Avon.

Williams, D. (1994). *Somebody somewhere.* New York, NY: Times Books.

Wing, L., & Gould, J. (1979). Severe impairments of social interaction and associated abnormalities in children: Epidemiology and classification. *Journal of Autism and Developmental Disorders, 9,* 11–29.

Index

Note: Page numbers in **bold** reference non-text material.

A

A-/an-/dys-, usage of, 149
   AAC. *See* Augmentative and alternative communication
Abduct/adduct, usage of, 146
Accept/except, usage of, 146
Access barriers, 322
Accountability, 28
Activities
   adults: group activities, 327
   children: group activities, 323–324
   children: social skills group activities, 334–336
   children: speech sound remediation, 373–375, **375**
   cultural consciousness activities, 160, 170
   lesson plan section, 197–200
Activity logs, 86
Activity records, 86
Activity/task section, lesson plans, 197–200
Adams, L., 322
Adduct/abduct, usage of, 146
Adults
   inpatient sample report for, 239–240
   language disorder sample goals and objectives, 241–242
   outpatient sample report, 226–230
   suggested group activities for, **327**
Affect/effect, usage of, 145
Age equivalent, of children, 268
Aided AAC communication, 390–391
Aids, augmentative and alternative communication, 389–391
Airborne transmission, **173**
Airway obstruction, 181–182, **181**
Allergic reactions, 183
Alphabet boards, **391**, 402
Alphabetic principle, **348**

Alternate/alternative, usage of, 145
American Sign Language (ASL), 383, **384**
American Speech-Language-Hearing Association (ASHA), 3, 4
   administrative support by, 10, **10**, 20
   affiliation status, 13–14, 18
   on bilingual service providers, 160, 162, 164
   Board of Ethics, 90, 117, 124
   Code of Ethics, 22, 35, 90–91, **91–94**, 94, 98, **99**, 104–108, 118
   confidentiality statement, 117–124
   on electronic communication, 132
   Frequently Asked Question file on website, 5
   on lesson plans, 194–195
   mentoring program, 82, 84nn1,2
   on play, 339–340
   practice portals, 5
   prevention and advocacy by SLPAs, 10, **11**, 20–21
   resources for SLPAs, 5
   service delivery to culturally and linguistically diverse clients and students, 156
   SLP scope of practice, 35
   SLPA duties and responsibilities, 7–9, **8**, **9**
   SLPA job description, 10–11
   SLPA minimal qualifications, 7
   SLPA minimum qualifications, 18–19
   SLPA responsibilities, 8–10, **9**, **10**, 11, **11**, 19–21
   SLPA responsibilities outside SLPA scope of activities, 7, **8**, 21–22, 253
   SLPA scope of practice, 4, 16–29, 35, 288
   SLPA scope of responsibility, 8–10, **9**, **10**, 11, **11**
   SLPA service delivery, 8–10, **9**, 20
   on SLPAs as interpreters/translators, 162

American Speech-Language-Hearing
Association (ASHA) *(continued)*
   *Speech-Language Pathology Assistant Scope
     of Practice* (2013), 4
   State Advocacy Team, 5
   on supervision of support personnel,
     109–111
   website, 5
Analyze portion, SOAP note, 275–277, **276,
   277**
Angelou, Maya, 355
Annual goals, 195
Antecedent-behavior-consequence
   sequence, 289, 305, 311–312
Appearance, 128–129
Apps
   for communications purposes, **392**, 408,
     409
   for speech sound remediation, 375
Argentina, 30
*Articulatory and Phonological Impairments:
   A Clinical Focus* (Bauman-Waengler),
   366
ASD. *See* Autism spectrum disorders
ASHA. *See* American Speech-Language-
   Hearing Association
ASHA Code of Ethics (2010), 22, 35, 90–91,
   91–94, 94, 98, **99**, 104–108, 118
ASL. *See* American Sign Language
Aspiration precautions, 184–186, **185**
Assessment of patients/clients, 194
   note writing during, 271–285
   oral peripheral examination, 252
   preschool initial speech-language
     assessment, 204–210
   vs. analysis, 276–277, **276, 277**
Assessment of speech-language pathology
   assistants
   competency assessment of, 11–13, **12,**
     61–65
   direct observation skills brief checklist,
     69, 70
   in educational setting, 70, 151–152
   journaling, 136, **137**, 279, **280**
   in medical setting, 69, 153
   self-assessment and self-improvement,
     135–138, **137**
   self-evaluation of intervention sessions,
     151–154

skills proficiency checklist, 71
technical proficiency checklist, 66–68
Assimilation, **360**
Assistive technology (AT), 382–383
   See also Augmentative and alternative
     communication
Associative play, 352
Audio recording, for speech and language
   sample, 260
Audiology associations, international,
   30–34
Auditory bombardment, **364**
Auditory prompts, 303, **304**
Auditory sensitivities, autism spectrum
   disorders and, 420–421
Augmentative and alternative
   communication (AAC), 312, 381–411
   aided communication, 390–391
   aids, 389–391
   assistive technology (AT), 382–383
   barriers to use of, 321
   children, **386**
   components, 387–395
   defined, 383
   devices, 389
   intervention guidelines, 394–396
   intervention, purposes of, 384–385
   medical conditions that benefit from
     AAC, **385**
   myths about, 385, **386–387**, 387
   sample goals and objectives, 242
   strategies, 392, **393**
   symbols, 387–389, **388, 389**, 392, **393**, 394
   techniques, 392, **393**, 394
   tips for, 397
   unaided communication, 389–390, **389**
   users, 383–384, **385**
   vocabulary selection, 396–397, **396**
Augmented input strategies, 394
Australia, 30
Austria, 30
Autism spectrum disorders (ASD),
   413–427
   behavioral supports, 425
   characteristics of, 415–424
   clinical definitions, 414
   collaborative teaming and, 424
   communication challenges, 417–419
   educational definitions, 414–415

Index **431**

foundational supports, 424–425
inclusion as supportive, 424
insider's perspective, 415
learning differences, 423, 425
movement differences and, 422–423, 425
nonverbal communication and, 416
passions, fascinations, and interests, 423–424
relationships and belonging, 424
rituals and, 424
sample goals and objectives, 242–243
sensory differences, 419–422, 425
social communication and, 414, 424–425
social differences and, 416–417

B

Balls, as therapeutic activity, **347**
Barriers, to use of augmentative and alternative communication, 321
Barron, Sean, 419, 421
Battle, D., 157
Bauman-Waengler, J., 366
Behavior code, 309–310
Belgium, 30
Benchmarks, 197
Bernthal, J., 357
Big Muscles! (group activity), 335
Bilingual individuals, 159, 164
Bilingual service provider, 160, 162, 164
Bilingual SLPAs, 45, 157–158, 160, 162
Biliterate person, 166
Bird, A., 357
Bishop, Elin, 55
Blackman, Lucy, 420
Blackstone, S., 381
Blind-review process, confidentiality and, 119
Blissymbol, 388, **388**
Blocks, as therapeutic activity, 347
Bloom, L., 346
Boardmaker choice icons, **395**, 400
Body jewelry, 129
Body language, 130, 416
Books, with print salience, 349
Bound morphemes, 418–419
Bowen, C., 357
Bowling, as therapeutic activity, 334–335, **375**

Boyce, S.E., 366
Bradley, D.F., 328
Brazil, 30
Bubbles, as therapeutic activity, **347**
Burda, A., 159

C

Cajun dialect, 157
Canada, 30
Cardiac arrest, 179
Cardiopulmonary resuscitation (CPR), 178
Cars, as therapeutic activity, **347**
Carter, E.W., 318
Cause-effect actions, 340
Cerebral embolism, 179–180
Cerebral thrombosis, 179
Cerebrovascular accident (CVA). *See* Stroke
Certificate of Clinical Competence, 23, 26, 76, 105
Chabon, S.S., 90, 94
CHD. *See* Coronary heart disease
Checklists
clinical note writing checklist, 279, **281**
in data collection, 249–251, **250**, **252**
direct observation skills brief checklist, 69, 70
skills proficiency checklist, 71
technical proficiency checklist, 66–68
Chest compression, 179
Children
age equivalent and MLU, 268
antecedent-behavior-consequence sequence, 289, 305, 311–312
augmentative and alternative communication (AAC), **386**
client-centered approaches, 289
cognitive development, 340, **340**
elementary school Individualized Education Plan, 211–218
inability to speak, statistics, 382
language disorder goals and objectives, 243–244
with limited language ability, 370
morphological features, 269
motivation, 291
outpatient sample report, 231–238
preschool initial speech-language assessment, 204–210

432 *Speech-Language Pathology Assistants: A Resource Manual*

Children *(continued)*
  private practice sample report for, 219–225
  sample group activities for, **323–324**
  social skills group activities, 334–336
  speech and language sample, 260–261
  speech and language screening, 251
  speech sound remediation, 360–379
  visual rules for posting, 328, **329**
  See also Play
Choice boards, **391**, 403
Classroom management principles, in
    group treatment, 328–331, **329**, **330**
Cleaning, of contaminated surfaces,
    177–178, 189–190
Client-centered approaches, 289, 305
Client information, confidentiality of, 35,
    98, 102–103, 105, 118
Clients
  clinical rapport with, 297–301
  clinician-client relationship, 290
  motivation, 290–291
  sitting position of, 292, **292**
  with special medical needs, 183–187
  See also Assessment of patients/clients
Clinical interactions, 301–315
  demonstration/modeling, 301–302, **302**
  directions, 301
  operant conditioning, 305
  prompts/scaffolding, 302–303, **304**, 305,
    332
Clinical notes. *See* Note writing
Clinical rapport, 297–301
"Clinical" service delivery model, 288
Clinician-client relationship, 290
Clinician-directed approaches, 289, 305
Clock communicator, 391, 404
Clothing, professional attire, 128–129
Cloze procedures, as scaffolding approach,
    345
CLSA. *See* Computer-aided language
    sample analysis
Cluster reduction, **360**
Co-articulation, **365**
Code-switching, 395
Cognitive development, of children, 340,
    340
Colleagues, confidentiality in relation to,
    103, 123–124

Comic strip, as group therapy tool, **323**, **325**
Common medical abbreviations, 131–132,
    141–142
Commonly misspelled words, 132, 150
Commonly misused words, 132, 145–149
Communication
  autism spectrum disorders (ASD),
    417–419
  body language, 130
  defined, 383
  disability-sensitive communication,
    132–133, **134**, 135
  electronic communication, 132
  non-verbal communication, 130
  scaffolding communication, 344, **345**
  verbal communication, 120–121, 129–131,
    138
  written communication, 131–132,
    141–144, 145–150
  See also Augmentative and alternative
    communication
Communication books, **391**, 400
Communication temptations, 343
Competency assessment, 11–13, **12**, 61–65
Computer-aided language sample analysis
    (CLSA), 263
Computers
  apps for communications purposes, **392**,
    408, 409
  eye-tracking device, 392, 410–411
Concrete operations, 341
Confidentiality
  ASHA confidentiality statement, 117–124
  of client information, 35, 98, 102–103, 105
  to record speech and language sample,
    260
  of recorded speech and language
    sample, 260
  in relationships with peers and
    colleagues, 103, 123–124
  research and, 118, 119–120
  rights of incompetent individuals,
    117–118
  student privacy issues, 122–123
  of treatment plans, 194
  verbal communication and, 120–121
  of written records, 121–122
Conflict resolution, 138–140, **139**

Consensus building, 94
Consent, to record speech and language sample, 260
Consequences, in treatment, 289, 311
Consonant clusters/blends, in development of speech, 358–359, **359**
Consonants, in development of speech, 357–358
Contact transmission, **173**
Contextual cues, **365**
Conversation ladder, **323**, **327**
Core vocabulary, 396–397, **396**
Coronary heart disease (CHD), 180
Corrective feedback, in treatment, 289, 306, **308**, 310, **311**
Cough etiquette, 178
CPR. *See* Cardiopulmonary resuscitation
Credibility, establishing, 127–128
Criteria, lesson plans, 197–199
Cues, 258, 303, **345**, 349, **365**, 416, 417
Cultural and linguistic diversity, 155–170
    augmentative communication and, 395–396
    ethnoculturally appropriate stimuli, 295
Cultural competence, 158–160
Cultural consciousness activities, 160, 170
Cultural informants, 160, 166
Cultural literacy, 159
Cyprus, 30
The Czech Republic, 30

D

Data, 197
Data collection, 247–269
    defined, 247
    efficiency/accuracy in, 264–265
    frequency counts/tally, 249–253
    group treatment, 331, **332**, 337
    position for, 293, **294**
    prompts during treatment, 303
    recording and describing behavior, 249–264
    response accuracy, 253–255, **254**
    response analysis, 253–259
    response independence, 256–259, **258**, **259**
    response latency, 255–256, **256**, **257**, 258
    speech and language sample, 259–263, **260**, **261**, **264**
    speech sound remediation, 375–376
    treatment sessions, 248, 375–376, 379
Data collection section, lesson plans, 197–198, 201–202, **202**
Data sheet
    for SOAP note, 283
    for sound speech remediation, 375–376, 379
Decision making, ethical, 94, **95**, 96–99, **96**, **100**–**101**, 112–116
Delayed echolalia, 418
Demographics, 155–156
Demonstration/modeling, 301–302, **302**
Denmark, 31
Descriptive praise, 309, **310**
Devices, augmentative and alternative communication (AAC), 389
Devoicing, **360**
Diagnosis, 252–253
Dialects, 157–158, 166
Dibble, S., 158
Dice Talk (group activity), 334
Differentiated instruction, 330–331
Digital audio files, for speech and language sample, 260
Digitized speech, 391, 406
Direct contact transmission, **173**
Direct selection, 392, **393**
Direct supervision, 27, 28, 74
Directions, 301
Disability, use of term, 133
Disability-sensitive communication, 132–133, **134**, 135
Disinfection, of contaminated surfaces, 177–178, 189–190
Disruptive behaviors, in group treatment, 328–330, **330**
Diversity. *See* Cultural and linguistic diversity
Documentation, 194
    See also Reports
Donnellan, A., 422–423
Donohue, J.S., 366
Douglas, Jeneane, 54
Dress, professional attire, 128–129
"Drill" activities, 289

E

"Drill-and-kill" method, 362
"Drill and play" activities, 289
Droplet transmission, **173**
DSM–5, autism spectrum order in, 414
Dynamic symbols, 387
Dys-/a-/an-, usage of, 149
Dysfluency index, 254–255
Dysphagia, aspiration precautions, 184–186, **185**

E

Ear training (perceptual training), 363–364, **364**
Early eight, 358, **358**
EBP. *See* Evidence-based practice
Echolalia, autism spectrum disorders and, 418
Educational setting
    Individualized Education Plan, 211–218
    sample reports for, 204–218
    speech-language pathology assistants in, 59–60, 70, 151–152
    See also Schools
Effect/affect, usage of, 145
Effectiveness, in treatment, 320
Efficiency, in data collection, 264–265
Effortful learning, 303, 305
Egypt, 31
Einstein, Albert, 127
Electronic communication, 132
Elicit/evoke, usage of, 146
Eliciting Sounds: Techniques and Strategies for Clinicians (Secord et al.), 366
Embolism, 179–180
Enable Eyes Control Bar©, 410–411
Encoding, **393**
English, dialects, 157–158, 166
Enumeration, 249
Environment
    for treatment, 291
    visual schedules, 312–313, **313**, **314**, 315
Environmental infection control measures, 178
Errorless learning, 305
Ethical conduct, 22–24, 35, 69–126
    ASHA on, 22, 35, 90–91, **91–94**, 94
    complaints, 124

confidentiality, 35, 98, 102–103, 105, 117–124
ethical decision making, 94, **95**, 96–99, **96**, **100–101**, 112–116
misrepresenting credentials, 103, 106–107
SLPA ethical dilemma scenarios, 125–126
supervision of support personnel, 109–111
Ethical decision making, 94, **95**, 96–99, **96**, **100–101**, 112–116
Ethical decision making worksheet, 112–116
Ethics, defined, 89
Ethnicity, 166
Ethnoculturally appropriate stimuli, 295
Ethnographic interviewing, 159
Ethnographic methods, 159, 166
Ethnography, 166
Evaluative praise, 309, **310**
Evidence-based practice (EBP), 247
Evoke/elicit, usage of, 146
Except/accept, usage of, 146
Expansion, 344
Expatiation, 344
Extension, 344
Eye contact, autism spectrum disorders and, 421
Eye gaze, **393**
Eye-gaze board, **391**, 401
Eye tracking, 392, 410–411

F

Face shields, for SLPAs, 177
Facepiece respirators, 177, **177**
Facilitator, in telepractice, 288
Fading, 302
Family Educational Rights and Privacy Act (FERPA), 102, 118
Farther/further, usage of, 145
Fay, W., 418
FCD. *See* Final consonant deletion
FCT. *See* Functional communication training
Feedback, 299
    corrective feedback, 289, 306, **308**, 310, **311**
    OK syndrome, 310–311

performance feedback, **307**
Feeding tubes, 186
Final consonant deletion (FCD), **360**, 370–371
Finland, 31
First aid, 178–179
Food, as reinforcement, 306
Foreign object obstruction of airway, 181–182
Formal operations, 341
Fox, R.A., 366
France, 31
Franklin, Benjamin, 171
Freilinger, J., 357
Frequency counts, 249–253
Functional communication training (FCT), 312
Furniture, for treatment, 292–293, **292**

G

Game mirage, 321
Germany, 31
Gestural assistance, 258
Gestures, as scaffolding approach, **345**
Gloves, for SLPAs, 174, 177
Goal-directed interaction, 320
Goals and objectives, lesson plans, 195, 197–199, **198**, **199**, 241–245
Goggles, for SLPAs, 177
GoTalk Express 32© (device), 406
Grammatical morphemes, 370–371
Grandin, Temple, 419, 420, 423
Greece, 31
Group dynamics, in group treatment, 320–322
Group treatment, 310, 317–337
  about, 317–319
  advantages and disadvantages, 319, **319**
  classroom management principles and, 328–331, **329**, **330**
  client interactions, 320
  data collection during, 331, **332**, 337
  group dynamics, 320–322
  role of clinician, 318–319
  sample group activities, 322, **323–327**
Group Treatment for Asperger Syndrome: A Social Skills Curriculum (Adams), 322

Group Treatment of Neurogenic Communication Disorders: The Expert Clinician's Approach (Elman), 322

H

HAIs. *See* Health care-associated infections
Hall, L., 418
Hand hygiene, 172, 174, **174–176**, 178
Hand, L., 357
Hand rubbing, 174, **174**, **175**
Hand washing, 174, **174**, **176**
Haskill, A., 377
Health and safety, 171–190
  clients with special medical needs, 183–187
  CPR, 179
  first aid, 178–179
  infection control, 171–178
  medical conditions and emergencies, 179–183
Health care-associated infections (HAIs), 172
Health care setting, speech-language pathology assistants in, 54–56
Health Insurance Portability and Accountability Act (HIPAA), 102, 118
Healthcare Infection Control Practices Advisory Committee (HICPAC), 178
Hearing screening, 251
Heart attack, 180–181, **181**
Hemorrhagic stroke, 179, 180
Heritage language, 166
High-road processing, 290
High-tech AAC systems, 391, **392**
Hoffman, P.R., 342, 343
Hungary, 31
Hypo-/hyper-, usage of, 149

I

Iceland, 31
Iconicity, 387, **388**
Icons, 394, **395**
IDEA. *See* Individuals With Disabilities Education Act
IEP. *See* Individualized Education Plan
I'll Be Your Server (group activity), 336

436 Speech-Language Pathology Assistants: A Resource Manual

Imitation, **365**
Immediate echolalia, 418
Incompetent individuals, right to confidentiality, 117–118
India, 31
Indirect contact transmission, **173**
Indirect selection, 392, 394
Indirect supervision, 27, 28, 74
Individualized Education Plan (IEP), 211–218
Individuals With Disabilities Education Act (IDEA), autism spectrum disorders (ASD) and, 414–415
Indonesia, 31
Infection control, 171–178
    cleaning and disinfection of contaminated equipment or surfaces, 177–178, 189–190
    cough etiquette, 178
    hand hygiene, 172, 174, **174–176**, 178
    personal protective equipment, 174, 177, **177**
    respiratory hygiene, 178
    standard precautions, 172
Infectious disease, 172, **173**
Informative feedback, **307**
Initial consonant deletion, **360**
Inpatient sample report for adults, 239–240
"Integrated" service delivery model, 288
Integrity, 89
Inter-/intra-, usage of, 149
International Association of Logopedics and Phoniatrics, 4
International Classification of Functioning, Disability and Health (World Health Organization), 361–362, **362**
International Phonetic Alphabet (IPA), 132, 143–144, 251, 262, 356
Interpersonal skills, conflict resolution, 138–140, **139**
Interpretation, 28
Interpreters, 159, 162, **163**, 164, **165**, 166
Intervention plan, 312
iPad, with Proloquo© app, 409
Ireland, 31
Ischemic stroke, 179
Israel, 32
Italy, 32
Its/it's, usage of, 146

J

Japan, 32
Johnson, W., 263
Joint book reading, as therapeutic activity, **348**
Journaling, 136, **137**, 279, **280**

K

Kanner, Leo, 416
Kennedy, C.H., 318
Korea, 32

L

Lahey, M., 346
Language
    code-switching, 396
    defined, 383
    heritage language, 166
    interpreters, 159, 162, **163**, 164, **165**, 166
    languages other than English in the U.S., 156, **156**, 160, **161**
    linguistic competence, 159
    modeling, 394
Language and speech sample, 259–263, **260**, **261**, **264**
Language difference, 158, 166
Language disorders, 158, 166
    goals and objectives, 241–242, 243–245
Late eight, 358, **358**
Latex gloves, 177
Learning differences, autism spectrum disorders and, 423, 425
Leary, M., 422–423
Lesson plans, 194–195, **196**, 197–200, **198–199**
    activity/task section, 197–200
    ASHA on, 194–195
    data collection section, 197–198, 201–202, **202**
    examples, 195, **196**
    goals and objectives section, 195, 197–199, **198**, **199**, 241–245
    materials/equipment section, 200–201
    prompts/modifications section, 201
Letter knowledge, **348**
Lewis, K., 377

Liability insurance, 24
Liability issues, 24–25
LightwriterSL40© (device), 407
Linguistic competence, 159
Linguistically diverse populations, 155–160, **156**, **158**, **161**
Lipson, J., 158
Liquid gliding, **360**
Literacy, 346
  print referencing, 348–349, **349**
  shared reading, 346, **348**
  speech sound remediation activities, **374**
Literacy intervention, 346, **347**, **348**
Lithuania, 32
Lof, G., 358
Long-term goals, 195
Low-road processing, 290
Low-tech AAC systems, 390–391, **391**
Lubbock, John, 287

M

Malaysia, 32
Malpractice, liability issues, 24
Malta, 32
Masks, for SLPAs, 177
Materials/equipment. *See* Activities; Tools
Materials/equipment section, lesson plans, 200–201
Maximal oppositions contrast, 368–369
McCready, V., 77
Mean length of utterance (MLU), 263, 268
Mechanical corrective feedback, 306, **308**
Medical abbreviations, 131–132, 141–142
Medical emergencies
  airway obstruction, 181–182, **181**
  CPR, 179
  first aid, 178–179
  heart attack, 180–181, **181**
  seizures, 182, **182**
  severe allergic reactions, 183
  stroke, 179–180, **180**
Medical setting
  inpatient sample report for adults, 239–240
  outpatient sample report for adults, 226–230
  outpatient sample report for children, 231–238

reports in, 226–240
speech-language pathology assistants in, 57–58, 69, 153
Medically fragile, 28
Mehta, Z., 159
Mentee, roles of, 80, **81**
Mentor, roles of, 80, **81**
Mentoring of speech-language pathology assistants, 80–83, **81**, **83**
Methicillin-resistant *Staphylococcus aureus* (MRSA), **173**
Mexico, 32
Microorganism transmission, 172, **173**
Middle eight, 358, **358**
Miller, Revonda, 55
Minimal opposition/minimal pair contrast approach, 368, **369**
Minimal pair method, **364**
MLU. *See* Mean length of utterance
MLU using words (MLUw), 263
Modeling, 302, **302**
Moon-Meyer, S., 319, 320
Morals
  defined, 89
  See also Ethical conduct
Morphemes, 263, 370–371, 418–419
Morris, J.F., 90, 94
Motivation, 290–291
Motor speech, goals and objectives, 244–245
Mouse control, eye-tracking device, 392, 410–411
Movement differences, autism spectrum disorders and, 422–423, 425
MRSA. *See* Methicillin-resistant *Staphylococcus aureus*
Multiple oppositions therapy, 369–370
Myocardial infarction. *See* Heart attack

N

Nametags, 129
Narration, language and speech sample, 259–263, **260**, **261**, **264**
Narrative sample, 262–263
Nasogastric (NG) tubes, 186
Netherlands, 32
New Zealand, 32
Nigeria, 32
Non-verbal communication, 130

Nonspeech oral motor exercises (NSOME), 371–372
Nonverbal communication, autism spectrum disorders and, 416
Nonverbal corrective feedback, 306, **308**
Nonverbal cues, 349, 416
Normal, use of term, 132
Norris, J.A., 342, 343
Norway, 32
Note writing, 271–285
  SOAP notes, 272–279
  tips for effective note writing, 279, **281**
NSOME. *See* Nonspeech oral motor exercises

O

Objective portion, SOAP note, 274–275, **274**, **275**
Objectives, lesson plans, 197–199, **198**, **199**
Observation, facilitating, 321
O'Connor, Lisa Cabiale, 17
OK syndrome, 310–311
Olfactory sensitivities, autism spectrum disorders and, 421
Opaque symbol iconicity, 387, **388**
Operant conditioning, 305
Operant principles, 308–309
Opportunity barriers, 322
Opportunity statement, 255
Oral-Facial Examination Form, 252, *252*
Oral peripheral examination, 252
Osler, William, 271
Outpatient sample reports, 226–238
Oxygen, use by client, 183–184, **184**

P

Pantomime, as scaffolding approach, **345**
Parallel talk, 344
Pathogens, 172, **173**
Patient information, confidentiality of, 35, 98, 102–103, 105, 118
Pauley, J.A., 328
Pauley, J.F., 328
PBS. *See* Positive behavioral support
Peek-a-boo, 339, **347**
Peer review, confidentiality and, 119

Peers, confidentiality in relation to, 103, 123–124
Percent correct method, 253, **254**
Percent Syllables Stuttered (%SS), 255
Perceptual training, 363–364, **364**
Percutaneous endoscopic gastrostomy (PEG) tubes, 186
Performance feedback, **307**
Personal protective equipment, 174, 177, **177**
Personnel/personal, usage of, 147
Perspective taking, autism spectrum disorders and, 417
Philippines, 33
Phonemes, 356
Phonemic awareness, **348**
Phonemic cues, 258, **345**
Phonemic inventories, 160
Phonemic/linguistically-based/phonologic approach, 361, 362, **363**, 366, 368–370
  maximal oppositions contrast, 368–369
  minimal oppositions/minimal pair contrast approach, 368, **369**
  multiple oppositions therapy, 369–370
Phonetic/motor-based/articulation approach, 361, 362, **363**–366, **363**
  perceptual training/ear training, 363–364, **364**
  sound establishment/sound elicitation, 364–366, **365**
  sound stabilization, 366, **367**
  speech homework, 366, 378
Phonetic notation, 131–132, 143–144
Phonetic placement, **365**
Phonological awareness, 370
Phonological processes, 359–360, **360**
Phonology, 361
  goals and objectives, 245
Photographs, as augmentative and alternative communication, 389
Piaget, Jean, 339, 340
Picasso, Pablo, 193
"Pictured" stimuli, 294–295
Place-Voice-Manner (PVM) chart, 357, **357**
Play
  ASHA on, 339–340
  associative play, 352
  creating communication opportunities, 343

determining level of play, 342–343
development of, 340–341
scaffolding communication, 344, **345**
shared reading as, 346
in speech-language treatment, 341–344,
344, **345**, 346
symbolic play, 341, 351
Westby's Symbolic Play Scale, 341,
351–353
Poland, 33
Portugal, 33
Positive atmosphere, for treatment,
320–321
Positive behavioral support (PBS), 298,
311–312
Positive reinforcement, 306
Positive reinforcer, 306
Practice play, 340
Praise, in group treatment, 328
Prediction, **393**
Preschool initial speech-language
assessment, 204–210
Pretend play, 351
Principal/principle, usage of, 146
Print knowledge, 348
Print referencing, 348–349, **349**
Print salience, 349
Privacy
confidentiality of client information, 35,
98, 102–103, 105, 118
student privacy issues, 122–123
Private practice sample report for children,
219–225
Professional attire, 128–129
Professional conduct, 127–154
appearance, 128–129
conflict resolution, 138–140, **139**
self-assessment and self-improvement,
135–138, **137**, 151–153
Professional organizations, international,
4, 30–34
Proloquo© app, 409
Prompts, 302–303, **304**, 305, 332
Prompts/modifications section, lesson
plans, 201
Proprioception, autism spectrum disorders
and, 419
"Pull-out" service delivery model, 288

Pumpkin decorating, as therapeutic
activity, 335
Punishment, in treatment, 305, 306, 308
Puppets, as therapeutic activity, **347**
"Push-in" service delivery model, 288
Puzzles, as therapeutic activity, **347**
PVM chart. *See* Place-Voice-Manner (PVM)
chart

Q

Quality of voice, autism spectrum
disorders and, 418

R

Rapport, with clients, 297–301
Real-object stimuli, 295
Recasting, 344
Recorded speech and language sample,
confidentiality of, 260
Records
confidentiality of written records,
121–122
weekly activity record, 86
Reflection journal, 279, **280**
Reinforcement, in treatment, 289, 305–306,
307, 308, 311
Remnant books, **391**
Reports, 194, 204–245
in educational setting, 204–218
in medical setting, 226–240
note writing for, 271–285
in private practice setting, 219–225
Research, confidentiality of data, 118,
119–120
Respiratory hygiene, 178
Response accuracy, 253–255, **254**
Response analysis, 253–259
Response cost, 306, **309**
Response independence, 256–259, **258**, **259**
Response latency, 255–256, **256**, **257**, 258
Response rate, 249
Rewards
social rewards, **307**
See also Reinforcement
Rituals, autism spectrum disorders and,
424

Robledo, J., 421, 422–423
Role-playing, 200
Rules and expectations, in group
    treatment, 328
Russia, 33

S

Sander, E., 357
Scaffolding, 303
Scaffolding communication, 344, **345**
Scanning, 394, 405
Schools
    cleaning and disinfection guidelines for,
        178, 189–190
    Individualized Education Plan, 211–218
    preschool initial speech-language
        assessment, 204–210
    See also Educational setting
Screening, 28, 251
Seating arrangement, for treatment,
    292–293, **293**, **294**
Secondary reinforcers, 306, **307**
Secord, W.A., 366
Seizures, 182, **182**
Self-assessment and self-improvement,
    135–138, **137**
    self-evaluation: intervention session in
        educational setting, 151
    self-evaluation: intervention session in
        medical setting, 153
Self-awareness, autism spectrum disorders
    and, 417
Self-contained classrooms, 318
Self-study, 200
Self-talk, 344
Sensory differences, autism spectrum
    disorders and, 419–422, 425
Sensory environment, for treatment,
    291–292
Sequencing, **393**
Service delivery model, 287–288
Severe allergic reactions, 183
Shaping, 302
Shared reading, 346, **348**
Shine, R.E., 366
Short-term goals, 197
Showing concern, autism spectrum
    disorders and, 417

Shriberg, L., 358
Simple enumeration, 249
Sinclair, J., 413, 427
Singapore, 33
Skills proficiency checklist, 71
Slovenia, 33
SLPAs. *See* Speech-language pathology
    assistants
SLPs. *See* Speech-language pathologists
Smit, A., 357
SOAP note, 272–279
    Analyze portion, 275–277, **276**, **277**
    data sheet for, 283
    Objective section, 274–275, **274**, **275**
    Plan section, 277–279
    samples of, 284–285
    Subjective section, 272–273
Social cognition, autism spectrum
    disorders and, 417
Social communication, autism spectrum
    disorders and, 414, 424–425
Social cues, 417
Social differences, autism spectrum
    disorders and, 416–417
Social initiation, autism spectrum disorders
    and, 416
Social networking, 132, **133**
Social reciprocity, autism spectrum
    disorders and, 416–417
Social rewards, **307**
Social skills group activities, 334–336
Software, for communications purposes,
    392
Sound elicitation, 364–366, **365**
Sound modification, **365**
Sound speech remediation, data sheet for,
    375–376, 379
Sound stabilization, 366, **367**
South Africa, 33
Spain, 33
Spanish-language service providers, 162
Speaking Dynamically Pro© (device), 408
Special need clients, 183–187
    dysphagia and aspiration precautions,
        184–186, **185**
    oxygen use, 183–184, **184**
    tracheostomy, 186–187, **187**
    tube feeding, 186
    ventilator use, 186

Speech, defined, 383
Speech and language disorders
    in autism spectrum disorders and, 418
    in linguistically and culturally diverse
        populations, 158, **158**
Speech and language sample, 259–263, **260,**
    261, 264
Speech-generating devices (SGDs), 391,
    392, 406
Speech homework, 366, 378
Speech intelligibility, 356, 361, 371
Speech-language pathologists (SLPs)
    bilingual, 162
    data collection, 248
    scope of practice, 35
    SLP to SLPA ratio, 26
    treatment plans, 193–194
    See also Supervising speech-language
        pathologists
Speech-language pathology
    associations around the world, 30–34
    lesson plans, 194–195, **196,** 197–200,
        198–199
Speech-language pathology aides, 29
Speech-Language Pathology Assistant Scope of
    Practice (ASHA), 4, 16–29, 35, 288
Speech-language pathology assistants
        (SLPAs)
    activity logs and records, 86, 87
    administrative support by, 10, **10,** 20
    in an educational setting, 59–60, 70,
        151–152
    appearance of, 128–129
    ASHA affiliation status, 13–14, 18
    ASHA Code of Ethics, 91–92, **91–94,** 94,
        98, **99,** 104–108, 118
    ASHA definition, 3
    ASHA minimum qualifications, 18–19
    ASHA on, 54
    ASHA SLPA Scope of Practice, 16–29, 35
    assessment vs. analysis, 276–277, **276,**
        277
    bilingual SLPAs, 45, 157–158, 160, 162
    in California, 40
    confidentiality, of client information, 35,
        98, 102–103, 105, 117–124
    cultural and linguistic diversity, 155–170
    data collection and, 248, **248,** 251–252
    a day in the life of, 10–11, 36–53

direct observation skills brief checklist,
    69, 70
duties and responsibilities, 7–9, **8, 9**
establishing credibility, 127–128
ethical conduct, 22–24, 35, 69–126
ethical dilemma scenarios, 125–126
expectations of, 19
in Florida, 48
goals of, 73
health and safety, 171–190
in health care settings, 54–56
international professional organizations
    for, 4, 30–34
as interpreters/translators, 159, 162, **163,**
    164, 165, 166
job description, 10–11, 57–58
liability issues, 24–25
in medical setting, 57–58, 69, 153
mentoring of, 80–83
minimal qualifications for, 7, 74
misrepresenting credentials, 103, 106–107
nametags, 129
placement in treatment room, 293, **293**
practice settings, 22
prevention and advocacy by, 10–11, **11,**
    20–21
professional conduct, 127–154
regulatory bodies for, 4–5
responsibilities of, 8–10, **9, 10,** 11, **11,** 19–21
responsibilities outside SLPA's scope of
    practice, 7, **8,** 21–22, 253
scope of practice, 16–29, 35, 288
scope of responsibility, 8–10, **9, 10,** 11, **11**
self-assessment and self-improvement,
    135–138, **137,** 151–153
service delivery, 8–10, **9,** 20
SLP to SLPA ratio, 26
in South Dakota, 52
state standards, 5, **6**
in Texas, 36
tips for establishing credibility, 127–128
training of, 17–19
treatment plans, 193–202, 204–245
in the U.S., 4
See also Assessment of speech-language
    pathology assistants; Mentoring of
    speech-language pathology assistants;
    Supervision of speech-language
    pathology assistants

Speech-language pathology technicians, 29
Speech-language treatment. *See* Treatment
Speech sound disorders (SSD), 355
Speech sound remediation, 360–379
   apps for, 375
   children with limited language ability,
      370
   final consonant deletion (FCD), **360**,
      370–371
   fun and motivational sessions, 373–375
   general treatment principles, 360–362,
      361, **362**
   grammatical morphemes, 370–371
   hierarchy of, **361**
   monitoring progress, 375–376
   nonspeech oral motor exercises
      (NSOME), 371–372
   phonemic/linguistically-based/
      phonologic approach, 361, 362, **363**,
      368–370
   phonetic/motor-based/articulation
      approach, 361, 362, 363–366, **363**
   phonological awareness, 370
   primary treatment approaches, 362–370
   sample activities, 374, **375**
   sample session, 362, **363**
   school-age children with SSD, 370
   selecting treatment materials, 372–373,
      372, **374**
   technology used for, 375
   tracking clinical data, 375–376
Speech sounds, 356
   classification of, 356–357, **357**
   consonant clusters/blends, 358–359, **359**
   consonants, 357–358
   development of, 356–359, **357–359**
   phonological processes, 359–360, **360**
   Place-Voice-Manner (PVM) chart, 357,
      357
   vowels, 359
SPM. *See* Syllables per minute
SSD *See* Speech sound disorders
Standard American English, 157
Standard precautions, 172
State law, confidentiality laws, 118
Stepanek, Mattie, 317
Stevens, Earl Gray, 3
Stevens, Wallace, 247

Stimuli, 255, 294–297, **296**
Stopping of fricatives, **360**
Stored speech, 391
Story retell, 262
Story retelling rope, **323**, **324**
Stroke, 179–180, **180**
Student privacy issues, 122–123
Student Teacher (group activity), 336
Subjective portion, SOAP note, 272–273
Supervising speech-language pathologists
   ASHA Code of Ethics and, 22, 23, 35,
      90–91, **91–94**, 94, 98, **99**, 104–108, 118
   ASHA paper, 35
   defined, 29
   documenting supervision, 27, 76–77, 85
   expectations of SLPA, 77
   feedback by, 27, 78–80, **78**, 132
   guidelines for supervision, 25–28
   minimal frequency and amount of
      supervision, 74–75, **75**
   qualifications of, 76, **76**
   role of, 80
   service delivery model, 288–289
   student privacy issues, 122–123
   supervisory conferences, 77–78
   supervisory relationship, 77
   supervisory role, 25
   training and credentials, 76
Supervision of speech-language pathology
      assistants, 73–80, 85
   absence of supervisor, 28
   after SLPA's first 90 days, 26–27, 74, **75**
   ASHA on, 35
   defined, 29
   direct supervision, 27, 74
   documenting supervision, 27, 76–77, 85
   expectations of SLPAs, 77
   feedback by supervisor, 27, 78–80, **78**, 132
   guidelines for, 25–28, 73
   indirect supervision, 27, 28, 74
   minimum requirements for, 26–28
   qualifications of supervising SLP, 76, **76**
   supervisory conferences, 77
   supervisory plan, 27
   supervisory relationship, 77
   within SLPA's first 90 days, 26–27, 74, **75**
Supervision of support personnel, ethical
      rules and guidance, 109–111

Support personnel, 29
  ethical principles for supervision of, 109–111
Swallowing, aspiration precautions, 184–186, **185**
Sweden, 33
Switch and button communicators, 391, 405
Switzerland, 33–34
Syllable deletion, **360**
Syllables per minute (SPM), 249
Symbol iconicity, 387, **388**
Symbol sequencing, **393**
Symbol stability, 387
Symbolic play, 341, 351
Symbolic Play Scale (Westby), 341
Symbols, for augmentative and alternative communication (AAC), 387–389, **388**, **389**, 392, **393**, 394
Synthesized speech, 391

T

Tactile-kinesthetic method, **365**
Tactile prompts, 303, **304**
Tactile sensitivity, autism spectrum disorders and, 419–422
Taiwan, 34
Tallies, 249–253
Tattoos, 129
Technical proficiency checklist, 66–68
Technology
  apps for communication purposes, **392**, 408, 409
  apps for speech sound remediation, 375
  eye-tracking device, 392, 410–411
Telepractice, 29, 288
Telesupervision, 27, 29
Texas, 36
Text-to-speech devices, **392**, 407
Than/then, usage of, 147
Their/they're/there, usage of, 145
Then/than, usage of, 147
Therapy in a group model, 319–320
Three-Step Response Plan, 329–330, **330**
Thrombosis, 179
Tic-Tac-Toe, with target words, **323**
Timeout, 306, **309**

Tokens, 263, **307**, 321
Tolbert, L., 377
Tone of voice, autism spectrum disorders and, 418
Too/two/to, usage of, 147–148
Tools
  for group therapy, 321
  for speech sound remediation, 372–373, **372**, **374**
Toys, in treatment activities, 346
Tracheostomy, 186–187, **187**
Training, 17–19
Transcription, of narrative sample, 262
Translators, 162, **163**, **164**, **165**, 166
Transparent symbol iconicity, 387, **388**
Travis, L.E., 320
Treatment
  assessment, 194
  client parameters, 290–291
  clinical interactions, 301–315
  clinical rapport, 297–301
  clinician-client relationship, 290
  data collection and, 248, 375–376, 379
  environment, 291
  feedback given in, 289, 299, 306, **308**
  furniture choice, 292–293
  group treatment, 310, 317–337
  implementing, 287–316
  note writing during, 271–285
  play in, 341–344, **344**, **345**, 346
  punishment in, 305, 306, 308
  reinforcement, 289, 305–306, **307**, 308, 311
  seating arrangement, 292–293, **293**, **294**
  sensory environment and, 291–292
  service delivery model, 287–288
  speech sound remediation, 360–379
  stimulus, 255, 294–297, **296**
  See also Activities; Treatment plans
Treatment goals, 195, 197–199, **198**, **199**, 241–245, 360
Treatment plans, 193–202
  confidentiality, 194
  documentation, 194
  Individualized Education Plan for elementary school, 211–218
  lesson plans, 194–195, **196**, 197–200, **198–199**
  observation prior to, 200

Treatment plans *(continued)*
reports, 194, 204–245
role-playing, 200
self-study, 200
TTR. *See* Type token ratio
Tube feeding, 186
Tuberculosis (TB), **173**
Turkey, 34
Turn-taking cues, **345**
Two/too/to, usage of, 147–148
Tyler, A., 377
Type I/II punishment, 306
Type token ratio (TTR), 263

U

Unaided communication, 389–390, **389**
United Kingdom, 34
United States
demographics, 155–156
languages spoken other than English, 156, **156**, 160, **161**
Universal precautions, 172
U.S. Bureau of the Census, 155, 156

V

Vancomycin-resistant enterococcus (VRE), **173**
VAS. *See* Visual analog scales
Vector-borne transmission, **173**
Vehicle-borne transmission, **173**
Velar fronting, **360**
Venezuela, 34
Venn diagram, as group therapy tool, **323**, **326**
Verbal communication, 129–131, 138
confidentiality of, 120–121
Verbal corrective feedback, 306, **308**, 310
Verbal cues, 349
Verbal model, 258
Vestibular system, autism spectrum disorders and, 419
Videotaping, for speech and language sample, 260
Vietnam, 34

Vinyl gloves, 177
Virgules, 356
Visual analog scales (VAS), 298–301, **300**
Visual prompts, 303, **304**
Visual scene display, 408
Visual schedules, 312–313, **313**, **314**, 315
Visual sensitivities, autism spectrum disorders and, 421
Vocabulary selection, augmentative and alternative communication (AAC), 396–397, **396**
Voice, autism spectrum disorders and, 418
Voice output, 391
Vowels, in development of speech, 359
VRE. *See* Vancomycin-resistant enterococcus

W

Ward, Matt, 420
Weekly activity log, 86
Weekly activity record, 86
Were/we're/where, usage of, 145
Westby, C., 159
Westby's Symbolic Play Scale, 341, 351–353
White, Darren, 420, 421
WHO Guidelines on Hand Hygiene in Health Care, 172
Williams, Donna, 420, 421
Words per minute (WPM), 249
World Health Organization (WHO), 133, 172
WPM. *See* Words per minute
Writing notes. *See* Note writing
Written communication, 131–132
commonly misspelled words, 132, 150
commonly misused words, 132, 145–149
electronic communication, 132
medical abbreviations, 131–132, 141–142
phonetic notation, 131–132, 143–144
Written records, confidentiality of, 121–122
Written stimuli, 295

Y

Your/you're, usage of, 146